HOW DO I K...
FIBROMYALGIA?

Patients suffering from fibromyalgia experience a variety of painful and debilitating symptoms, including chronic fatigue, joint and muscle pain, chronic bladder and vaginal infections, depression, insomnia, and disorientation.

WHAT WERE THE TRADITIONAL
REMEDIES?

Recognized as a disease by the World Health Organization in 1993, fibromyalgia has been treated in the past with medications, including antidepressants, analgesics, and narcotics, to relieve symptoms. These remedies have not worked for everyone.

WHAT'S SO SPECIAL ABOUT
GUAIFENESIN?

Guaifenesin is an inexpensive medication used in over-the-counter cough medicines. But in his studies, Dr. St. Amand discovered that this drug, taken in the proper dosage, is the first effective treatment for reversing fibromyalgia—with no known side effects. Recently, the drug has become more available in new formulations and dosages—sold, in some cases, over the counter.

WHERE CAN I TURN FOR MORE INFORMATION—AND SUPPORT?

Dr. St. Amand is the country's foremost expert on this subject and is himself a past sufferer of the disease. Drawing on Dr. St. Amand's firsthand experience and filled with the latest research on the subject, this book also offers complete and newly revised and updated appendices that include Internet user groups and dozens of support organizations for people with fibromyalgia and for those using guaifenesin.

"Dr. St. Amand's unique approach to fibromyalgia gives patients who have run out of treatment options a new hope... A revelation to fibromyalgics."
> —Miryam Ehrlich Williamson, author of *Fibromyalgia: A Comprehensive Approach* and *The Fibromyalgia Relief Book*

"Offers a clear road map out of the wilderness of fibromyalgia pain and fatigue."
> —Kendall Gerdes, MD, former president, American Academy of Environmental Medicine

"I've been using guaifenesin and the protocol in this book in my practice for seven years. The results have been amazing! If you have fibromyalgia I strongly recommend you buy this book and begin treatment immediately."
> —C. Ronald McBride, MD, assistant clinical professor of medicine, UCLA Medical Group

WHAT YOUR DOCTOR MAY NOT TELL YOU ABOUT™

FIBROMYALGIA

The Revolutionary
Treatment That Can
Reverse the Disease

3rd Edition

R. PAUL ST. AMAND MD,
CLAUDIA CRAIG MAREK

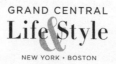

GRAND CENTRAL
Life & Style
NEW YORK · BOSTON

Grand Central Life & Style
Hachette Book Group
237 Park Avenue
New York, NY 10017

www.HachetteBookGroup.com

Printed in the United States of America

RRD-C

First Edition: May 2012
10 9 8 7 6 5 4 3 2 1

Grand Central Life & Style is an imprint of Grand Central Publishing.
The Grand Central Life & Style name and logo are trademarks of Hachette Book Group, Inc.

The Hachette Speakers Bureau provides a wide range of authors for speaking events. To find out more, go to www.hachettespeakersbureau.com or call (866) 376-6591.

The publisher is not responsible for websites (or their content) that are not owned by the publisher.

Library of Congress Cataloging-in-Publication Data

St. Amand, R. Paul.
  What your doctor may not tell you about fibromyalgia : the revolutionary treatment that can reverse the disease / R. Paul St. Amand and Claudia Craig Marek. — 3rd ed.
     p. cm.
  Includes bibliographical references and index.
  ISBN 978-1-4555-0271-4 (pbk.)
  1. Fibromyalgia—Popular works. 2. Fibromyalgia—Treatment—Popular works.
I. Marek, Claudia. II. Title.
  RC927.3.S73 2012
  616.7'42—dc23
                                                              2011038119

Contents

Preface

The first edition of this book was written with some hesitation. The focus of my practice had always been on helping the patients who came to me directly. In the past, I avoided publicity for my work because of the controversy I knew would arise from treating a no-name illness that other doctors didn't believe existed. Because of this, I even hesitated to discuss this strange illness with my colleagues and the large medical group I headed. But I soon realized that I had no choice but to ignore their skepticism, because results are what really count in medicine—and I was getting them.

In those early days, however, I was on my own. I drew sketches to help my patients better understand their disease and the course of treatment I recommended. The "fibrofogged" needed something written to facilitate understanding and to placate long-suffering families. So I wrote a few descriptive papers that got copied and circulated again and again. I didn't anticipate how many people they would reach. Patients began coming from different parts of the United States, even from around the world.

When the name *fibromyalgia* was coined about twenty-seven years ago, I gratefully adopted this classification—misnomer though it was! A terribly common illness that had previously existed only in obscurity suddenly had a name. The term was not immediately embraced, but it gained acceptance from rheumatologists and open-minded members of the medical community. This emboldened me to more militantly champion the illness. Although my approach might have seemed unconventional, I had already been using it for more than twenty-three years.

Slowly, a consensus party line of preferred treatment emerged, but it has always ignored our successful protocol. A few physicians tried to follow our program, but mostly got lost trying to teach patients how to avoid myriad sources of salicylate. (You'll learn about this hideous, ongoing problem soon enough!) I was increasingly asked to speak and write about fibromyalgia. Patients told us about their experiences and we listened. We learned about associated conditions, most prevalent being hypoglycemia (or low blood sugar). The sickest ones certainly had a depth of knowledge about their disease spectrum.

As I studied and learned more about this newly named fibromyalgia, I realized that I also had it. Later, I was able to identify the condition as one of my father's legacies. It was he who wielded the gene(s) passed on to my two sisters and me. I, in turn, passed it on, and each of my three daughters developed serial symptoms. Illnesses take on special significance when they strike near to home. Probably my family's health concerns sharpened my skills; fine honing became mandatory.

Over the ensuing years, I'd found four effective medications. Their side effects kept me looking for something safer, which is what we now have in the compound guaifenesin. Imagine how success with the very first medication would stir me to ask why it worked. This "why?" led to possibilities and then to theories, which I occasionally modified, and will continue to do. Of course, a theory is merely a supposition based on as much fact as can be garnered. This search keeps me poring over esoteric papers—finally some of our own—looking for insights into cellular physiology to test and embellish our hypotheses. Please appreciate the fact that whatever errors might exist in my theories don't diminish the efficacy of the treatment. Perhaps a simpler statement is: What works, works. In fact, the heart of my approach is so basic that it can be stated in a simple quartet of phrases:

1. There is an inherited disease known as the fibromyalgia syndrome (FMS)—a misnomer because of what the title doesn't describe.
2. There exists an effective, safe treatment using a very common medication, guaifenesin.
3. The inability to generate sufficient energy for body-wide requirements explains the entire illness.
4. Hypoglycemia, or low blood sugar, is a frequent co-condition.

This book was first written and is again being revised from the stimuli of both despair and dedication. Initial despair originated from the cries for help, pleas for understanding, and for some type of answer. Years later, we're no longer desperate. In fact, we're optimistic as we are finally yielding data that will steer us to a diagnostic blood test. Dedication is paying off as we can now document some of the effects of guaifenesin. We've been reassured by the thousands of patients who got well. Though the picture is yet incomplete, we can confidently disseminate information to the millions who've never had the chance to validate their symptoms. Yet we still must shed a tear for those who'll never know what curse they carry.

Most of my life has been spent treating fibromyalgia, and I must now ask all patients to accept two responsibilities: (1) to complete their own disease reversal, and (2) to promote the protocol and assist others. As with any chronic illness, it's unrealistic for patients to lean totally on doctors without helping themselves so we're sharing our protocol with those who want to listen and have a true desire to succeed.

Critics cite that our guaifenesin protocol has not been subjected to a successful, double-blind study. Any technically skilled individual has wondered how we dare postulate so much altered biochemistry and simultaneously implicated multiple genetic mutations in fibromyalgia. Additional skeptics still feel that we're utterly simplistic in recommending a seemingly unsophisticated protocol for treating such a terribly complex disease.

Let me respond to this. We did attempt to show the success of our treatment with a double-blind study. Failed results from the Oregon Health and Sciences University were reported in 1995. I was the consultant for the project, and too late, I spotted errors we made in the study. I knew little about the dermal absorption of salicylate; the academic staff failed to identify and eliminate hypoglycemic participants. Both mistakes quite thoroughly doomed the project. It's now obvious to me that a double-blind study will not likely succeed. We'll discuss why in succeeding chapters. Yet despite the depressing failure, it redirected our focus onto seeking the defective biochemistry and genes underlying fibromyalgia.

We can now arm the reader with enough new data, the kind of stuff demanded by my peers. You no longer have to bow your head when saying you're on our protocol. You can be humbly militant in urging your physician to read our patient-vindicating, scientific publications. Those papers and two others now in progress give credence to overcome "just theories" leveled at our earlier editions. We have the right to demand a change in negative attitudes: There's now considerable science, not just our own, backing our earlier assumptions about fibromyalgia.

Lastly, let's address previous concerns of the medical sophisticates. The science we invoke is up to date only as we write this edition. Our current research and that of others will make sizable revamping in the time just ahead. Argue as anyone might, there is ample, well-documented evidence concerning the dearth of chemical energy (ATP) in fibromyalgia.

We'll continue trying to discover why that's so. Our genetic and chemistry findings are added to data from other researchers and our goal, the Holy Grail: A diagnostic test is the only thing that will finally soothe the continual angst of my medical colleagues.

Altogether too many new Band-Aid medications are being prescribed for fibromyalgia. Doctors are overwhelmed by the choices; patients are, too. This is a major reason for writing this edition. The array of drugs is bad news. When first asked to do this revision, I said, "I won't do it!" Too many hours go into revisions. Then Claudia said, "It's time to man up, boss. We've got to discuss what the drugs do and don't do to patients. On top of that, you've always said this was a genetic illness and that's being confirmed by our research." I agreed: Proof is showing up in blood and in the deformed genes sneaking out of various chromosomes. She shamed me into the rewrite when she added less aggressively and more poignantly, "Patients all over the world deserve to know that they have reasons for feeling as bad as they do." How do you fight a cogent argument? You don't!

Further inspiration arises from the realization that there will ever remain multimillions of untreated people with fibromyalgia. Which of us, including you, is going to get to them? Thankfully, our success rate has improved as we've learned from our patient-teachers. Their perceptions of seemingly insignificant nuances and their eagerness to share their experiences have proved invaluable. This book is in large part dedicated to them. They were and are the flesh and blood of my concepts of fibromyalgia, hypoglycemia, and their conjoined "fibroglycemia." They've been the affirmation of our protocol. Please give them well-deserved kudos for helping you resurrect your health.

If you've met us before, welcome back. Also, welcome if you're new to our description of fibromyalgia and its treatment. Much of this book has been rewritten because we've learned so much more since its last publication. We've accumulated larger numbers for our statistics concerning most symptoms of fibromyalgia. Some of you are familiar with our previous editions and will easily get through some of the descriptive material, but please don't flip pages too quickly for there's quite a bit that's changed. We're offering some subtle, but necessary maneuvers in the treatment protocol. A noun like *fibromyalgia* doesn't kill, but an adjective like *sedentary* does. Please learn why that's true and let's get you into the script. Come right along then. The game is indeed afoot.

R. Paul St. Amand, M.D.
Associate Clinical Professor
Medicine/Endocrinology
Harbor–UCLA

Acknowledgments

I bow to my nurse and coauthor, Claudia Marek, who has filled this book with her intelligent perceptions. She has provided years of inspiration, not only for me, but also through her dedication to our patients. She has done this with her caring and deep-seated knowledge of these illnesses. In the book world, I must thank Mari Florence for her wisdom and expertise in helping me simplify often complicated medical jargon. Diana Baroni, our editor at Grand Central, labored with skill and enthusiasm to help us, and we appreciate all her efforts. There's not enough room to express gratitude to all of our friends and families, especially Janell, Lou, Malcolm, and Sean, who patiently added their art and observations while allowing us to steal monumental time from our relationships. Lastly, another stands out as a mighty contributor: my secretary, Gloria Martinez, who has efficiently and uncomplainingly assumed many mundane and technical duties that freed nurse and doctor to pursue this endeavor.

Part I

The Plan for Conquering Fibromyalgia

In my fifty-five years as a practicing and teaching internist/ endocrinologist, I've devoted fifty to the diagnosis and treatment of fibromyalgia—even before it supposedly existed. I've found there is only one safe and effective treatment protocol for the condition, one that I had to follow myself. The illness entered my life when I was in the armed services in 1945. I was hospitalized with the diagnosis of "possible rheumatic fever" because of my red, swollen leg joints and painful muscles. All my tests came back normal. After six weeks, everything cleared spontaneously. Cycles of various symptoms appeared sporadically over the ensuing years but with much lighter intensity. I was hit in earnest in my early thirties with many new symptoms including joint pains, but never again with the earlier swellings. I had no idea why this developed; I had never been taught about such a ridiculous condition. I assumed I was not emotionally geared for the stresses, long hours, and general tribulations of private medical practice. I tried to pace myself and relax as best I could. That didn't help, of course, so I was convinced I needed to work harder at it! Only after I stumbled onto and began treating patients with what was later named fibromyalgia did I realize that theirs was a misery I shared. I simply began treating myself. Who else was going to do it?

Over the years, I've explored the many facets of this illness mainly through observation and compilation of data from my patient-teachers. They willingly joined me in our trial-and-error approach that lacked any other scientific credentials. It has taken me many years to reasonably grasp the full extent of this illness and to comprehend just how insidious, infuriating, and debilitating it can be.

Part I of this book is an invitation to learn about fibromyalgia. We're presenting you a compilation of facts gleaned from several thousand patients who have described how they've felt over the years. Patients don't all come in with the same complaints and certainly not in the same order. We'll tell you how we reassemble those statements, blend them with the physical findings that confirm the diagnosis, and channel that mix into an effective treatment.

Many of our readers already know they have fibromyalgia. Others are suspicious and in using this book will make their own diagnosis and perhaps see their doctors for confirmation. It's certainly not like it was twelve years ago when we first wrote this book since the illness is far better known and earlier diagnosed. In the end, you'll decide for yourself if you're a candidate for our protocol. Even if you opt out, you'll at least learn considerably about your illness and why it so devastatingly ravages your life.

We will also devote several pages to describing the medication we use, and what you may expect as you start treatment. So many fibromyalgics have carbohydrate intolerance that we have written a full chapter describing low blood sugar or hypoglycemia. Though there is no particular diet for fibromyalgia, you'll grasp why you might feel considerably better by avoiding sugars and starches.

The last chapter in this part will provide a concise step-by-step explanation of our protocol. We understand that many fibromyalgics have what's been labeled "fibrofog" and will have difficulty understanding, let alone remembering, what they've just read. For that reason, we've tried to keep our explanations and advice simple and to the point. We've also intended this as a reference book that can be consulted when particular symptoms arise.

Chapter One

An Invitation to Join Us and
Find Your Way Back to Health

Most people don't really understand fibromyalgia. Most of my friends only know that it hurts a lot, but they don't really know what that means. Most of my doctors don't really know what to do for me. It's hard when the doctor doesn't really believe me because of the pain being disproportional to the problem.

—Nina, West Virginia

I<small>T CAN START</small> off subtly: a bit of muscle pain, along with some generalized aches and stiffness. Then there are periods when concentration is impossible, a day or two of overwhelming fatigue, and maybe a little dizziness, heart palpitations, irritability, and anxieties. Symptoms come and go at first, and it's easy to chalk them up to a mild case of the flu that never quite fully develops. You, like most individuals, tend to blame stress or overexertion for these strange little complaints.

Then, one day, you realize one part or another of your body always hurts. You're often confused, short of memory, unable to concentrate, and you're always stressed and feeling as if you're at the end of your rope. You wake up tired every morning no matter how much sleep you've had. Your symptoms begin to worsen, and you notice new ones: depression, numbness and tingling of the hands, leg cramps, headaches, abdominal pains, cramps, constipation taking turns with diarrhea, or bladder infections. Now you notice that you can no longer sleep through the night. Sometimes pain keeps you awake; most of the time, though, you don't know what causes the insomnia or what keeps waking you. And what causes your craving for sugar and starch? Why is it that you haven't changed your eating habits, but you still gain weight? You've accumulated enough bad omens that you aren't too surprised when bad days outnumber the good ones. Eventually you just cycle from bad to worse. When you look back, nature gave you ample warnings.

> It feels like coming down with the flu, yet it never manifests fully. It's like being fluish, achy and tired, and embarrassed and discouraged about it because you don't know why or what you can do to make it better or what you did to make it worse. Everyone gives advice but they don't have a clue as to what it's really like. Having people tell you to eat differently and exercise more and not focus on your health makes you just want to isolate yourself because you've already experimented with every possible food plan, supplement, and idea.
>
> —*Miki K., Hawaii*

You become increasingly immobile and unconsciously you stop making plans with family and friends because you don't know how you'll feel the next day—or the day after. Go supermarket shopping? You're kidding. That's just one of the many chores you've come to dread. At least you now have the time to review the long list of doctors you've visited. Each time your hopes have been dashed despite the number of tests you've taken and the many tubes of blood you've sacrificed. Sure enough: Results are normal. Increasingly, doctors are making the diagnosis despite the unrevealing tests and a sequential array of drugs; some will escort you out of the office and point to the nearest psychiatrist; a few will admit that nothing much will help you. Predictably, you've subsidized your neighborhood health food store by taking a variety of supplements.

Your life has entered a downward spiral into more pain, depression, and fatigue. Some of you may be nearing rock bottom. You reproach yourself for everything. Your lament includes a review of all of your inadequacies and poor coping abilities. You put yourself on trial for repeatedly letting down family and friends. You feel as though you've certainly damaged their lives and your own.

Wounded relationships are the most damaging side effect. You're not the person your spouse married, and you know it. You fret and sputter about your fragilities, but you can't seem to correct them. You're depressed especially when you look at your children and the parental deprivations they suffer. Suicide may have crossed your mind, but you know that's not the solution. Okay, enough already with the remorse!

> It feels like everyone around me is normal and happy and having a good time and I'm so different. I want to have a few normal days. I don't fit in anywhere because no one understands. People laugh and say, "You look fine," but I'm dying inside and I can't explain it to them. I'm so tired of pretending I'm okay when I want to scream. I have kept a positive attitude for so long but it's exhausting and I just can't do it anymore. I wish I could just go away somewhere and hide.
>
> —*Susie, California*

Fibromyalgia is prevalent in all ethnic groups in all parts of the world. In North America, it's estimated that about 5 percent of the adult population suffer from it. Since the early cases are not being diagnosed, we feel that over 10 percent of women and 2 percent of men are affected. Using our guess, some twenty million Americans suffer from fibromyalgia, 85 percent women. Fibromyalgia is the most common disorder seen by rheumatologists.[1] It's further thought that chronic fatigue syndrome affects twenty-five million people. I and many other physicians consider the two the same disease. Blending the entities into one would augment the percentage of people with fibromyalgia. We'll develop the thought later on, but we have enough observations to conclude that today's fibromyalgia is the prelude to tomorrow's osteoarthritis, something that affects nearly 40 percent of older people. Adding up combinations of those numbers would lead us to conclude that nearly one third of our population will, however mildly, suffer some symptoms akin to fibromyalgia in their lifetime.

> My rheumatologist told me I was too old to have FMS. At that time I was fifty-four, never mind the fact I had had symptoms most of my life. The disease had become "full blown" when I was about fifty-one...After another year of suffering, I diagnosed myself via the Net. My DO (doctor of osteopathy) sent me back to the same rheumatologist because he is the only board-certified one in our area. At that time he told me I was too old to have FMS, but even if I did, there was nothing that could be done...I have since been diagnosed with FMS by three other doctors, all of whom have told me the only thing they could do was treat my symptoms. I was as good as I would ever be and would get much worse.
>
> —*Betty, Texas*

In 1843, Dr. Robert Froriep outlined the condition we now call fibromyalgia. He described it as "rheumatism with painful, hard places," which he could feel in many locations on the body. Unfortunately, the word *hard* (swollen) is being ignored nowadays and replaced by a search for *tender points*. In the early 1900s, Sir William Gowers in London studied his own lumbago and symptom clusters in his patients, and dubbed this disease *fibrositis*. (This name stuck for the next eighty years or so despite the fact that it was subsequently revealed that the inflammation the name implies was not present.) Dr. Gowers observed that his patients were also exhausted and that the disease was "so painful it would make a strong man cry out." He tried everything he could think of in an attempt to relieve this pain, including injecting cocaine into the tender points (it didn't work very well). He also gave his patients a newly discovered drug, aspirin, and noted that it didn't work very well, either.[2]

Fibromyalgia, a coined word that suggests "pain in muscles and fibers," has now replaced the previously popular names *fibrositis* and *rheumatism*. On New Year's Day 1993, the World Health Organization (WHO) as part of the Copenhagen Declaration officially declared fibromyalgia a syndrome.[3] It was described as the most common cause of widespread chronic muscle pain. Because of this action, the illness was given an ICD code (International Statistical Classification of Diseases and Related Health Problems), further validating the entity. Henceforth, doctors could credibly bill insurance companies or even declare patients disabled if worst came to worst. The WHO also incorporated the American College of Rheumatology's 1990 distinguishing features of fibromyalgia as penned by Drs. Muhammad Yunus, Hugh Smythe, Frederick Wolfe, and others.[4] They sought the eighteen most frequent locations of tender points dispersed over the bodies of fibromyalgics. They opted for a symmetrical distribution of nine such on each side, some in all four quadrants. The criteria they created was that at least eleven should be represented and that multiple symptoms suggesting fibromyalgia should have existed for more than three months.

But the World Health Organization went a little farther.

The Copenhagen Declaration added: "Fibromyalgia is part of a wider syndrome encompassing headaches, irritable bladder, dysmenorrhea, cold sensitivity, Raynaud's phenomenon, restless legs, atypical patterns of numbness and tingling, exercise intolerance, and complaints of weakness." It also recognized that patients are often depressed.[5]

Today, thousands of medical articles later, fibromyalgia is almost universally recognized as a distinct illness. Sadly, there remain a few uninformed and increasingly rare doctors who still tell patients that it's just a catchall name for symptoms shared by a bunch of neurotic women. Were that true, I would have long since gone fishing! Despite much research and speculation, fibromyalgia remains poorly understood. It's a complex and chronic disease that causes widespread pain and profound fatigue. Its range of symptoms makes simple, everyday tasks daunting or difficult, and often impossible.

> I remember: turning on the bathroom sink and forgetting to turn it off, completely flooding the bathroom; eating half a piece of toast and throwing the other half out because it was too much work to chew it; trying to read the newspaper and reading the same sentence over and over again because I couldn't comprehend it; lying on the couch in a zombie-type state all day long before going to bed; lying on the floor in pain. I remember not getting any diagnosis or any help at all from the medical field and being completely terrified, thinking I was going to die.
>
> —*Cheryl K., Canada*

Patients with fibromyalgia generally share the same complaints since symptoms appear from widely disparate parts of the body. This makes it difficult for doctors to find the connection between a foggy brain, pain in the neck, bladder infection, brittle fingernails, hives, and diarrhea, just to mention a few. Yet they must see the relevance if they are to properly treat a patient for one illness and not several, disparate conditions.

People who enjoy semantics will argue whether we are dealing with a condition, illness, syndrome, or disease. If you are unwell, you have a condition that causes your illness. Disease suggests lack of ease. Fibromyalgics are certainly qualified to wear that name. Symptoms and findings that regularly appear together often enough are regularly grouped in medical terms as syndromes. Lucky you: Fibromyalgia is that, too. Use any of those according to your preference or simply acknowledge that you're sick.

Many publications have listed the symptoms of fibromyalgia, most of them incompletely. Despite this, it remains a phantom illness with very few physical findings according to medical literature though not so to a trained examiner. The breadth of symptoms and unreliable physical targets greatly deter diagnosis. Though we're closing in, there are no validating laboratory, X-ray, or scanning techniques to give physicians a sound diagnostic footing. By ignoring what we've preached for fifty years, fibromyalgia is still being called an "invisible disability."

A well-conducted history, all by itself, will uncover the cyclic and progressive symptoms that point directly to the diagnosis. The recommended physical examination, a poking finger style, is far from perfect and totally falls apart in someone with a high pain threshold. We've far more successfully used our own technique long before the illness had a name. We make patient "maps" by sliding our hands along body surfaces looking for any swollen joint, muscle, tendon, or ligament. There are plenty of them!

I had watched my mother disintegrate. She died at ninety-four, never knowing what was wrong. No one ever explained why

her muscles hurt, why she could not move her bowels naturally, why she had constant headaches, etc. She wanted to die,
yet she lived to be just short of ninety-five, suffering terribly.
I could not help her. I had no idea what was causing all her
symptoms. Then I read Dr. St. Amand's book. By chapter 2,
I thought I knew what was wrong. And when Dr. St. Amand
diagnosed my daughter, he was also diagnosing the rest of the
people in my family that were suffering with FMS.

—*Bonnie J., Florida*

Although fibromyalgia is not a terminal illness, it is a demoralizing and debilitating one. The symptoms can be unbearable—
so much so that the so-called Suicide Doctor, Jack Kevorkian,
helped a few patients end their suffering. In 1997, one of these
fibromyalgics was forty-year-old Janis Murphy. After her death,
her father spoke out about his daughter's struggles with her illness. "Over the years, I've seen my daughter experience intractable and unrelenting pain," he said. He hated losing his only
child, but "there are things in this world worse than death."
Such a solution is not acceptable—not when something can be
done. Our purpose in writing this book as a new edition is to
continue clarifying the only treatment that works. We will also
tell you about our exciting new findings, along with those of our
research colleagues.

Although few patients can tolerate doing even a token
amount, many physicians advise exercise. That suggestion usually comes with the offer of chemical Band-Aids to temporarily soothe or block the ever-growing list of symptoms. Medical
professionals unwittingly promote eventual disability when
they prescribe ever-stronger medications that, sooner or later,
further deplete energy and deepen the mental haze. They have
nothing else to offer and justifiably defend the practice because
they can't sit idly by and watch people suffer.

Something bad is getting worse since long-term disability

insurance companies have entered the mounting fray—and they're hardly disinterested parties. It's to their advantage if they can get a fibromyalgic diagnosed as a psychiatric case via the depression and the anxieties. They do have growing difficulty in finding a psychiatrist or other professional who will ignore fibromyalgia. Yet because the vast majority of insurance policies do not cover mental disability, the companies keep trying.

Since there's a great deal of money at stake, other ploys are regularly used. They hire physicians who call the patient's doctor and quote him or her only in part. They end up reporting what is slightly twisted in favor of their employer. In some mysterious way, patients are given a dictum: "Your disability will end on [date]," and enforce it no matter what the personal physician writes. In other words, "We won't pay you anymore." The implication is, "Go get a lawyer if you want to fight." Insurance companies defend themselves by pointing out that fibromyalgia cases have reached epidemic proportions and are fully assaulting their bottom line. It's also true that this same virus-like intrusion is plaguing our other systems: U.S. Social Security, state disability, workers' compensation, and accelerating litigation. As many as 25 percent of American fibromyalgia patients have received some form of disability or injury compensation.[6]

We are the first to agree that the country can ill afford to swell these ranks. Indeed, when compensation has been granted, we want to get that patient motivated to heal and reenter the workforce. Yet neither can we turn our backs on very real suffering. We see only one solution to this dilemma: Get to the sick ones much sooner, and get them well.

The basic problem for patients and physicians is that there is no consensus regarding the cause of fibromyalgia. Considerable amounts of time and money have been spent, and few experts agree on anything. However, there is an answer. The purpose of this book is to present mutual findings, those of our patients and our own. As we've already stated, fibromyalgia is mainly an inherited problem that can be variably triggered. We'll discuss our theory and our recent findings that mutations exist on a few genes. Any of those aberrations can lead to faulty renal excretion and, hence, retention of a compound known as phosphate.

The vast majority of physicians are skillfully trained, well intentioned, and dedicated to their oath-driven principle of trying to help patients. Fibromyalgia is such a system-wide illness with so many seemingly unconnected, rapidly shifting complaints that doctors are understandably confused. Add to that the professional frustration they experience when they're stymied at every turn no matter what they prescribe. They eventually respond by referring patients to another doctor who should know more than they do about some "new" symptom. In the process, patients receive a fast-track medical education as they go from specialist to specialist.

It's also no wonder that most of our colleagues consider fibromyalgia incurable. All they can do is relieve symptoms as best they can often by prescribing the latest drug promoted by a drug company. With no known cause to treat, it makes total sense to attack individual symptoms with whatever may ameliorate them. Polypharmacy soon emerges, making use of NSAIDs (nonsteroidal anti-inflammatory drugs), various analgesics, antidepressants, sedatives, tranquilizers, and ultimately narcotics. The process is unstoppable. Patients get sicker and are forced by their medications into a far worse limbo state than before treatment. For many, the picture is truly bleak.

What do you do when fibro is causing your whole life to come apart? Your money situation has gone from bad to worse because you can't work and you can't think well enough to budget. You forget to make a deposit or your lights get turned off because you forgot to pay. Your husband wants to know when you'll get better because he feels lonely when all you can do is drag yourself through the day let alone make passionate love all night. Your kids are having trouble in school and you can't help them because you can't think. Neither can you skate with your daughter or play basketball with your sons. You look at your laundry piled up and you can't imagine sorting it let alone carrying it over to the laundry room. I can't think, can't talk, can't feel. I feel dead.

—Debbie, California

Over the years, we've used several different drugs to treat fibromyalgia. In the past, we exclusively prescribed gout medications that were thoroughly effective. Unfortunately, each had certain side effects that left a small group of patients in a treatment limbo. In 1992, our search led us to try guaifenesin, a widely available medication. It is well tolerated and has no known side effects. It's available over the counter without prescription both in long- and short-acting formulations that we'll later discuss. Prices vary among these preparations, and despite the fact that the cost has gone up in recent years, the drug is still relatively inexpensive.

We use guaifenesin as the mainstay of our treatment protocol. It actually addresses the basic disturbance caused by our defective gene(s) and doesn't just mask resulting symptoms. This book is the culmination of five decades of research and hands-on examinations. We've treated thousands of patients who have traveled from all over the world seeking relief from this enervating disease. With our approach, symptoms and pain reverse and often completely disappear in most patients if joints have not been damaged. Most individuals resume normal lives with minimal residual problems. Recovery is not immediate: We have to find the effective dosage of guaifenesin and try to clear out what it took years to accumulate. There are other crucial factors that we will stress.

In order for guaifenesin to work, it must have unrestricted access to receptors in the kidneys. These are like little garages where the medication must park and unload its contents before it will effectively work. Many ingredients in the products we use every day—pain medications, lipsticks, muscle balms, nutritional and herbal supplements, skin care products, toothpastes, deodorants, sunscreens, and even the sap of plants—contain a chemical known as salicylate. That little devil hogs all of the parking spaces in the kidney receptors and, like a union picket on strike, won't let guaifenesin work. This was not surprising for us since all of our previous medications faced the same problem. You'll find that we stress, again and again throughout this book, that the main demand of our protocol is that patients strictly avoid all sources of salicylate.

Approximately 30 percent of female fibromyalgics have hypoglycemia, or low blood sugar, with symptoms that greatly overlap those of fibromyalgia. For complete success offered in this book, both conditions must be addressed simultaneously. If this connection is overlooked and patients fail to make required dietary adjustments, fatigue, cognitive, and intestinal symptoms of hypoglycemia will persist even though fibromyalgia overlaps will reverse on guaifenesin.

As we will expand on in this book, our protocol must be followed very carefully if patients are to achieve the positive results we describe. You can imagine our frustration when we hear, "Oh, I tried this treatment and it doesn't work." We've heard too often from patients and physicians alike who missed the mandatory step of cleaning out all sources of salicylates. We would like to take up twenty pages of bold print with caps repeating the mantra: Don't Use Salicylates! Enough said?

We will share our knowledge of fibromyalgia throughout this book. We know firsthand the nature of the disease: the cognitive distress, the unrelenting exhaustion, and the pains that cumulatively induce deep depression, and finally even suicidal thoughts. We know how hard it is to be understood in a healthy world, where perfectly healthy people are all around you, when friends and even family say (dare we repeat?), "You don't look sick!" We've poured our hopes into yours in the succeeding chapters. We'll try to explain simply and discuss clearly all of the important lessons you must learn if you plan success. We'll stress what you must change, because most of you need more than just a pill to get fully reenergized and relatively pain-free. Patients of any age can follow our protocol, which is designed to reverse fibromyalgia in far less time than it took to develop the illness. Despite damage in later years from osteoarthritis that guaifenesin cannot reverse, clear thinking, full energy, and bowel and bladder functions can be restored.

Believe us, the guaifenesin protocol is not yet accepted in mainstream medicine. We have not provided the coveted double-blind study, but we now have published papers in medical journals for those willing to decipher their contents. Word of our protocol is spreading thanks to grassroots support of our healing patients. Thereby, many physicians and other practitioners are using the protocol, but we don't know how many are enlisted in this growing infantry. We frequently get e-mails and some letters from people who've either recruited their physicians or been urged by them to adopt our protocol. In addition to face-to-face, hands-on training with doctors who've come to us, Claudia and I have spoken at medical meetings, patient-doctor mixed groups, guaifenesin support groups worldwide, and even participated in occasional television and radio interviews to deliver our simple message. During these events, we regularly extend invitations to join us in fighting the battle. In short, we've been preaching to anyone who'll listen. Whether through this book or in person, we keep repeating, "Guaifenesin works, but we plead with you to follow our instructions!"

I have never contacted an organization or a website for any reason so I'm not sure what I'm doing. I just hope you receive this. I do not know what else to do. I'm divorced, single mother of two daughters, sixteen and ten. I've been through some extremely stressful years while trying to work, raise my girls, and go to numerous doctors, some of which claim they specialize in fibromyalgia. I don't know what to say next except I'm hoping you can help me. I'm forty-two years old, and for the past few years, I feel like I'm seventy-two. I'm always exhausted, experiencing pain, irritable, dizzy, issues with my bowels, skin problems...I've always lived my life feeling that no matter what was handed to me, my glass was always half full, but now it feels like my glass is empty. I want my life back. I want to be the person I was in the past.

—*Lisa, Maryland*

Why preach to the choir? You surely know that you must take charge of your own illness. Physicians will never spend the time to look for salicylates in products other than prescription drugs. They're not going to shop at cosmetics counters using magnifying glasses to scan labels. No one will hover nearby to slap your hand when you reach for a piece of pie if you're hypoglycemic. But look at it this way: Not reading labels or cheating on the diet will obviously harm you, but will also discourage your doctor, who's observing you and hoping for your success if only to acquire a method for treating other patients. Even practitioners who've feigned disinterest and only allowed that guaifenesin can't hurt you will become attentive as you begin to feel better. Since you're reading this book, you must still be motivated to try again despite all of your previous setbacks. That speaks volumes. For each one who picks up this book, we know that there are some who'll put it down because it "looks too hard" and "I'm too sick to try this." It is truly your loss.

Eleven years ago this evening I took a deep breath and swallowed my first half-pill of guaifenesin. I had been following all the standard treatments—antidepressant for pain and sleep, pain meds for pain, sleeping pills for sleep, following a very rigid schedule of waking and sleeping and activity every day, avoiding stress whenever possible, and meditating for half an hour morning and evening. But I got sicker and sicker anyway. At night, I would hear somebody scream in my sleep, and wake up to realize it had been me, crying out in pain when I changed position. I was sure within six months I would lose my job and never be able to work again. I was planning to commit suicide before I became totally incapacitated. But I had decided that first I would give the guaifenesin protocol a try.

—*Anne L., Minnesota*

We invite all fibromyalgia sufferers (and their loved ones) to embark on the journey to improved health. Let us be your tour directors. We're passionate about providing you with the information you need. We've both done it, paid our dues, and are eager to share what we know. Realize up front that this trip is not for the faint of heart. For most of you, the road back to good health will seem long, with days of discomfort living in a cognitive wasteland. In the beginning, this may be more intense than what you have suffered to date. But the destination is gold-laden; grasp for it.

This treatment is designed to flush the body of the metabolic debris that's clogging up your energy-producing factories, tiny mitochondria buried deep inside all your cells. While that's happening, your emotional and physical pain will most likely increase. But with time, you'll notice symptoms easing and you'll soon find that you have some good hours, eventually better ones, and ultimately great days. You'll actually bounce back after an illness, injury, or hard work, just as you once did. Most welcome is the ability to participate in activities with the energy and enthusiasm that have eluded you for years. By following our treatment regimen to the letter, along with your doctor's advice, this is all within your reach. We want you to resume living your life to the fullest. The best definition of happiness we've ever heard is: "Happiness is freedom from pain." Wipe out mental anguish and constant pain, and life is a joy.

Chapter Two

The Fibromyalgia Syndrome

An Overview of Symptoms and Causes

Fibromyalgia is real, Fibromyalgia hurts, and Fibromyalgia intrudes into lives and relationships in a real way. The two basic challenges that face a newly diagnosed patient are the following: learning about your illness so that you understand it and then explaining it to everyone else in your life so that they do as well.

—*Claudia Marek,* Fibromyalgia Is Real

WHAT IS FIBROMYALGIA? Twenty-seven or so years after the condition was given a name, the medical community and patients are still looking for that answer. My coauthor, Claudia, asked her son, Malcolm Potter, that question when he was about ten years old. His response was, "It feels like all my muscles want to throw up!" That intuitive response still seems as descriptive as anything else that's been offered. Another one is: "the irritable everything syndrome," coined by Dr. Hugh Smythe of Toronto, Ontario. From ten-year-old boy to prominent researcher—two phrases that pretty well cover it, wouldn't you say?

Fibromyalgia is different from other illnesses. If we were to describe thyroid diseases, diabetes, or rheumatoid arthritis, for example, we could easily recite their distinguishing characteristics. Most conditions have a single set of lab tests to help confirm the diagnosis. Often, one major organ or gland is the culprit. That's not so with fibromyalgia, because it doesn't pick on just a single type of cell or limited body part. Instead, it shows up with myriad seemingly unrelated symptoms in endless combinations. At first glance, the only thing these complaints seem to have in common is that they coexist in a single human being. Symptoms don't neatly fit into diagnostic categories. Perversely, they spill profusely over the borders that define any particular medical specialty. You just can't quite tuck it in. It remains elusive, treacherous, troublesome to pin down, and taxing to treat.

Though there is no set pattern, fibromyalgia assaults enough systems to raise a warning flag to the alert physician. The same amalgam of characteristics drives patients to seek help from whatever specialist they deem best suited to handle the chief complaints. Specialists, by definition, work in somewhat limited spheres. That narrow focus may not allow a panoramic view where all the symptoms are displayed. Thinking within their particular fields, they find it difficult to expand perspectives to include minutiae into an all-encompassing diagnosis. So they end up treating just a few symptoms as if those represent the entire disease. Therefore, irritable bowel syndrome, interstitial cystitis, vulvar pain syndrome, chronic fatigue syndrome, chronic candidiasis, and myofascial pain syndrome are treated as separate entities though they represent facets of fibromyalgia. Often, physicians in family practice, internal medicine, and rheumatology, who more routinely perform complete patient evaluations, are more adept at identifying the many outlying symptoms.

I've already described the environment in which I practiced in my early years. I was visited by patients with numerous complaints, who had seen many doctors, and had taken many medications. They still weren't well, but certainly more frustrated.

Their family doctors had examined and tested them, often in memorable detail. The conclusion: "Everything's normal; it's just your nerves." Family and friends eventually echoed those words and accepted the fact that their loved one was just a neurotic who was cracking up under stress. I equally fell into that trap because I was taught that methodology and had no evidence to contradict it.

What we were all missing was the connecting thread among patients. Glaringly obvious was the sheer volume of complaints. Sure, many patients found it difficult to pinpoint exactly when their symptoms had begun. Most had great trouble discerning the order in which they appeared. They wilted under questioning as if they were being cross-examined and a wrong answer would result in condemnation. Migraines, fatigue, depression, muscle aches, dizziness, nasal congestion, gas, diarrhea, breaking nails, numbness, bladder infections, and on and on. Shouldn't someone have caught on sooner? All of them were repeating the same things!

Some mornings I would wake up and feel so lethargic it was all I could do to make it to work. For several years, I'd attributed my muscle pain to the few fender-benders that I'd been in. I'd thought the migraine headaches were hereditary. And I would tell myself I'd caught a "bug" when the dizziness and fatigue became a problem. The strange thing was the symptoms seemed to get worse as time went on, not better, despite the treatment I'd received from traditional M.D.s, chiropractors, holistic practitioners, acupuncturists, masseuses, and herbalists.

About a year ago, I was so frustrated I rattled off all my recurring symptoms to my [previous] doctor and demanded, "I've been here before with these problems. What's wrong with me?" To which she replied with annoying frankness, "I don't know."

— *Michelle, California*

Not unlike other illnesses, the severity and impact of fibromyalgia differ from patient to patient. Some are able to lead relatively normal lives. Often they live with a number of irritating symptoms for years when suddenly the hesitation is over and the full-blown, unrelenting disease hits. Others become considerably debilitated early on or even homebound. There are those who feel well until traumatized by an accident, surgery, extensive dental work, infection, or emotional stress. They single out those events as triggers that precipitate their illnesses. In most cases, when taking a more detailed history, we can elucidate many, much earlier complaints. But for the vast number of people, symptoms sneak up insidiously, wax and wane, gradually intensify, and eventually never go away.

In addition to the physical complaints, the vast majority of patients also have difficulties with memory and concentration—cognitive difficulties that have been nicknamed "fibrofog." This embarrassing entanglement often takes a heavier toll on patients than do the aches and pains. It raises fear of serious brain deterioration, and begs reassurances that it isn't the embrace of premature Alzheimer's. You can appreciate the alarm invoked by the neurological involvement upon reading the following description.

> I sit at a computer at work with a headset on, answering calls from people about computers of all types...I have to solve their problems, at the same time "teach" them. Many times I have found myself not knowing who I am talking to (man or woman?) and what we were talking about. It is like just waking up from a dream. So I have to keep notes of what I'm doing on my calls, or just plain ask the person to repeat what they just said. This will eventually cost me my job...I don't know what my future holds. I've gotten in my car and forgotten how to turn the lights on, or where the windshield wipers

are. Sometimes I can laugh about it, later. But it's getting more frequent and I'm not laughing anymore.

—Cyndi S., Arkansas

At the beginning of my medical career, I knew of no disease that could encompass the weird symptoms expressed by this group. The sheer number of people reciting the same litany of complaints made it ever more likely there was some undocumented disease. The depth of cycling and rapid shifting from good to bad days didn't quite fit into the description of neurosis. I also noticed that sick days were not always related to tensions and stresses at home or work. Neurotics are neurotic and don't usually experience great days out of nowhere. The fact that my patients were inexplicably better at times despite living under identical conditions made me more attentive to the repetitious nature of their symptoms.

There was no doubt that these patients were emotionally upset, frequently at the end of their rope. They complained of varying degrees of pain, at least some stiffness, affecting many parts of their body. That seemed pretty tangible and at least represented specific locales for me to start probing. I kept trying to find some palpable abnormalities in the designated, painful areas. Eventually I did feel them: very detectable swellings scattered pattern-like everywhere on these people. I soon made the connection that worse-pain days meant worse-everywhere complaints. It wasn't long before I realized that the entire symptom cascade was interrelated. It became obvious that pain hurts whether it stems from an emotionally floundering brain or from a gut in spasm, a burning and irritated bladder, or a headache. It was indeed one great big mess! I was literally feeling my way and reinforcing my ever-growing conviction that everything was linked and had to have a single cause. What on earth could it be?

THE SYMPTOMS OF FIBROMYALGIA

By and large, fibromyalgia symptoms can be grouped into the following categories: central nervous system, eye-ear-nose-and-throat, musculoskeletal, dermal, gastrointestinal, and genito-urinary. There are a few other, isolated problems that don't fit easily into any classification other than miscellaneous. We'll look at all of those affected areas and present you with a tableau of fibromyalgia. Each of these biological systems earns its own chapter later in this book. We'll separate them just to make the full ramifications of the disease more comprehensible. But please remember, they are all very much connected, all stem from the same cause, and are all equally restored by one medication, guaifenesin.

Cerebral—Fatigue, irritability, nervousness, depression, apathy, listlessness, impaired memory and concentration (fibrofog), anxieties and suicidal thoughts, insomnia, frequent awakening, and nonrestorative sleep.

Musculoskeletal—Pain and generalized morning stiffness in the involved muscles, tendons, ligaments, and fascia that may arise from such structures surrounding the neck, shoulders, upper and lower back, hips, knees, inner and outer elbows, wrists, fingers, toes, and chest as well as from injured or old operative sites. Pain can assume any form and intensity, such as throbbing, burning, stabbing, stinging, grabbing, or any combination of these. Joints may be swollen, red and hot, or just painful as in the temporo-mandibular joint (TMJ). Numbness of the extremities or face and tingling anywhere arise from contracted structures pressing on nearby nerves. Facial and head pains spring from the neck or skull bone connections (sutures). Tiny parts of muscles often twitch, and the restless leg syndrome makes it impossible to find a comfortable position. Patients also complain of feelings resembling electrical impulses in their muscles, and a feeling of general weakness. Leg and foot cramps are common.

Dermal—Undue sweating; various rashes may appear with or without itching: hives, red blotches, acne, tiny red or clear bumps, blisters, eczema, seborrheic or neurodermatitis, and rosacea. Nails are often brittle, or they peel or chip. Hair is of poor quality and either breaks or falls out prematurely, sometimes in bunches. Strange sensations are common, including cold, heat (especially of the palms, soles, and thighs), crawling, electric vibrations, prickling, hypersensitivity to touch, and flushing that is sometimes accompanied by a somewhat pungent and irritating sweat.

Gastrointestinal—Irritable bowel syndrome, leaky gut, spastic or mucous colitis, fibrogut. Transient nausea, gas, pain, bloating, constipation alternating with diarrhea, mucus in stools, and sometimes hyperacidity with reflux.

Genitourinary—Pungent urine, frequent urination, bladder spasms with very low (suprapubic) abdominal aching, burning urination (dysuria) with or without repeated bladder infections or so-called interstitial cystitis. Suspected vaginal yeast infections without the usual cottage cheese discharge are mimicked by vulvodynia (vulvar pain syndrome), which includes vulvitis (painful, irritated, burning, and sometimes raw vaginal lips), vestibulitis (same symptoms deeper into the opening), vaginal spasms or cramps, burning mucous discharge, increased menstrual-uterine cramps, and painful intercourse (dyspareunia).

Head-eye-ear-nose-and-throat—Headaches that are labeled "migraines" when they're severe enough. Others, less intense, could be in the back of the neck and head only (occipital); front only (frontal), which are often erroneously blamed on the sinuses; one-sided only (hemicephalic); or generalized (entire head); dizziness, vertigo (spinning), or imbalance; dry eyes as well as itching and burning with or without a sticky or gritty discharge (sand) first thing in the morning; blurred vision; excessive nasal mucous congestion and postnasal drip; painful, burning, or cut tongue; abnormal tastes (bad or metallic), scalded mouth; brief ringing (tinnitus) or lower-pitched sounds in the ears; ear and eyeball pains; sensitivity to light, sounds, and odors. Late-in-life-onset asthma and hay fever are sometimes related.

Miscellaneous—Weight gain; low-grade fever with night sweats; lowered immunity to infections; morning eyelid and hand swelling from water retention that slowly gravitates to the lower extremities and by evening stretches tissues, impinges surface nerves, and causes the restless leg syndrome.

TENDER POINTS

It took years to happen. It was not until I turned sixty-three that I became totally aware of the fact that my body was breaking down. Before that I had plenty of indications that my health was disintegrating; eighteen years of chiropractic adjustments, visits to many nutritionists, and a kitchen cabinet filled with at least twenty different homeopathic remedies purchased from people who charged me for their alternative practices. I tried that route because my mom, who had similar symptoms, had had no success with regular doctors. Researching FMS took me to Devin Starlanyl's book *Fibromyalgia and Chronic Myofascial Pain*. I was relaxing on the beach, reading her book, and saw a diagram of the tender points. I found all eighteen on me. And then I knew what I had.

—*Bonnie J., Florida*

Ever since the 1840s, when "painful hard places" were described in certain patients with rheumatism, doctors and patients have been fascinated by them. These sensitive spots are now referred to as *tender* or *trigger points*. The latter designation is used for the so-called myofascial pain syndrome. The official American College of Rheumatology (ACR) criteria for the diagnosis of fibromyalgia are based to a degree on finding tenderness in eleven out of eighteen predetermined sites when appropriate, finger pressure is exerted. Such spots have been mapped, poked, prodded, biopsied, injected, and scanned. They're frequently assessed using a contraption called a dolorimeter, a spring-loaded device that measures the pressure load when a patient cries out or flinches.

When questioned, most patients confirm tender areas throughout their bodies. Most are located on muscles, tendons, and ligaments. Pain complaints move around a lot, but tender sites don't vary all that much. In reality, the most painful spots of the day take precedence and drown out the others. Swelling changes with fluid content, and pain is determined by how much pressure squeezes neighboring nerves. That's why small swellings can sometimes hurt much more than the bigger ones. Pain sensitivity is largely inherited and varies in a spectrum of tolerance.

The tender-point concept has always seemed arbitrary to us and to a growing number of rheumatologists. What do we do with someone who has all the symptoms of fibromyalgia but only nine tender points in the locations we're supposed to check? What if a patient has limited numbers in the predetermined sites, but has twenty in undesignated areas? People with high pain thresholds may feel no tenderness or only negligible sensitivity anywhere on the body. That's not uncommon, especially in athletes. The obvious question is what to do with a nontender individual who's loaded with swollen tissues, has all of the fatigue, cognitive, bowel, and urinary tract symptoms of fibromyalgia? The lack of tender points is what is used to shift such persons out of the proper diagnosis and into the realm of chronic fatigue syndrome.

We find the the tender-point concept is unduly limiting. After taking a patient's history, we begin our search for any involved tissue in a process we call *mapping*. This manual examination turns up many large and small spastic zones, sometimes involving an entire muscle bundle. These areas are distinctly swollen, not always tender, so we simply call them the lumps and bumps of fibromyalgia. We record each of these, noting its location and size on a sketch of the body. (See chapter 7 for a description of our technique and a blank body map.) Some patients can barely be touched; others can be prodded with little concern. Our examination doesn't rely on what a person feels: They've already told us about their pain distribution. We are purely objective and record only what we can feel without added input from the patient.

WHAT CAUSES FIBROMYALGIA?

Given the broad spectrum of bodily functions and tissues affected by fibromyalgia, it's only natural to wonder: What kind of pathology would affect so many, diverse systems of the body? Can brittle nails and migraines really be connected? Why haven't we found abnormalities in the customary diagnostic tests? Such issues have perplexed physicians and patients alike. Those of us who've studied fibromyalgia for years still don't agree on the answers, but luckily the enigma is breaking up, as you will learn.

There are controversies in the medical community about the nature of fibromyalgia. I've seriously studied the proposed concepts, and I disagree with them. I've long ago joined in and expounded my own theory. Luckily, I have a lot of data: firsthand experience and much gleaned from basic science, as well as published results from our own research. The current treatments being offered don't hold up well and mainly mask the developing disease. Before delving into details, here is my authentication. I've gathered firsthand evidence examining more than ten thousand patients and from their follow-up visits. I add to those numbers daily and I've examined every single one of them personally. For the past ten years, I have only treated fibromyalgia. Therefore, I hardly feel pompous saying "in my experience." What we're about to recite makes the most sense from the perspective of physiology, biochemistry, and clinical medicine. We continue expanding on a concept that fits, and a treatment that works.

Here we ask you to bear in mind that a theory is nothing more than a set of assumptions based on many accumulated facts. Encountering a theory, immediately recognize that it undoubtedly contains errors and oversights. This edition of the book will tell you how we are improving it by actively delving deeper into the biochemical and genetic factors we've always thought were at the root of fibromyalgia. We're totally satisfied that the illness responds well to guaifenesin. Our recently published papers give a glimpse into the effects of the drug. The truth is revealing itself at last. Please remain patient with us. Our theories are undergoing rigorous testing and so far so good!

We wish we could choose a more descriptive name for the disease that would fit all of its symptoms. *Fibromyalgia* is a Latin term meaning pain in muscles and fibers, but that's clearly inadequate to define the rest of the illness. *Chronic fatigue syndrome*, the second most commonly used moniker, focuses mainly on brain exhaustion and malfunction. For most patients, both labels apply at various times during their illness but can't be easily combined into one classification. At times, the symptoms of one condition are prevalent and tilt the scale to one or the other diagnosis. However, it just takes a careful history and appropriate examination to make it very clear that we're dealing with one and the same condition. It's merely a matter of tissue sensitivity, disease intensity, and individual pain threshold.

For these reasons, fibromyalgia badly needs a new name— not that this is likely to happen. We proposed *dysenergism syndrome* (faulty energy) in our first edition. Since then, a learned Greek colleague invoked his native language to suggest *energopenia*, meaning "dearth of energy." That would cover it well, but it's not being accepted. Indeed, our treatment restores vitality by lifting the biochemical blockade we're about to describe. That done, the symptoms of the illness recede. I use myself as an example. At age eighty-four, I'm able to do some things I couldn't do in my thirties. Sadly, however, much as we'd love to change the name, at this time we'll go along with common usage and stick with *fibromyalgia*.

THE MALFUNCTION JUNCTION OF FIBROMYALGIA: A BIOCHEMICAL THEORY

What in the world could be the metabolic difficulty that springs up to cause such a body-wide failure? The stack of symptoms we've listed above strongly signals that many bodily functions have gone on strike and often at the same time. You and your doctors may have been just looking at the surface effects of fibromyalgia. There certainly has to be some type of fundamental breakdown. Aches and pains arise from spasms; the brain is obviously too tired to remain functionally alert. But why do the bladder, skin, intestinal tract, eyes, nose, throat, and more structures all join in? All of those parts are nothing but a bunch of cells that should work harmoniously. There must be some altered chemistry behind all this—a truly basic connection.

We believe that fibromyalgia is caused by an excess of a specific biochemical substance that enters individual and intercommunicating cells. This process begins at birth and accrues until the body's safety nets are overstretched and become porous. The time from birth until the symptoms appear varies with the individual's genetics. We think there's an inherited malfunction in a specific area of the kidneys that allows the buildup of something in the body that, in normal people, is excreted. We strongly suspect inorganic phosphate. There is a saying in medicine that either too much or too little of a given element will interfere with function. Not surprisingly, cells work within a very narrow range for each of their chemical contents. Logically, to preserve itself, the body distributes surplus concentrations among a variety of cells. However, there is a critical level that, when exceeded, induces a malfunction—in this case, an energy deficit.

Every bodily function needs energy—not only in moving, running, exercising, and speaking, but also simply growing hair, breathing, digesting food, fighting illness, and, especially, using the brain. Eighty to 90 percent of our food must be converted to fuel. All cells produce a currency of energy known as adenosine triphosphate (ATP). Every chore we've just listed and whatever else a body does all depend on this vital compound. That's even true for anything else that's alive: plants, bacteria, and all animals large and small. This process involves extremely complicated biochemical mechanisms. Many of the compounds and enzymes that play significant roles in energy production are already known.

In order to understand how fibromyalgic cells malfunction, we need to study how energy is produced. In properly functioning cells, the concentration of all the substances integral to energy formation is meticulously maintained. Tiny power stations called *mitochondria,* where raw materials are processed, are where our story is now focused. These are present in all cells of the body, but they're stacked especially high in brain and muscle cells. They're complex little factories that convert 80 percent or more of our foods into adenosine triphosphate—three phosphates (tri) hooked onto a single molecule of adenosine. When a cell must perform a function, it rips one high-energy phosphate off adenosine, and expends it for the chosen activity. Such chemical reactions provide most of the energy required by living tissue. Almost magically, electrons are released in these bursts and are somehow directed to the right place to do the right job at precisely the right time. Then it's somewhat like the gasoline in your car's tank: ready for burning. It's also like plugging in an electric cord: The energy's been there all the while, just waiting for a signal to connect. Electrons flow through cells, charge up various enzymes, and run electrical currents in tissue "appliances." In healthy bodies, cells seem to have an almost unlimited supply of ATP. In fact, within thousandths of a second, cells can produce new energy from a series of reservoirs.

So how does an energy deficit occur in fibromyalgia? We know that this is the problem. It had been suggested much earlier, but a study reported in 1989 actually measured ATP levels in tissues of fibromyalgics.[1] Two Swedish researchers, Drs. Bengtsson and Henriksson, found a 20 percent reduction in muscle biopsies taken from such sites. They sampled bits from the swollen and tender trapezius, a muscle located at the top of the shoulder. Adjacent, normal tissue was also biopsied and studied but showed no similar ATP deficits. A few years later, low ATP levels were found in red blood cells of affected individuals. These studies, along with the more technical magnetic resonance spectroscopy that can probe inside living cells (see the Technical Appendix), support our theory of inadequate energy as the cause of fibromyalgia.

We like having our theory validated, but the question still arises: Why this depletion? What has interfered so stressfully to suck out ATP? The body is superbly geared to prevent such an occurrence, since major losses would mean cellular death. Obviously, that doesn't happen in fibromyalgia. Something must be lacking or have entered and accumulated to gunk up or idle the generators.

It's well known in physiology and biochemistry that phosphate excesses in the inner core of mitochondria, the matrix, slow down these power stations. Eventually, this not only eats up surplus ATP, but slows basic production as well. Blocking ATP generation means there won't be enough high-energy phosphates available for the cell to do any real work beyond simply surviving. Cells with the highest activity are the first hit and worst affected by this shortage. The more cells are pressed into service, the more seriously are they affected. So it's a small wonder that brain and muscle are the heaviest hit! Optimal function is permitted only when energy is sufficiently replenished. Is any of this news to a fibromyalgic?

But phosphate is not the only problem. It can't pile up indiscriminately inside cells without causing permanent damage. Because each phosphate ion carries two negative charges, electrical equilibrium can only be sustained by a counterbalancing (buffering) with an element that sports two positive charges. Enter calcium, the preferred companion for phosphate. Whenever and wherever phosphate goes, so does calcium.

Calcium normally sits quietly inside storage bins, known as the endoplasmic reticulum, and mitochondria, or lurks just outside the cell's wall. When a stimulus arrives, the command is given to the endoplasmic reticulum to release stored calcium into the fluid chamber of the cell, the cytosol. The amount released is just enough to perform the desired task, no more and no less. If more is needed to amplify the signal, liberal amounts can be imported from the readily available external pool. Focus on the fact that calcium is the final battery terminal—the ultimate messenger that commands any cell to "Get going and do what you're told!" (See figures 2.1 and 2.2.)

Calcium won't stop its demands for performance as long as it sits in the cell's liquid interior, the cytosol (known as the sarcoplasm in muscles). So the poor cell must strive to keep working as instructed until it's relieved of duty. To interrupt go-ahead signals, calcium must be either pumped back into storage within the endoplasmic reticulum, or totally pushed out from the cell. (Enzyme pumps exist that are used just for this purpose.) As you've learned, any function performed by the body uses up ATP for energy; the pumps need the same

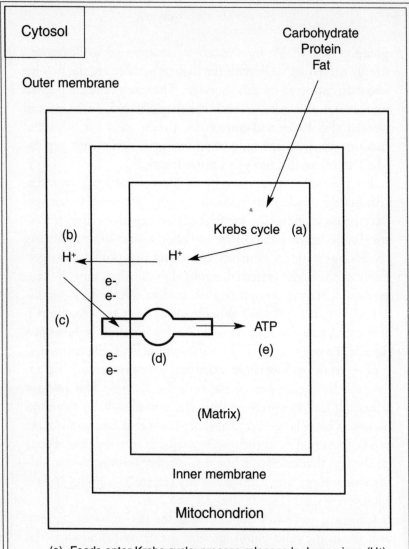

(a) Foods enter Krebs cycle; process releases hydrogen ions (H+).
(b) H+ is driven out to the outer chamber.
(c) H+ enters space within inner wall of mitochondrion and releases electrons (e-).
(d) H+ is driven through proton pump back into the matrix.
(e) Process produces ATP.

Figure 2.1

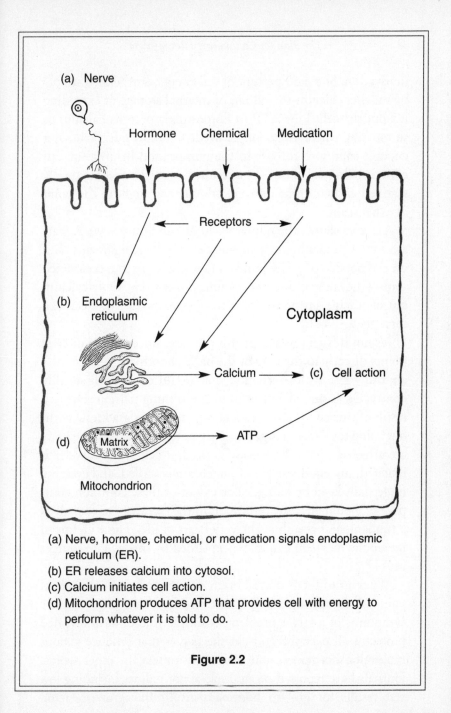

(a) Nerve, hormone, chemical, or medication signals endoplasmic reticulum (ER).
(b) ER releases calcium into cytosol.
(c) Calcium initiates cell action.
(d) Mitochondrion produces ATP that provides cell with energy to perform whatever it is told to do.

Figure 2.2

motivation. Some 40 percent of cell energy is expended simply by moving calcium in and out of internal storage or extruding it from the cell. Low ATP in fibromyalgia permits calcium to sit too long where it's no longer needed. Simply put, there's not enough energy to fully man the pumps, and insufficient calcium is being baled out. As a result, tissues affected are totally strained and continue to overwork day and night to the point of exhaustion.

As we've stated, the numerous lumps and bumps we palpate are found predominantly in muscles, tendons, ligaments, and on the outside of a few joints. These areas are in a contracted state—they're working twenty-four hours a day. Only calcium out of storage sitting in the cytosol (sarcoplasm) of a cell can force that.

It's not difficult to accept this premise, since patient distress points directly to the core of the basic abnormality. There isn't anything else we can surmise that would cause such steadily contracted tissues. There is an overwhelming tension state as a result of this condition. Readers with fibromyalgia know without being told how many seemingly unrelated parts of the body are affected. "My whole body is tired, it aches, my bladder is irritated, my gut doesn't work, my brain is addled, and even my fingernails keep breaking." The extent of these common complaints should alert my profession to the fact that the malady is a fundamental assault at the very heart of life. The widespread metabolic mayhem can all be explained by inadequate sources of ATP.

We tend to focus on the brain deficits and musculoskeletal pains of fibromyalgia and ignore the facts that they, too, are symptoms of a larger problem. Multiple studies have revealed problems all over the body in the tissues that produce various molecules, hormones, and neurotransmitters. In other words, journals have reported on multiple abnormalities including low test results for growth hormone, insulin-like growth factor, serotonin, certain amino acids, and free urinary cortisol. These and numerous other results have still failed to produce a single accurate diagnostic test for fibromyalgia despite the dedicated efforts of many researchers.

Energy deprivation is certainly at the root of this illness. No matter what findings pop up in the future, the shortage of ATP will continue to explain the disturbance. Many capable M.D. and Ph.D. investigators are looking for a culprit and findings are finally emerging, things new to this edition. Any new theory would need to propose a similarly debilitating disturbance, serious enough to destroy what was once a well-functioning body. But only restoration of normal ATP production can give back to patients their mental and physical energies.

In genetics, polymorphisms speak of multiple variations in a single gene. We're now certain that there is more than just one of these variations scattered in various chromosomes in fibromyalgia. We defended this position early on because we had treated several patients under the age of five, but also many individuals who displayed neither the symptoms nor characteristic findings until later in life—even one who began at the age of seventy-four. That last observation suggested the presence of one or more less-destructive genes. The addition of kinder (recessive) genes to less gentle (dominant) ones permits all sorts of combinations (permutations), which in turn determine how intensely and when the illness is first expressed. If both parents have such defects, their mutual children will, too.

In our first edition, I erroneously predicted that the X chromosome would be the likely site for the major genetic defect. When we wrote a book about childhood fibromyalgia, Claudia realized that prior to puberty we had equal numbers of boys and girls (ninety-three to ninety-four, respectively). So why is it that, postpubertally, women make up 85 percent of the fibromyalgia population? It dawned on us that bones and muscles require huge amounts of phosphate to sustain rapid growth.

That timing put to rest the myth of "growing pains." They occur mostly in the preteen years of relatively slow growth and usually disappear during the spurt that signals puberty. Testosterone-fed male tissues beef up and sustain lifelong phosphate requirements. Such buffering offers men partial protection from fibromyalgia, but does not eliminate them as genetic carriers.

The human genome has now been mapped, and though there are yet slots to fill in, we and others have identified some mutations. So many people have fibromyalgia that geneticists might at first consider the variations as normal subtypes. We and our patients remain involved in an ongoing study with a premier research institute in Southern California, the City of Hope. I personally suspect that our adverse traits encode defective enzymes that are normally dedicated to precision control of phosphate or other ions. They would be less responsive and would neglect the retention or elimination of phosphate that should accommodate to bodily needs. Initially, the defects would still allow the body to tuck retained excesses into receptive sinkholes, particularly in bones. The daily retention would be minute, but we believe that "tuckability" is eventually exceeded. Other cells must take up the slack even though they get sick doing it.

Had enough of the technical explanations? It's time to discuss our treatment for reversing fibromyalgia.

Chapter Three

Guaifenesin

How and Why It Works

> I will consider changing my medications, my physical therapies, and even my exercise routine, but I will not consider going without guaifenesin, nor will I take anything that might block its effect. It's too important to my well-being.
> —*Devin Starlanyl, author of* The Fibromyalgia Advocate

As OFTEN HAPPENS in medicine, I stumbled upon the treatment for fibromyalgia quite by accident. I was young and naive, but I was lucky. It all began with a patient's chance observation.

In 1959, long before our illness had been defined or officially named, a patient came to see me on a revisit. He suffered from gout and for two years had taken the only drug available at that time, probenecid (Benemid). He was feeling fine but unexpectedly said, "Hey, Doc, does this drug take tartar off your teeth?" He then scraped off bits and pieces of tartar (clinically referred to as dental calculus) and flicked them onto my office floor. Though I was not particularly pleased with his newly discovered skill, I responded the way a poised physician should. I harrumphed appropriately and said, "I don't think so." Yet my curiosity was piqued, and I began to reflect on this finding. I awakened two nights later asking myself what this flaking might indicate.

My knowledge of dentistry was limited so I consulted a textbook that had a page or two devoted to dental calculus. I learned that the mineral backbone of tartar was 75 percent calcium phosphate in a chemical structure called apatite. Tartar develops from saliva, which in turn derives from the serum of blood. Water, all varieties of minerals, proteins, abundant calcium, and phosphate are secreted from blood plasma into the salivary glands. These glands modify and manufacture their own proteins, such as mucus and digestive enzymes. They then mulch and concentrate such things with the above elements to make saliva. My search taught me that salivary phosphate concentrations were four times that normally found in blood. The level of salivary calcium, on the other hand, is just about equal to what's inside the bloodstream. Chemically speaking, this makes for a very unstable solution. We multiply the calcium level by that of phosphate and produce a number called the solubility constant. Sufficient instability caused by too much or too little of either element allows crystals to form deep under the gums and on the teeth; that's what is called *tartar*.

Though dental calculus can wreak havoc on the gums, teeth, and oral hygiene, that was all the information I could find. Not everyone creates dental calculus, and some people produce the stuff at variable rates. My quest was to learn what was metabolically different about tartar formers. I began by looking more closely at people with gout, since it was a gout medication that let my patient chip tartar off his teeth.

I'd been interested in gout and suspected that there was more to the illness than merely joint pains and swelling. I reread the original description written by Thomas Sydenham almost three hundred years before, in 1683. He described gout as a disease with joint pain and one manifested by "great mental torpor," "suffusion of the sinuses," generalized flu-like aching, and malaise or fatigue, along with many other complaints, all in the dramatic language of his day. In other words, there were

Gout—A metabolic disease unrelated to fibromyalgia. Diagnosis is helped if a high plasma uric acid level is discovered. Aspiration of a gouty joint will show needle-like, uric acid crystals. Gout is treated with two types of medications: uricosuric drugs such as sulfinpyrazone and probenecid, which cause the kidneys to excrete excess uric acid; and more commonly used nowadays, allopurinol or febuxostat, which inhibit the formation of uric acid. Gout has many symptoms, but the most diagnostic is a red, hot, or swollen joint usually located from the knee down. It is inherited, and ten times more common in men than in women and then only after menopause.

Uric acid—A waste product from the breakdown of nucleic acids in body cells; it is also produced in the digestion of some foods. Most uric acid passes by way of the kidneys into the urine and is excreted, although some is passed through the digestive tract. When the kidneys do not excrete uric acid properly, high levels can build up in the body. This can lead to gout or, to a lesser extent, kidney stones.

system-wide effects that were often overshadowed by the pain and throbbing of the joints.

Gout is usually inherited, and we know the cause. In susceptible individuals, accumulations of uric acid crystallize and form deposits in certain joints. Sydenham's description of systemic symptoms preceding a joint attack made me wonder if there might be a gout syndrome. In this scenario, people would have all of the preliminary symptoms of gout without an acute arthritic attack. The condition would appear in cycles owing to minideposits in certain tissues such as the brain and the gastro-intestinal tract. Muscles would be slightly affected and joints spared altogether until very much later in the disease. An elevated plasma uric acid level would be the only way of alerting a physician about such a syndrome.

I soon found a few patients whom I thought might have these pregout symptoms: cyclic bouts of fatigue, irritability, nervousness, depression, insomnia, anxieties, loss of memory and concentration. They also described generalized, flu-like aching and stiffness (mainly in muscles), headaches, dizziness, numbness and tingling of the extremities, and leg cramps as their most prominent complaints. Indigestion with a sour stomach, gas, and flatulence completed the picture. Blood tests revealed higher-than-normal levels of uric acid (urate). When I treated these patients with gout medication, their uric acid dropped to normal. I was exhilarated by the fact that their symptoms also disappeared. Oddly enough, although patients quickly felt better, they still relapsed off and on: They suffered less often and intensely during each subsequent attack by staying on the medication. I'd always known that lowering the blood uric acid actually precipitated acute attacks of gout. As uric acid crystals are pulled from joints, they cause the pains just as they did going in. My gouty-syndrome patients indeed suffered reversal symptoms similar to those they experienced before treatment. It was exactly the same as Sydenham had described—except, I must stress, that there was no joint involvement. This was surely gout at its inception, before there was gout!

Flushed as I was with success, my confidence in my new "gout syndrome without gout" was soon shaken. Here came another group of patients who had all of the symptoms suggesting my new creation. Yet no matter how many times I tested, they never showed an elevated uric acid. Their aches and pains emanated from the entire musculoskeletal system and only mildly in joints. They had tenderness and swelling in tendons, ligaments, and especially muscles, structures that are not usually affected by gout. I decided to try gout medication anyhow. Oddly, they began recycling symptoms the same as did the high–uric acid group. I grew suspicious that they were clearing something different out of affected tissues since uric acid wasn't in the picture. They improved in the same way: Gradually, cyclically, and progressively, they accumulated more good than bad days; ultimately, some went on to complete clearing and also remained well if they stayed on the medication. In short, results were identical in all three groups: those with the classic symptoms of gout (red, hot, and swollen joints); those without joint symptoms—the gouty syndrome; and now this no–uric acid condition. The same drug was effective for all three, but what in the world was the cause of this third thing?

I tried to concentrate on what was different about the last group. They suffered from many aches and pains, but their fatigue was more overwhelming and constant. Women greatly outnumbered men whereas gout predominantly affected men. (Gout in women is almost nonexistent before menopause.) I thought it unlikely there was a connection with gout or the uric acid group except in the similarity of symptoms even though probenecid worked to reverse both conditions. My sleeping brain must have been mulling this over, and I woke up one night with the thought: Could there be an entirely new disease that acts like the gouty syndrome and is somehow connected to my patient's tartar?

I found it difficult to stop thinking about this idea. There existed no name for such an entity. *Fibrositis* had fallen into disuse and *fibromyalgia* wasn't yet born. I, too, had dismissed these patients, considering them hypochondriacs. I'd been well taught about these psychological misfits, the anxiety neurotics. In school, we were drilled to look for unbalanced hormones, unhappy marriages, empty-nest syndrome, inadequate upbringing, or just plain social maladjustment. When I lingered to elicit all the symptoms, I became fascinated by how similar their stories were. If psychosomatic, how could all these women invent closely identical complaints? There were pain, fatigue, emotional and cognitive defects, spastic colon, cramps, numbness and tingling of various parts of the body, and insomnia. And that's the short list.

They didn't know each other; they represented every ethnic group; they came from all over the world and from widely disparate socioeconomic demographics. Yet their recitation of symptoms seemed choreographed! Some were stoic, some slightly militant, but most just psychologically whipped. Their lips twitched and they sometimes sobbed a bit when one by one I extracted their unpredictable complaints. They usually recalled good and bad days in the earlier phases of their disease. Most remembered what happiness was before they succumbed despite having the same marriages, same children, ugly dogs, stress, and anticipated fun times. I knew it was ludicrous to continue in my belief that all of this was due to their nerves, no matter what psychiatry books iterated. I knew I might as well accept it: There existed a prevalent, unidentified, unexplored, but very real disease.

When I first used the gout medication, probenecid, I had variable success. The first two patients began the cyclic reversal I had learned to expect in the gouty syndrome. My enthusiasm was soon dashed when I failed with the next three patients. After some initial teeth gnashing (mine), something told me to try a higher dosage. I did so, and the rewards were swift: All three patients began the hoped-for reverse cycling. It now seemed even more likely that there actually was a tartar, or apatite crystal, syndrome—as I first named it. Equally obvious was the fact that uric acid had no part in the condition, since I could never detect abnormal levels in any of these people.

I found progressively more patients who fit the mold. So

many, in fact, that I knew I was looking at a very common and major illness. This was a debilitating disease that inexorably consumed energy and ultimately destroyed the quality of life. Vast numbers of these patients soon swelled my practice; I learned a great deal from them. Besides learning its parameters, I soon realized the illness was familial. The oldest related their own horror stories with a longer litany of complaints. Many of them were now contending with the added discomfort of osteoarthritis.

I was routinely touched by the years patients had suffered. Nuances in their stories made each one different, but left no doubt they were ill with the same sickness. It would have helped to have had such a thing as an electronic tablet to record the number of prior physician visits, tests, surgeries, and oddball diagnoses. Any of my readers can add to this list: "It's a bad menopause," "you're depressed," "inner ear disorder," "defect in your neurotransmitters," "rheumatoid arthritis," "migraine syndrome," "early lupus," or "multiple sclerosis." It was only a matter of time before most women were told: "It's all in your head; you need a psychiatrist." Some had seriously considered suicide, so compromised was the quality of their lives. They were frustrated and guilt-ridden about not being able to care for their families. They fiercely resented being different from other people. When I told them they suffered from an honest-to-goodness illness, I had to hand many of them the Kleenex box.

I have had fibro since I was a little kid but I did not know that I was ill—at least not beyond the allergies, migraines, etc., that I had accepted as part of my family heritage. Our first child came when I was twenty-one. It did not take me long to realize that I was different from other young mothers. They got more done than I did. They were not sick all the time like I was with almost weekly migraines and multiple bouts of bronchitis. Even when I was not sick, I did not get to the end of my work before I crashed, just out of steam. Even with all of that, I often thought I could cope if I could just think straight, but I couldn't. I would forget things that I knew. I lost important things. I couldn't remember people's names. My husband became so disgusted with my behavior that he avoided me more and more rather than trying to help. He worked odd shifts and I was pretty much left alone to tend to myself and the kids...My husband was slow to believe the diagnosis. It was just another "excuse" for substandard behavior as far as he was concerned.

—*Mary Lee, California*

New uricosuric medications appeared over the years: Anturane, Flexin, and Robinul. Each acted at a well-defined kidney level to increase uric acid excretion and was effective for gout. Strikingly, each also worked for our gouty syndrome and for fibromyalgia. But remember, fibromyalgia is not connected to uric acid. Several articles and books have printed that I believe uric acid is involved. I have consistently denied that I ever believed such a thing. There are similarities, but something other than uric acid is being extruded. Whatever genetic defect manifests at that location, it is mitigated by guaifenesin as well as the uricosuric drugs.

With treatment, many patients began flicking tartar. That wasn't much help to us since too many healthy people can do the same. Nevertheless, those early observations had put me on the right track. The successes forced me to suspect that the body was improperly handling either calcium or phosphate. Patients also commonly described chipping and peeling of their fingernails in cycles. Nail minerals are predominantly calcium and phosphate—the same as tartar. I theorized that nails were also cycling and depositing similar excesses at their roots. Compare this to the concentric rings of trees created as they grow. They reflect fibromyalgia and make defective layers during adverse cycles.

Calcium was not the problem. Our gout medicines worked on the negatively charged urate part of uric acid (sodium urate). Calcium, unlike urate, is an ion with positive charges. If I could eliminate calcium, logically I could suspect its companion in tartar, phosphate. There were ample biochemical reasons that pointed to phosphate. Like urate, it carries negatively charged ions. Calcium tablets sometimes helped patients feel slightly better. It bound chemically to phosphate in the intestine, decreased its absorption, and helped eliminate it into the stools. Kidney reabsorption or excretion into the urine is handled in about the same area as uric acid. I wish we could treat fibromyalgia so simply, but calcium just isn't enough help.

Although the drugs I was using to treat fibromyalgia were successful, they did have side effects. Sulfinpyrazone could raise stomach acidity enough to cause ulcers. Probenecid is a sulfa drug, and if allergy develops, the resulting hives could last for weeks. Robinul causes dry mouth or eyes (dangerous in glaucoma), nausea, abdominal pain, and increases fatigue or feeling spacey; it may also cause major urinary retention in men with an enlarged prostate.

Due to these limitations, I was always on the lookout for a more effective, better-tolerated medication. In 1991, more than thirty years after I began my initial research, I got lucky. My nurse's ten-year-old son, Malcolm Potter, had been on our treatment for fibromyalgia since the age of seven. As he grew, he needed somewhat larger amounts of his medication, sulfinpyrazone (Anturane), to continue his reversal. As mentioned above, this drug causes hyperacidity and gastric upsets in 8 percent of patients. As my young patient grew taller, we finally raised his dosage to a level too toxic for him, and sure enough, his stomach began to hurt. I didn't want to try the other medications since I worried about their particular side effects. Remember, this was a kid who would need some drug possibly for the rest of his life. So I intensified my search for a safer substitute.

Luckily, it wasn't long before I recalled a little clipping about another drug that could ever so slightly lower uric acid. I was able to confirm this in a newer edition of the *Physicians' Desk Reference*. The effect of this medication on uric acid is far too weak to successfully treat gout.[1] But you'll recall that anything I'd used so far with that effect had also worked for fibromyalgia. A bit later, I came upon a corroborating article in an old copy of the *Journal of Rheumatology*.[2]

The FDA-approved use of guaifenesin is for producing and loosening mucus in various respiratory infections. Thus, it's found in many cold preparations. It originated somewhere around 1530 as a boiled tree bark distillation called guaiacum and, believe it or not, was widely used for rheumatism.[3] It was even used to treat gout. In 1928, a medical paper extolled its virtues for treating growing pains in children. It also relieved several symptoms we would now recognize as fibromyalgia related. Guaiacum was later purified to guaiacolate, and made its first appearance in cough mixtures about seventy years ago. It was eventually synthesized and about thirty-five years ago was pressed into tablets and named guaifenesin. Its original use isn't completely ignored, however. In the *PDR for Herbal Medicines*, *Guaiacum officinale* remains a liquid medication indicated for rheumatism.[4]

The standard guaifenesin dosage for creating looser phlegm in bronchitis, asthma, hay fever, nasal and sinus congestion, is two tablets (1,200 mg) in the morning and two in the evening (2,400 mg per day). For many years, guaifenesin was a prescription drug in the form of 600 or 1,200 mg tablets. The drug is now available over the counter and is sold in differing strengths without prescription, making it widely accessible and affordable. It's available in 200, 300, and 400 mg strengths, as well as combined short- and long-acting 600 or 1,200 mg tablets sold under the brand name Mucinex. There are liquid forms with

100 and 200 mg per teaspoon, which we've used for children who could not swallow tablets. We've also recommended the sprinkles, which are in capsules that can be opened, allowing minigranules to be disguised in applesauce for kids. Guaifenesin is quite well absorbed from the intestinal tract at rates that differ among preparations.

Guaifenesin (gwy-FEN-e-sin) is an expectorant that thins mucus and helps to loosen phlegm. Guaifenesin is quickly absorbed from the gastrointestinal tract, and is rapidly metabolized and excreted into the urine. Guaifenesin is also known to lower uric acid levels. No serious side-effects have been reported.[5]

—Physicians' Desk Reference

To learn more about guaifenesin, go to such sources as www.drugs.com or bring it up in your computer through your search engines. Your pharmacist could copy a printout for you. But the newer *Physicians' Desk Reference* (*PDR*) book no longer describes it because it is over the counter.

Let's go back to my willing test subject, Malcolm, who had been off his original medicine for some time because of his irritated stomach. I surmised that I'd see some kind of reversal symptoms within a few days if guaifenesin was effective. Luckily for all of us, sadistically for Malcolm, on the second morning after beginning guaifenesin, he stumbled out of his bedroom moaning, "Mom, I can't walk—even the bottoms of my feet hurt!" So pervasive were his stiffness and aching that we knew we'd struck therapeutic gold! Indeed we had stumbled upon the safest and most potent weapon against this terrorist disease.

Since guaifenesin has no significant side effects, his symptom onslaught could only mean that we were purging his fibromyalgia. Unconvincingly for him during his full-blown torture, he was to lead us all back onto a safer road to recovery!

HOW DOES GUAIFENESIN WORK ON FIBROMYALGIA?

Do you remember our discussion in chapter 1 about the lumps and bumps of fibromyalgia? We find them on every single patient with the disease. We transpose each onto a body caricature, or map, for future tracking. These swollen places are for the most part tender. They're located in tendons and ligaments, but mostly in muscles. Ninety to 95 percent of the swelling is simply water that has collected under considerable pressure. We suspect this fluid has been sent into cells because of the presence of a slight excess of phosphate, calcium, and probably other constituents such as sodium and chloride. Bodies dispatch water to these areas and dilute these ions, keeping them from crystallizing inside cells. This keeps the tissue accretions in solution. Cells survive, but at the expense of losing some normal functions. The worst part of this process is that swelling presses on nerves and they transmit messages of discomfort to the brain, the only organ that can feel pain. Only when each ion is tucked into safe storage areas is some of the water allowed to leave. That actually reduces the size of the bump and somewhat eases pain.

Why did his getting worse actually tell us that Malcolm was improving? The answer is reversal pain, the opposite of what happens when the disease develops. The body can't pull concentrates out into more diluted areas because this would defy some chemistry and the body's dictum of equilibrium. When reversal begins, water has to reenter the ailing cells, wherever clearing is about to start. That extra fluid again causes swelling and pressure on nerves to renew pain messages. When guaifenesin initiates purging, the newly retained fluid reverses direction and is extracted from cells and takes some of the phosphate, calcium, and other excesses that had accumulated. Expanded cells shrink down a bit and ease some of the miseries of fibromyalgia.

When cells do their cleaning, they sweep the rejected phosphate and its fellow travelers back out into the bloodstream. Varying with the amount of waterborne material being extracted, the blood undergoes a miniflooding with the same debris it just tried to hide. This time the phosphate flows into the kidneys for excretion. But the kidneys can't immediately process all of that sudden inflow. You'll recall our theory that fibromyalgia occurs because the kidneys are sluggish when it comes to expelling phosphate. Since the urine is the only elimination route, the waste backs up waiting its turn for elimination. The blood is impatient and, meeting renal resistance, responds by stashing minideposits into temporary staging areas all over the body. Muscles absorb up a fair share, which causes generalized, flu-like aching. The brain also cooperates and stores enough debris to intensify fatigue, cognitive impairment, irritability, depression, anxiety, and insomnia. It's as if the disease were heading entirely in the wrong direction. In fact, it seems worse than ever, since purging is moving detritus out of cells at least six times faster than it had been allowed to enter. The difference this time, however, is that the kidneys are now working in the right direction, thanks to guaifenesin. They're in overdrive at full capacity trying to eliminate the unacceptable excesses. As you'd expect, symptoms of fibromyalgia worsen until the kidneys catch up.

What pours out under treatment are the accumulated chemical energy blockers that induced fibromyalgia. Guaifenesin will pull out some excess phosphate in small batches with help from the kidneys. During this purging, along with the above symptoms, patients also describe unpleasant tastes, scalded mouth, bad breath, burning perspiration and urine, as the body dumps the acidic phosphate into all bodily fluids. Even tears and vaginal secretions may sting. During this leaching-out period, people often notice small amounts of particulate matter or bubbles in the urine. Each cycle ends when that's all that can be done metabolically for the time being.

Between reversal cycles, relative rest periods follow. They could last for just a few hours, sometimes days, or even weeks. During more peaceful periods, it's still likely that some reversing is going on at a subliminal level. What patients experience varies greatly since so much depends on individual pain thresholds and ability to cope. Only one thing is sure: It soon becomes clear that the next attack is under way. Over time, these symptom onslaughts gradually diminish in intensity and frequency. The severity of symptoms lessens, and patients gradually get ever closer to restoring their health. Reversal symptoms, however intense, should reassure the patient that guaifenesin is working because the drug has no known side effects. Given to a normal individual, even in large amounts, no symptoms appear. These attacks and body map improvements tell us that restoration is under way.

My daughter was diagnosed with FMS after two years of searching for what was wrong. That year she missed over seventy days of school. Then I found the information about guaifenesin. I took it to my doctor, who had heard of it and didn't know if it would work. Together we followed the directions.

Now, for the first time in over five years, my daughter was able to go on a vacation and not be afraid of the pain. She was able to go to school without fear and went outside and played with her girlfriends! When school started this year, teacher after teacher stopped her and asked her what had changed over the summer; she looked so good and different! She is thirteen years old and in junior high…to be pain free and to be able to go out on the soccer field with her friends without the fear of the pain has been amazing.

—*Irene, California*

We commented earlier that we've had five totally different chemical compounds that worked for fibromyalgia. They had nothing in common except for where in the kidney they exacted their effect. Each urges the kidney to excrete a lot or a bit of uric acid. We've already explained that fibromyalgia has nothing to do with urates. I had measured the urinary output of phosphate, calcium, and urate before and during treatment using probenecid in the early years of our protocol. Later we appropriately retested patients using guaifenesin and got virtually the same results. We found a 60 percent increase in phosphate excretion and a lesser (30 percent) unloading of oxalate and calcium with both drugs. But whereas the gout medications significantly increased uric acid excretion, only a minimal discharge occurred with guaifenesin.

How does guaifenesin purge phosphate from the body? It's somewhat like opening a spigot that lets the kidneys drain out the problem. Think of your home water system. You open the tap, and water flows out of the faucet from the pipes that connect to the main line, which pulls from a larger source. Ultimately, the reservoir to which your pipes are connected gets lowered by the amount you've used at home, no matter what is the distance between the two locations.

We can use this analogy to explain our version of fibromyalgia. Those of us with one or more defective genes have otherwise perfectly normal kidney function. We think the problem arises because our inherited trait produces some slightly crippled proteins called enzymes. Healthier, top-quality specimens normally allow well-controlled opening of the spigot whenever the bloodstream offers up waste for renal filtering. Our theory suggests that affected kidneys badly direct the fate of inorganic phosphate (symbol: P_i). Our genetic malfunction causes fibromyalgia because it doesn't let the tap open fully; phosphate still leaks out, but somewhat sluggishly. There may be considerable daily variability, but that back-damming effect will eventually accrue P_i and redistribute it throughout the body. Different tissue susceptibilities determine which ones will best scoop up the excess phosphate.

Metabolic by-products are blood-borne to the kidneys for filtering. No-longer-needed substances and water are extracted to form urine. Major interfaces of blood and kidney occur at places called glomeruli. Flushing through such structures are surplus minerals, chemicals, and water in concentrations almost identical to those of the blood—with some notable exceptions such as inorganic phosphate (P_i). Huge amounts are absorbed from our foodstuffs and mainly used to make cellular energy. But like most other body ingredients, there are leftovers. Our activities exact tolls in the power molecules locked inside cells in the form of a chemical makeover named high-energy P_i. A lot of it is recycled, but there are some losses that get extruded from cells and ultimately into the blood. That excess baggage is what's sent downstream to the kidneys for possible elimination.

The kidneys are the command centers when it comes to designing urine. At some point, cells lining the walls of the renal tubules make decisions. They solicit nerve or hormonal advice before releasing filtered products such as phosphate into the bladder. Impulses can arrive from multiple sources requesting urgent need for extra P_i. Tubules are capable of reabsorbing it into the circulation for distribution wherever needed. Cells lining the millions of kidney tubules face the developing urine stream on one side, and the blood capillaries on the opposite end. That's where choices are made concerning many urine-borne products including P_i. They can open side gates to retrieve P_i and slither it through to the blood side for retrieval.

Depending on the incoming signals, they can also keep them closed, deny access, and thereby direct partial or total excretion. You can see in figure 3.1 how this works.

So phosphate has two ways to go. Both are through the bloodstream's capillary walls. The first system shoves it directly into the fluid that's about to become urine. The second extracts it from the blood straight into the tubule-lining cells from one side and ejects through the other side into the urine. While this sounds like an unnecessarily duplicated effort, these two venues are under different yet synchronized control. Phosphate concentrations are sensed; nerve and hormonal suggestions are respected to please the body's requirements. *If you're soaking in* P_i, *get rid of it. You need a bit extra? We know how to get it, and we'll absorb some for you.* It sounds simple, but these activities count on enzymes responding correctly to the body's needs. In fibromyalgia, it is probable that one or more of the involved enzymes are genetically defective or malformed. This would fit with our theory: Fibromyalgics just can't get rid of enough phosphate.

Now we can choreograph the whole scene. Cells work so we can live, and require a huge amount of energy in the process. Most of our food is expended to create ATP in the many mitochondria that sit inside each cell. Once formed, this adenosine triphosphate can flip off attached, energized phosphates one at a time and make metabolic things happen. It's highly energy-expensive to keep body parts functioning. Normal wear and tear of cells adds more waste phosphate into the dietary surpluses not earmarked for immediate use. All of that is dispatched to the kidneys for the sorting out we've just discussed.

The body won't tolerate P_i accumulation in the blood, because it's a reciprocal to calcium. This means that when phosphate rises, calcium must fall. There are four parathyroid glands in the neck that won't permit such an imbalance. They pour out hormones that protect calcium levels. So phosphate can't escape in the urine, and it isn't even allowed to linger in

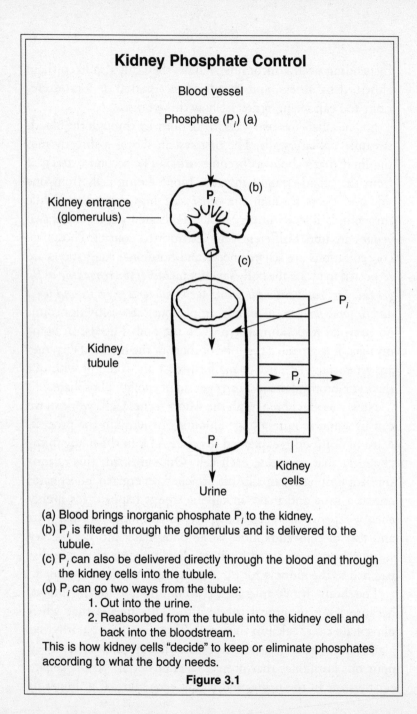

Kidney Phosphate Control

Blood vessel

Phosphate (P_i) (a)

Kidney entrance
(glomerulus)

P_i

(b)

(c)

Kidney
tubule

P_i

P_i

P_i

Kidney
cells

P_i

Urine

(a) Blood brings inorganic phosphate P_i to the kidney.
(b) P_i is filtered through the glomerulus and is delivered to the tubule.
(c) P_i can also be delivered directly through the blood and through the kidney cells into the tubule.
(d) P_i can go two ways from the tubule:
    1. Out into the urine.
    2. Reabsorbed from the tubule into the kidney cell and back into the bloodstream.

This is how kidney cells "decide" to keep or eliminate phosphates according to what the body needs.

Figure 3.1

the bloodstream. Now the quandary: In some predetermined pecking order, certain tissues must accept phosphate as inmates and help clear the blood. Bones are the most adept at tucking it in, but eventually they become saturated and refuse to soak up any more. Muscles and sinews should help, and they do. The process drives inorganic phosphate back into cells willing to accept the responsibility. At some point, P_i excesses slow down the mitochondrial generators and energy production starts lagging. It's chemically necessary that water enter affected cells to keep incoming phosphate and its fellow traveler, calcium, in proper concentration. Sodium and chloride surf along to permit such mandatory dilutions. Those cellular visitors cause swelling and produce the lumps and bumps of fibromyalgia. In turn, that squeezes nerves and sends distress signals to the brain. There, the problem is interpreted to express the symptoms of fibromyalgia: pain, burning, crawling, tingling, and numbness. The brain itself isn't immune to the process so add fatigue and cognitive impairment. We've sketched this sequence in figure 3.2.

Earlier we explained how excess phosphate interrupts energy (ATP) production in mitochondria and causes the symptoms of fibromyalgia. We can solve the problem by helping the kidneys back into efficiency. Purge excess phosphate and, no surprise, watch the body's cells eagerly produce all of the ATP we need. Calcium that's been tied up by P_i is also siphoned out of overladen stores. Rid of misplaced calcium, cells get out of overdrive and can relax. Such restoration predictably reenergizes our systems to their full capacity. We believe guaifenesin to be the best and safest agent to prod reluctant enzyme spigots to open wide and let us get on with the business of robust living. (See figure 3.3.)

A very difficult aspect of treatment is what patients must go through during reversal. They've already been too often disappointed by promises of cures that never materialized. They

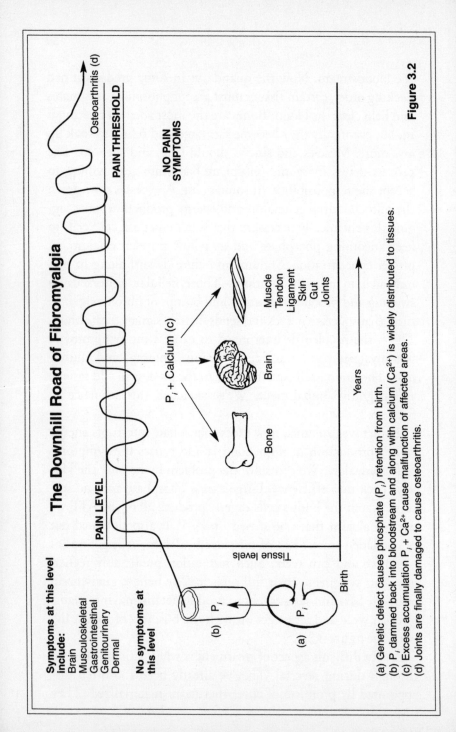

The Downhill Road of Fibromyalgia

Symptoms at this level include:
Brain
Musculoskeletal
Gastrointestinal
Genitourinary
Dermal

PAIN LEVEL

Osteoarthritis (d)

PAIN THRESHOLD

NO PAIN SYMPTOMS

No symptoms at this level

Tissue levels

P_i + Calcium (c)

Muscle
Tendon
Ligament
Skin
Gut
Joints

Brain

Bone

Years

Birth

P_i

P_i

(a)

(b)

(a) Genetic defect causes phosphate (P_i) retention from birth.
(b) P_i dammed back into bloodstream and along with calcium (Ca^{2+}) is widely distributed to tissues.
(c) Excess accumulation P_i + Ca^{2+} cause malfunction of affected areas.
(d) Joints are finally damaged to cause osteoarthritis.

Figure 3.2

The Road Back from Fibromyalgia

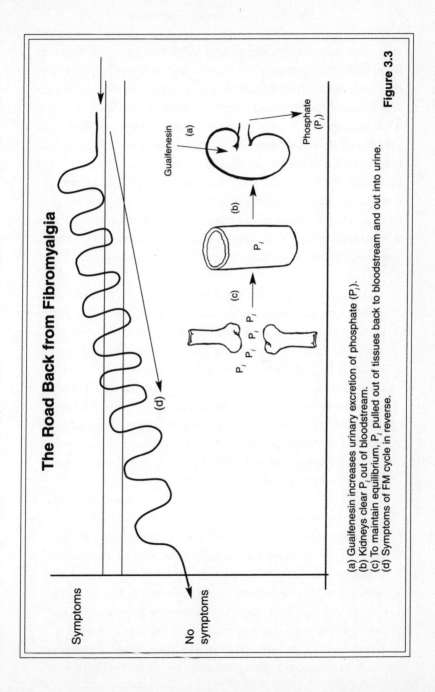

(a) Guaifenesin increases urinary excretion of phosphate (P_i).
(b) Kidneys clear P_i out of bloodstream.
(c) To maintain equilibrium, P_i pulled out of tissues back to bloodstream and out into urine.
(d) Symptoms of FM cycle in reverse.

Figure 3.3

enter the initial recycling phases desperate for a glimmer of hope flashed by getting a few decent hours. We tell our patients that such inspirational moments will be their assurance of success ahead. Once the body provides a few better hours or days, it's signaling that it can do so on a permanent basis. But until people feel that first pain-free moment, they can only believe in help from guaifenesin. It takes guts and perseverance to keep faith when confronted by sometimes intense, early reversal symptoms. Later cleansing cycles are also tough, but by then patients have had a taste of recovery: a series of good days with diminished pain and fatigue. That makes coping a lot easier. Even so, the next reversing cycle raises former concerns.

> And then, one day, when you have been on guai properly for some length of time, you will stop whatever you are doing, and try to figure out what is different. It will feel as if the world got quiet and peaceful, and you realize that you don't hurt anywhere. It feels like someone turned off a pain faucet. Pay very close attention to that, because it is your body saying, "I'm not permanently broken. Remember what this feels like. I am getting fixed." Then the pain or anxiety or fatigue or everything will come back again. So write the feeling down immediately in colored letters, big and bold in your diary, so you can find it and know it was real.
>
> —*Bonnie J., Florida*

I was diagnosed in 1987, when it was called fibrositis, while in physical therapy school. I was lucky to be where I was because my diagnosis was quick but I was in no way prepared for the destruction this new entity would have on my life. From the day of my diagnosis until the present, I have studied and searched for anything that would help me have a more functional life. It has been hit or miss at best, from consuming shark cartilage to applying magnets to my body. There have been chunks of time taken away from me where the only thing I wanted to do was stay in bed. I have been limited as a mother of two boys and as a wife and at times felt totally inadequate at both.

Two years ago I found Dr. St. Amand's book and began the protocol. A year ago I went on the liberal diet. I began running, although told a long time ago that was a big no-no. I just turned forty-five and I have gone from fibromyalgia to 5K. In the last year, I have completed five 5Ks and just came in first in my age group, winning a medal. I am still on my medication but feel nothing can stop me now. I am more active and have more energy. Enjoying life is now my priority, not my fibromyalgia. In my wildest dreams, I would have never guessed I would be where I am now.

—*Cheri M., California*

A common reaction from patients is to suspect that their bodies are different from those of other fibromyalgics. They have trouble overriding the fear that their case is too far gone to get sustained benefits. But as treatment progresses, confidence mounts, and relatively soon they become old pros at the ins and outs of their disease. They know good days will return in greater numbers, attacks will be milder, more bearable, and leave progressively fewer areas to purge. Though the initial reversal cycles might have attacked ten or twenty places at one time, later reversals work on only one or two sites simultaneously. This alone greatly diminishes the severity of subsequent attacks. In addition, purging phases get progressively farther apart, making setbacks minor by comparison.

Every patient asks: "How long will it take for me to clear?" There's no easy answer. It depends on several things: the duration of the illness, genetic makeup, and the dosage of guaifenesin required for response. Low-dose patients (300 mg twice a day) are fastest, but clear with intense and almost constant attacks. Slower-responding patients need larger dosages and have reversal rates spread over a spectrum of possibilities. We rely on a well-tested rule that the slowest people clean out one year of fibromyalgic debris every two months. The clock doesn't start ticking, however, until they've found the proper dosage and become totally salicylate-free. Yes, it's gradual for some and unbelievably fast for those lucky ones. Slow responders can go faster under a doctor's guidance by raising the dosage using either longer- or faster-acting guaifenesin. Just don't lose heart.

I have been on guaifenesin for seven and a half months. I have had painful FMS symptoms since July 1991, following whiplash and a concussion during an auto accident. Since being on guai, my quality of life has greatly improved. I have less pain overall, even when cycling. I used to have trouble riding in the car, even for a few miles, because the vibrations felt greatly magnified to me. This has lessened slightly. The severity and frequency of my headaches have diminished significantly. My MPS (myofascial pain syndrome) is gone. I have periods that my skin doesn't hurt when someone touches it lightly; I used to hurt all the time from a soft touch or rub. I am capable of doing much more day-to-day things like loading the dishwasher and watching our children during the day. I need to rest quite a bit less...I have had a full three weeks with virtually no pain. This is the first time in seven years that this has happened. This treatment is our one great hope.

—J.M., Texas

Another patient who went through years of hardship with fibromyalgia and had difficult cycling during treatment, recounts her experience:

I want to brag about my second thirty-mile bike ride. I am very proud of myself. I want you to know how far I've come. I am forty-eight years old and suffered all my life with progressively more and more pain and depression. I have been on most of the powerful painkillers and antidepressants over the years. I closed my business and quit working in 1994. My mind was worthless, the fatigue and pain made getting out of bed impossible on most days, and I had horrid insomnia for years. The symptoms would come and go, and most of the time I "looked normal," although I put on a lot of weight. Life has always been a fight against body and mind pain. In February of 1997 I was hit hard. My entire body swelled, my skin burned all over, my mouth burned badly, and I salivated constantly. My stomach contorted. My mind went crazy. Most of my muscles were in spasm. I couldn't move without sweating profusely.

—*G.M., California*

FREQUENTLY ASKED QUESTIONS

Before we leave the subject of guaifenesin and end this chapter, let's deal with some of the questions most commonly asked.

Does guaifenesin have side effects?

Other than infrequent and transient nausea in the early treatment stages, guaifenesin has no known side effects. Even that sensation is such a frequent part of the irritable bowel that, most times, we can't blame the drug. Also, upset stomachs may be just part of cycling. Some people have difficulty with any medication. We urge them to buy or cut tablets into sizes that will fit into gelatin capsules, which can be purchased in any pharmacy or health food store. Since the stomach can't digest gelatin, the capsule slips the drug into the small intestine, where it's released. Very rarely, we've seen individual sensitivities to some filler in the tablets or to an added dye. Pharmacists can suggest different brands that are dye-free and contain different fillers. The pain, numbness, and host of other symptoms you might feel while taking guaifenesin are due to the anticipated reversal process. Even occasional hives or other rashes are almost always part of the disease and are due to purging of the skin, not to allergy. All of these cleansing symptoms are great clues that guaifenesin is at work.

Which guaifenesin should I use?

Guaifenesin is an ingredient in many cough mixtures and decongestants. These items contain too many other substances that either block the kidney actions of the drug or will make you even sicker. Any pure guaifenesin free of added medications such as pseudoephedrine and dextromethorphan will do just fine as long as it is a longer acting or timed release compound. We've restricted our use of liquid guaifenesin to children, since the concentrations are too low for adults unless they're willing to drink nearly a bottle a day.

Can I get guaifenesin over the counter?

As stated earlier, guaifenesin is available in 200, 300, 400, 600, and even 1,200 mg tablets. Currently, all are being sold over the counter. Some are twelve-hour acting (600 and 1,200 mg), and others are short acting (400 mg or less). Powders are also available but we do not recommend these because often they have lost potency before being pressed into tablets or while being stuffed into capsules owing to excess handling. There are numerous brands, but none can claim the twelve hours of Mucinex (also bottled by ProHealth—available online). All 400 mg tablets are short acting and must be taken on a more frequent schedule. Short acting can impact symptoms heavily as we warn in the preceding text.

We don't particularly recommend self-treatment unless there's no alternative. There are many symptoms in fibromyalgia that could easily mask some other condition. It's certainly best to exclude these before starting our protocol. Once that's done, you're correct in expecting physicians to consider the diagnosis of fibromyalgia and knowing how to confirm their suspicions by physical examination. However, not enough doctors know about our protocol. You the patient could help educate them. If you luck into a doctor who knows how to find the lumps and bumps of the disease, work on the reversal together. We'll soon tell you about selected parts of the body that regress within one month, and quickly help identify the correct dosage. If your doctor knows how to palpate these areas, it will provide you great reassurance in the early stages of treatment. Furthermore, you might need professional help down the line if strange symptoms pop up. Assistance is also essential should you stop improving or actually regress and need help in finding some hidden source of salicylate.

Are there any special instructions for storing guaifenesin?

The medication should be stored in an area that has a temperature between fifty-nine and eighty-six degrees Fahrenheit, not in the refrigerator or in a very warm room. Avoid getting your supplies wet. Tightly pressed tablets have a longer shelf life than capsules, and powder has the shortest shelf life of all. If you're filling capsules in your own home, make sure you purchase the powder in small amounts; freshness maintains potency.

Do I need to drink lots of water with my guaifenesin?

That's not necessary. Pushing fluids is mainly urged when taking guaifenesin for lung or sinus problems. Extra fluid helps loosen mucus. We're interested in its kidney effects.

Should I continue my other medications when I start guaifenesin?

Guaifenesin mixes safely with anything so your doctor will undoubtedly want you to continue other medications. But even trickles of salicylate block renal effects of guaifenesin though it will liquefy mucus. To name a few: avoid Soma Compound (replace with plain Soma), Fiorinal (replace with Fioricet), Empirin, and Percodan (replace with Percocet). It's best if you can avoid potent drugs and make do with Tylenol (acetaminophen) with or without nonsteroidal anti-inflammatories (NSAIDs), such as ibuprofen and naproxen. We'll tell you more about such things as Pepto-Bismol, toothpastes, Bengay, and others in chapter 4. Don't discontinue or change dosages of prescription medications without consulting your physician.

Some people refer to the guaifenesin protocol as detoxification. Is that correct?

There are no toxins in fibromyalgia. Our new research, which we describe in this edition, and past testing found none. Whatever causes FMS doesn't appear to be something foreign to the body. It mounts no inflammatory response or antibody attack. We think fibromyalgia is caused by customarily friendly phosphate—there's just too much of it in the wrong places. Since there are no toxins, guaifenesin does not "detox."

Is it beneficial to cleanse the body of yeast or parasites before starting guaifenesin?

We don't ascribe to the concept of chronic candidiasis as currently defined, which uses plasma antibodies or stool cultures for diagnosis. Antibodies are usually our friends and are present because we've encountered a particular infection or toxin in the past. They're poised to pounce on the offender at any time it tries to reenter the body. Also note that the so-called anti-yeast diet is the very one we prescribe for hypoglycemia. Most people feel better on low carbohydrate intakes since the blood sugar does not rise and fall at various times of day, not because of a theoretical effect on candida. Similarly, parasites are too often blamed for fibromyalgia. It's not something we've observed. "Herbal cleansing" ingredients block guaifenesin. If you feel you must, get it over with before attempting our protocol.

Remember that the immune system is slightly depressed in fibromyalgia, and therefore permits more infections.

Is guaifenesin safe to take if I get pregnant?

Guaifenesin has actually been used to help women get pregnant. It was thought to be helpful solely for its ability to liquefy the mucous plug that normally sits at the opening of the uterus. Later findings identified spermatocidal qualities of this mucus in some women, a defect that is corrected using guaifenesin. We suggest each woman discuss this issue with her own doctor. We advise our pregnant patients to totally stop all medications before attempting to become pregnant. With the permission of your obstetrician, you may resume treatment after the sixth month of pregnancy since the baby is fully formed by then. This way, fibromyalgic women can avoid the sudden burst of symptoms that often follow delivery.

Am I at greater risk of osteoporosis when taking guaifenesin?

The calcium excreted by guaifenesin is limited to the inappropriate surplus temporarily locked within your cells. So you don't have to worry about causing osteoporosis. Remember, the medication is more than four hundred years old in some form or other. Problems would have shown up by now.

Can guaifenesin cause kidney stones?

No, there are no connections with kidney stones, guaifenesin, or fibromyalgia. Most stones are calcium oxalate, some are sodium urate, and others complexes of calcium-clutching phosphates and carbonates. We repeat, guaifenesin has been used for years and never implicated with kidney stones. One tiny study found a possible connection, but as confirmed by the authors, affected patients were not taking pure guaifenesin. They were abusing combinations of guaifenesin and pseudoephedrine. The latter is the drug used in the unlawful manufacture of methamphetamine. That drug was the likely suspect, and the patients were not endangered by guaifenesin.

Is it okay to drink colas while taking guaifenesin?

We have not had to restrict colas though they do contain phosphoric acid. Phosphate is what we're trying to purge from the body, but guaifenesin overcomes that added load rather easily. It also handles amounts contained in plant foods.

If I have asthma, can I take guaifenesin?

Guaifenesin is frequently used for asthma. It's actually marketed as being "mucolytic." That helps cells produce a lighter mucus, making it less tenacious, and easier to raise. Anyone with added medical conditions should always ask their physician for permission to add any medication.

Are you ready to move on and learn about the protocol? The next few chapters will describe lots of things that will help you understand and successfully treat fibromyalgia.

> After the initial onslaught of the illness, there was disbelief. I sat in my chair for hours not believing I could possibly be living in such a broken body. The pain came in waves, rendering life an unpredictable nightmare of perceived uselessness and anger. I gave up my role as a wife, a mother, a daughter, and a therapist. I had loved each of those roles. [The depression began] so long ago I don't even remember. I prayed to God. Then I quit praying. No strength for it. I gave in and gave up and spent most of the time doing nothing. It is so easy to get stuck right there doing nothing, not caring, not wanting to live, hoping not to die. It is hard work to be sick. It's harder work to get well...but getting well is the best thing there is, and guaifenesin is the way to do it.
>
> —*Gretchen, South Carolina*

Generic "Mucinex" Guaifenesin Now Available

Just prior to the publication of this book, we received good news regarding a generic version of guaifenesin. This information is meant to update the formulations information in this chapter.

In December 2011, Perrigo Co., a manufacturer of many generic over-the-counter medications, won a judgment that will allow it to produce 600 mg Guaifenesin Extended-Release Tablets, a generic version of Mucinex tablets. Perrigo received FDA approval in December 2011 and expects to launch the product within ninety days. Other companies are expected to follow suit.

Since 2002, it has been almost impossible to find generic guaifenesin, as the many brands were taken off the market following an FDA ruling. The generic guaifenesin was replaced on the shelves by the more expensive, but over-the-counter, Mucinex. While many of our patients take Mucinex, it is prohibitively expensive for others.

Chapter Four

The Fly in the Ointment

Aspirin and Other Salicylates

You can manage to get by without salicylates. In the beginning, if you are unsure and too confused to understand, just use fewer products. It's funny that we do without so many things when we are sick, but then want to argue about giving up mint toothpaste. There's no point in reading the book and getting guaifenesin and hoping that you'll get better if you don't do your homework about salicylates. There are many resources to help you and now there are even companies that make special products.

—Gloria, California

CRITICS SAY OUR protocol is difficult because it's hard to avoid salicylate by its many names. We've written this chapter to prove that it's not, especially when compared to living with fibromyalgia. It takes time to teach patients how to avoid salicylates but it is worth the effort. This book will guide you, and this chapter will help you better understand why it is so important. Resources on www.fibromyalgiatreatment.com are kept updated, and the online support group will walk you through the process of avoiding salicylates. It might be a bit stressful at first but it's a lot better than being sick every day of your life. Compared to that, reading labels whenever you buy something new seems barely an inconvenience. We think you'll agree when you have your first good day.

A BRIEF HISTORY OF SALICYLATES

All five of the medications we've used over the years to treat fibromyalgia have one thing in common. In each case, the compound *salicylate* has blocked their chemical activity at the precise kidney location where we need help.

We must stress that there are no known drug interactions between guaifenesin and any other medication. Mixing guaifenesin with salicylates will not make you ill. Guaifenesin will still help liquefy your mucus, and make a cough more productive, but the action we need to treat fibromyalgia will be totally neutered—or blocked. There won't be any outward manifestation of this blocking effect; that's both good and bad news. You won't feel sick if you make a mistake, but it also means that you won't be able to tell by how you feel if your medication isn't effective. In time, of course, you'll suspect the blocking situation when your body map gets worse and you start to feel ill more of the time. That's why it's so absolutely necessary to read and review this chapter until you understand what's written here. **Unless you successfully avoid salicylates, no amount of guaifenesin can do *anything* to heal you.**

Salicylates have been used medicinally since as early as 1500 BC, when a pain-relieving recipe using dried myrtle leaves was recorded by ancient Egyptians. In the fifth century BC, Hippocrates, affectionately known as the father of medicine, promoted juice extracts from the bark of willow trees for treating aches and pains. Other diverse cultures such as the Native Americans made the same discovery and used barks and meadow grasses to prepare topical or internal preparations for the same purposes. During the late Middle Ages, a willow bark concoction to alleviate pain and fevers was so popular in Europe it had to be outlawed as the trees were being cut down faster than they could be replanted—almost destroying the wicker industry. That law was repealed in 1806 because the alternative drug, quinine from Peru, couldn't reach Europe because of Napoleon's blockade.

Whenever plants are found useful in treating disease, a search begins to find the active chemical that's responsible. Then it can be extracted, purified, and made into doses that are uniform in potency. So in 1823, the chemical salicin was successfully extracted from the bark of a willow tree and named for its Latin moniker: *Salix*. Later it was extracted from meadowsweet and many other plants.

Once the chemical was identified, a race was on to synthesize the molecule—that is, to make it from scratch in a laboratory. It was hoped that this process would be less laborious, less expensive, and result in a successful capitalistic venture. No longer would entire trees be sacrificed just to extract a few milligrams of drug. In 1853, this was accomplished, but soon abandoned because the substance proved too acidic for humans to tolerate.

A few years later, a German chemist, Felix Hoffman, decided to search for a stomach-friendly, less-toxic salicylate in order to alleviate his father's arthritic pains. He was successful and convinced his employer, Bayer, to market it, and in 1899, aspirin was born in the form of a prescription powder. A tablet soon followed, and in 1915, it was made available without prescription as a condition of the Treaty of Versailles, which ended World War I.

Aspirin's full effects on the body are still being explored. Its pain-relieving aspects are enhanced by reducing the internal production of prostaglandins and clipping their role in inducing inflammation and nerve sensitivity to pain. Aspirin also lessens the adhesive tendencies of blood platelets and so cuts the risk of a repeat heart attack and certain types of strokes in men and older women. It has actions that might help lessen the risk of colon cancer and possibly cataracts. It costs very little because it's so inexpensively produced. It has wide applications such as the concentrate, salicylic acid, used to remove warts and corns; more dilute in cosmetic creams and lotions for treating acne and dandruff; chemical skin peels made with weaker concentrations to achieve a mild exfoliation. It's inserted into sunscreens for UVA protection even though that does not provide protection against the rays that cause skin cancers.

HOW SALICYLATES BLOCK GUAIFENESIN

Why do salicylates cause such problems for our protocol? The answer isn't very complicated. There is a particular area in the kidneys where guaifenesin must be allowed access to work unimpeded. Unfortunately, it's precisely the same location where salicylates attach to targeted cells: in the renal tubules. These cells have surface areas that house thousands of receptors. It's easy to visualize the process if you think of each receptor as a custom-made garage designed for use only by a certain specially shaped car. Each garage will allow parking only for cars that fit perfectly.

In the human body, every receptor on every cell is precision-made to accommodate only a specific hormone or chemical. For any medication to succeed, it must find and neatly fit into that receptor, which is always a space that was designed for a natural molecule. This is what the science of pharmacology is all about. Drugs are manufactured to occupy an existing receptor that will either trigger or block an action.

Unfortunately, guaifenesin and salicylates compete for the same receptors, but salicylates are a better fit and so get preferential parking. Even small amounts of salicylate can occupy all the available sites, leaving none for guaifenesin. In a manner of speaking, once the parking garage is full, it shuts down. As an aside, even with abundant circulating salicylates, guaifenesin still successfully liquefies mucus because it continues to fit into the altogether different receptors in tissues other than the renal tubules. But its benefit for fibromyalgia is nonexistent.

We've worked since the beginning with this problem we call *blocking* because we didn't discover it. We already knew patients would have to avoid aspirin. Salicylate's blockade of uricosuric compounds is well documented in medical literature, and the older gout medications all carry a printed warning on their bottles. So we knew that guaifenesin wouldn't work to reverse fibromyalgia when taken with aspirin. But we had a lot to learn about other forms of salicylate and what potent effects they had.

There are many studies that have demonstrated the ability of skin to absorb salicylates. Skin biopsies showed that salicylate topically applied directly at the top of one shoulder muscle (trapezius) was found within one half hour in almost equal concentration in the opposite side. Clearly it was absorbed into the bloodstream and transported effectively throughout the body. It's well known that topical creams applied for muscle pain easily penetrate into underlying tissues and provide relief. But initially we had no idea how quickly and thoroughly they did so or how well the salicylates were moved throughout the body. Once we began observing patients with worsening symptoms and mappings while using Bengay and Aspercreme (methyl salicylate), we were alerted.[1]

These days we're accustomed to topically applied medications, none of which existed when we first began using guaifenesin. Nicotine patches, migraine sprays, hormone gels and patches, pain patches, etc. Now it's accepted that drug delivery through skin has advantages. It makes for lower dosages, direct delivery into the bloodstream, bypassing the intestinal tract, and avoiding degradation by digestive juices.

There are still skeptical physicians who consider it inconsequential when we expound on how small amounts of salicylate can block guaifenesin. To this we simply say that we know it's true: We've created thousands of maps on our patients that graphically illustrate what we have found. Ignore any and all voices to the contrary; salicylates block with devastating efficiency.

Sensitivity to blockage is genetically determined, but since none of us knows the level of our personal susceptibility, each of us should meticulously abide by the protocol as written. To our readers, we plead—do your job and give guaifenesin a fair chance. Go to our website for help if you need clarification. If you don't do the protocol properly, you'll never know whether or not guaifenesin would have worked for you. Don't miss this chance to get well.

AVOIDING SALICYLATES

Even before medical school, I had a love affair with medicine. Yet I have to admit that over the years, that affection has been strained by the torment of ferreting out the source of salicylate that's blocking a particular patient. It's certainly been a learning curve! We daily counsel patients on how to scan all their products. And it's not as simple as not using aspirin or Pepto-Bismol. Even our best efforts have not prevented errors by intelligent and diligent people.

My first visit with a new patient begins predictably. I take a medical history and complete my examination, which produces a body map displaying the patient's lesions. After that, I make a sketch as I unfold a story—our version of fibromyalgia. I run through the details of how I began to treat it, thanks to an observant man who flicked tartar off his teeth. I move through the metabolism of calcium and phosphate as I believe it relates to fibromyalgia. I dwell a bit longer on the cyclic but progressive nature of the illness and what we are learning from our current research. Next I spend considerable time explaining the role of guaifenesin in correcting our faulty chemistry, offsetting our genetic problem. Patients grimace a bit when I get to my description of the reversal process. I explain that it's fully anticipated that they will see great swings in symptoms. They'll cycle quickly or gradually from worse-than-ever to better-than-in-a-long-time. Patients handle this information quite well—so far, so good.

I always brace myself when I move into the next part of my explanation. Now I must address the issue of the salicylates they'll have to avoid in topical products and the herbal medications they must discontinue. We've actually had a few patients dump both us and guaifenesin rather than give up a cherished item. One actress came out and said that the protocol was "too hard" and then simply failed to appear for her next appointment. Believe it or not, we've also heard: "I'd rather have fibromyalgia than give up my lipstick!" It can be equally difficult to convince patients to part with their Juice Plus+, liver cleansers, or herbal laxatives. At this point, we remind patients that were those things effective, they would have saved themselves the expense and time involved in visiting our office. But of course, there are also those who immediately say they'd give up anything at all to feel better!

> Over the years I've tried so many things from avoiding chemicals and certain foods. I've done elimination diets and stopped using gluten. None of them made my condition better. Now I have to check products for salicylates and I don't see a problem with reading more labels. And I know I have to do it right but I'm up for a challenge. I just want to get well.
>
> —*Alecia, Oregon*

SYNTHETIC SALICYLATES

We'll start the discussion with the easiest group of salicylates to identify: the synthetic or pure chemical form. Since salicylate or salicylic acid is exactly what you can't use, obviously that's the first thing you should look for on product labels. Simply put: If you see the word *salicylate* or *salicylic acid* on the label of any product you take as a medication or use on your skin—you must discontinue that product in order for your guaifenesin to be effective.

The most common salicylate is good old aspirin or acetylsalicylic acid. It may appear on labels by that name or by the abbreviation name *ASA* (a common designation especially in Canada). Many pain medications contain aspirin. Examples include Anacin, Excedrin, and Fiorinal. Their aspirin-free counterparts (Aspirin Free Excedrin, Excedrin PM, and Fioricet) pose no problem.

It's slightly more difficult to spot the compound when it's blended into a long chemical name. Sunscreens may list octisalate or homosalate; other examples include Pepto-Bismol (bismuth subsalicylate) or methyl salicylate (Listerine and Bengay). Many pain and anti-inflammatory medications list ingredients by chemical name. For example, sodium salicylate, choline salicylate, and magnesium salicylate. Look for salsalate, choline magnesium trisalicylate, and salicylsalicylic acid. Notice how easily you can spot *sal* buried within those names? When you see it, dump the product.

You'll also find salicylates in topical products that employ an acid to work. That's why acne soaps, dandruff shampoos, and corn-removing products may contain salicylic acid. It's also used to treat psoriasis and seborrheic dermatitis of the face and scalp, and to remove calluses. Plantar and common warts are treated with varying strengths of salicylic acid. Chemical peels should not be used if they contain salicylic acid but any other acid (lactic, glycolic) would be no problem.

Overzealous patients sometimes confuse silicate or sulfate and think they're potential blockers. Not so. We repeat: The three telltale letters are *s-a-l*.

There are several other chemicals that are also salicylates. These are derivatives of camphor and menthol and can be easily spotted because they contain the syllables *camph* or *menth*. No matter how long a chemical name—even if it has twenty-five letters—if it doesn't contain those syllables—*sal*, *camph*, or *menth*—you can use it. *Meth*—as in methyl paraben—is safe. Without the *n*, it is safe to use.

As mentioned earlier in this chapter, sunscreens often contain a salicylate. But none of the ingredients you need to avoid are the ones that protect against skin cancer or photo-aging. It's true that effective sunscreens are more expensive than those that don't actually protect you from anything other than sunburn, but it's important to use them. Look at it this way: You'll save on wrinkle creams later! The ingredients to avoid in your sunscreen are spelled a little differently but here they are: octisalate, homosalate, mexoryl, or meradimate.

Prescription and Over-the-Counter Medications Containing Synthetic Salicylate

Aspirin	Fiorinal
Excedrin	Disalcid
Anacin	Pepto-Bismol
Excedrin Migraine	Doan's Pills
Bufferin	Ecotrin

Common Topical Products That Contain Synthetic Salicylates

Buf-Puf Acne Cleansing Bar with Vitamin E
Clearasil Clearstick Maximum Strength Topical Solution

Compound W Fast Acting Gel
Freezone
Gold Bond Triple Action Medicated Body Powder
Occlusal-HP Topical Solution
Oxy Clean Medicated Pads
Sebex-T Tar Shampoo
Stridex Super Scrub Pads
Wart-Off Topical Solution

NATURAL SALICYLATES

All plants make salicylates.[2] The publication of the article
proving this, in 1984, was a defining moment for the guaifenesin protocol, as well as a missing piece of the puzzle. What had
been hazy and not quite appreciated was suddenly clear. Just
as the realization many years before that there was a condition
called hypoglycemia had hit me like a ton of bricks, this head-
line was staggering. It took a few more years, some refinements,
and some missteps, but an important piece of information had
suddenly dropped into our laps, and we knew it the minute we
read the article that was published in the journal *Science*.

It required no great leap of faith that if taking aspirin—or
acetylsalicylic acid—would block guaifenesin, then so would
taking white willow bark, which harbors the natural salicylate,
salicin. Once past the mouth, these chemicals—because they
are identical—fit the same receptors and have the same diverse
effects on the body. Only the source is different. So, then, if
all plants make salicylates, then all herbal medications contain
them. And because herbal medications are concentrates, then
they would contain substantial amounts of salicylate. Medicinal herbs, like all medications, are designed to deliver the active
chemical(s) into the bloodstream in sufficient quantities to
alter some kind of body function. They are designed to over-
ride the body's own natural defense system.

In the early days of the protocol, herbal medications were not as commonly used. The supplement market was almost nonexistent except for a few multivitamins. Self-respecting patients back then didn't take alfalfa, borage seed oil, wild Mexican yam, or bioflavonoids. But as time passed, everything old was becoming new again. People who wouldn't dream of taking eight aspirin a day would take white willow bark with a passion, commenting that it was natural and could not hurt them. Women who wouldn't take horse estrogens or synthetic (another nasty word) hormones saw no problem with taking black cohosh or yam, which contain other forms of steroids. Exotic juice extracts like gogi and acai and seemingly strange herbal names like *dong quai* have suddenly appeared on the shelf in every market. Asking what was natural about taking grape seed or seaweed extracts in concentrations that didn't exist in nature was suddenly a very politically incorrect question. And of course, the herbal pain preparations helpful for fibromyalgia quite simply work because they contain the highest levels of natural salicylate.

NATURAL SALICYLATES AS MEDICATIONS

These are found in dietary supplements. Gather everything you take as a medication that you have not yet discarded because they did not contain the chemical salicylate, camphor, or menthol. Look for the words *oil*, *gel*, or *extract* with a plant name. In nature, only plants make salicylates so you can use anything you can identify as not being a plant. Simply put: If it's not the name of a plant, you can take it. For example: calcium, magnesium, and zinc. Not plants, no problem. Glucosamine, 5-HTP, malic acid, fish oil…again, not plants so they can't block guaifenesin. On the other hand, ginkgo biloba, green tea extract, valerian, evening primrose oil, flaxseed oil, or wild yam are plants and so they do block guaifenesin. Also check for bioflavonoids (quercetin, hesperiden, or rutin), which are concentrated plant pigments and will block guaifenesin. (Don't forget to recheck labels when replacing a product to make sure there have been no ingredient changes.) It's simple: If it's the name of a plant or contains bioflavonoids, don't use it.

Make sure you check the labels on all your vitamins—look for plant names such as rose hips or ginseng and bioflavonoids. Vitamin C or multiple vitamins that contain vitamin C are common culprits. Ingredients such as lutein or lycopene that are not the names of plants are okay. Hormones are fine; hormones are not plants. But you can't take the whole plant (such as saw palmetto or yam extract) to get the hormone. Use the purified form.

NATURAL SALICYLATES IN TOPICAL PRODUCTS

Gather up everything you use on your skin: shampoo, conditioner, bubble bath, body lotions, deodorants, lip balms, face cleansers, bar soap, eye makeup removers, nail polish remover, massage oils, cuticle creams, makeup, and so on. You're going to have to check the ingredients in all of these. If you have products without labels (or the packaging that had the ingredients printed on it), then set the product aside. You'll have to do a little more research to check these.

Once you've made sure that the syllable *s-a-l, camph,* or *menth* isn't listed, it's time to look for plant oils, gels, or extracts with a plant name. Coconut or macadamia nut oils, chamomile extracts, arnica, or aloe gels are examples of what you can't use on your skin. Remember that natural salicylates are found only in plants, but not in animal or mineral products. Thus, mineral oil, vitamin E, or emu oil and lanolin are all safe to use. We make an exception for products like hair coloring that are only used once every six weeks or so, but be careful with this leniency. Exposure to salicylates is cumulative: A little here, a little there, and eventually you'll have crossed the line and blocked your guaifenesin.

Check everything. All topical products including lipsticks, mouthwashes, suppositories, chewing gums, cortisone creams, nasal sprays, breath mints, toothpastes, razors, as well as shaving creams have the potential to block guaifenesin. Some of these products contain camphor, menthol, or castor oils; others add mint: spearmint, peppermint, or wintergreen oils, which easily provide enough salicylate to block guaifenesin. There are strips coated with aloe adjacent to the cutting edge of many disposable razors. The salicylates in the aloe slide into the tiny cuts made by shaving legs, underarms, or faces and readily block guaifenesin. Don't forget that you must check any product that contains a sunscreen (SPF) for octisalate, homosalate, mexoryl, or meradimate.

Plant ingredients in most products are not difficult to identify. Witch hazel, lavender, arnica, rosemary, ginseng, chamomile, and aloe vera are some of the well-known ones. Bark, stem, leaf, root, and flower are tip-offs that you're dealing with a member of the plant kingdom. Less commonly recognized names such as jojoba, castor, and yucca can be identified just using a dictionary or online at www.dictionary.com.

Unfortunately, there's a small group of plant names that are more difficult to find in standard reference books. Since the basic ingredients in all cosmetics are similar, manufacturers search for unique-sounding additives that will set their product apart on labels and in advertisements. Rain forests and tropical islands are being raided for cajeput, quillaja, bibia, padauk, and other native plants. These exotic but obscure substances can sometimes be defined using specialized sources. The easiest way to identify them is with the aid of an online search engine such as Google, Bing, or Yahoo. You don't need Wikipedia or Chemfinder; all you need to know is if the funny name on the product label is actually a plant. Not all of them are. You don't need to locate the molecular structure or learn where the plant grows in its native form. If it's a plant name coupled with oil, gel, or extract—don't put it on your skin.

I was forty-two years old when I started guai and pretty much homebound and bed bound. I'd stagger to the couch just so my son would know he had a mom. We farm, and my husband still thought meals on the table and clean laundry [were] possible. Life was very hard. I bought my guai at a discount store and took my skin care down to the basics. Just something to get clean and a lotion were all I used at the beginning. A great thing for me (living a half hour from a store) was using drugstore.com. I could SEE the ingredient lists and order everything my whole family needed with the click of a button. In my jammies. Easy. AND my UPS man carried the box to the door. Five years later, I'm living the best life I've ever had!! Now both my kids are on guai as well. Being sal-free is our life.

You can do this alone!

—*Joyce, South Carolina*

Medicinal Products Containing Natural Salicylates

CortiSlim Control Weight Loss Formula (green tea extract, bitter orange peel extract, banaba leaf extract, etc.)

Gas-X (mint oil)

GNC Herbal Plus (saw palmetto, ginkgo biloba extract)

GNC VA-Z Vitamin C 2000 (rose hips)

GNC Fast Flex Multi-Action Joint Formula (rosemary, white willow bark extracts)

Health Plus Super Colon Cleanse (fennel, peppermint, papaya, rose hips, and more)

ProClinical Hydroxycut Fat Loss Support Formula (lady's mantle extract, wild olive extract, wild mint extract)

Super Flex Joint Formula (ginger root, turmeric)

Topical Products Containing Natural Salicylates

Absorbine Jr. (calendula, echinacea, wormwood extracts)

Carmex Lip Balm (camphor, menthol)

Colgate 2 in 1 Toothpaste and Mouthwash Icy Blast
(mint oil)

Coppertone SPORT Sunblock Lotion SPF 30 (aloe extract,
jojoba oil)

Got2B Foot Polish (mint oil, ruby grapefruit oil)

Herbal·Essences Shampoo for Normal Hair (aloe, chamomile
extract)

Huggies Supreme Care Baby Wipes (aloe)

Kleenex Menthol Tissues (menthol)

Paul Mitchell Tea Tree Styling Gel (jojoba oil, rosemary
extract)

Preparation H Ointment (eucalyptus oil)

Stridex Daily Care Alcohol Free Sensitive (aloe, eucalyptus,
witch hazel extract)

Vicks VapoRub Ointment (camphor, eucalyptus, menthol,
nutmeg oil)

Products Without Listed Ingredients

When you bag up your products to check, you'll find things
without listed ingredients. This can be because they were listed
on the packaging you threw away or because it was on the display at the store. Luckily it's not too difficult in most cases to
retrieve them.

If you're checking a medication such as, say, Midol or Pepcid, you can ask a pharmacist or a doctor for the chemical (or
generic) name. You can also simply put it in your search engine
on your computer. This will give you the information you
need. Midol's own website shows pictures of each package so
you can check the one you are using and each shows you what

the active ingredients are. For example, Midol Extended Relief is naproxen sodium, not salicylate, so you can use it. Pepcid is famotidine—also not a problem with guaifenesin.

Many websites list the ingredients for products they sell. At www.drugstore.com, you'll find the ingredients in most of the products you generally buy in drugstores. For higher-end products, you can try www.beauty.com or www.sephora.com. Most companies have their own website, and while they don't all list ingredients, there's always a "contact us" button you can use to submit a query. Always ask for the list of ingredients; don't allow them to check for you. Trust only your own eyes! If a company won't give you the ingredients, don't use the product.

My motto: When in doubt, throw it out.

—Char M., California

Dental Products

What sits in your mouth is really topically applied. Nicorette gum, sublingual nitroglycerin, and orally disintegrating migraine tablets are examples of medications that can be quickly absorbed into the bloodstream. Guaifenesin can be blocked by oral hygiene products that contain salicylates. Some contain salicylate by name (the first ingredient in Listerine is methyl salicylate) but more commonly the blocker is some form of mint. All mint is methyl salicylate whether synthetic or extracted from the natural plant. If you smell or taste mint in a product, it will block your guaifenesin. It will also block even if it's there but you can't taste it.

Most mouthwashes and toothpastes celebrate mint (Fresh mint! Mint blast! Cool mint!) or menthol—the more powerful, the better. We're accustomed to the tingly potent flavor that makes our mouths feel cool and thus fresh. The presence of mint oil, salicylic acid, or methyl salicylate are often not listed separately but included in the word *flavor*. Unlike fluoride, no law says the individual ingredients of flavors need to be listed.

Because by law, toothpastes don't need to list ingredients, it's best to stick with those we know won't block guaifenesin. The Cleure brand of dental products, designed by Dr. Flora Stay, D.D.S., are all salicylate free. Tom's of Maine voluntarily reveals all their ingredients including the flavor components so these can be checked by reading labels. Alternatively, simply dip your toothbrush in baking soda. You can also sprinkle it with hydrogen peroxide or use a peroxide gel such as Arm and Hammer that contains no flavor.

Don't ignore dental floss, breath strips or sprays, cough drops, lozenges, gum, or hard candies. Fruit and cinnamon flavors are fine, but beware of mint that is hard to taste because of other strong flavors. Dr. Flora Stay, D.D.S., has a number of products and suggestions on her website (www.cleure.com). There you'll find such products as salicylate-free tooth whiteners, fluoride gel, mouthwashes, and a question-and-answer board for personal assistance. Our website (www.fibromyalgia treatment.com) also contains product lists and updates.

Dietary Salicylates

No foods need be avoided when taking guaifenesin except for the mint family. Even those with higher salicylate content, such as berries, fruits, colored vegetables, cooking herbs, and spices, won't block if eaten in normal quantities. Salicylates in foods are diluted and partially destroyed by digestive processes. They're further neutralized metabolically when the liver degrades some of their effects by tagging them with glycine.

Salicylate levels can be measured in the blood and in the urine. The average daily intake from foods is in the range of 10 to 20 mg. Experiments with various diets have supported conventional wisdom that foods add insignificant amounts into the urine and, therefore, presumably, into the bloodstream.[3]

One does not have to avoid small amounts of herbs used to flavor a recipe. But we do need to mention one of the often overlooked blockers—tea. Teas are leaves and leaves come from plants. Teas have been studied and most contain high levels of salicylate so we now ask our patients not to drink tea. Coffee contains none, and sodas such as root beer won't block.

WHAT AREN'T NATURAL SALICYLATES

Just having a plant name doesn't mean something can keep your guaifenesin from working. A single chemical is acceptable as long as it isn't salicylate, camphor, or menthol. Here's a list of safe examples: alpha hydroxyl acid, sodium cocyl isethionate, oleoresin, cocamidopropyl, caprylic triglycerides and glycerides, capric acid, beta-carotene, squalene, shea butter, cocoa butter, coconut fatty acids, starch, sucrose polycotton-seedate, and bromelain (an enzyme isolated from papaya and used to aid digestion). These are all chemicals and not a problem. Some chemicals are readily identifiable as having a plant source (coconut acid) and some are not (sodium laurel sulfate). But that's more than you need to know. The above ingredients are all made in chemical factories and are not the whole plant anymore.

Salicylates and Cosmetics

This protocol is not a quick fix. It's a long-term thing. And you get well one day at a time. And if you make a mistake, you get back on track and keep going. It's kind of like trying to lose a lot of weight or dealing with an alcohol problem. You have to learn to be patient with yourself. I have never been a patient

person. I think I have developed more patience on this protocol because I needed to. I was too sick to do anything else. If
you spend all your time worrying that it might not work for
you, you are wasting your healing energy. Your body is stressed
to the limit with being sick. Using your energy to worry means
that your energy can't be used in healing. So...follow the
directions to the letter. Titrate your dose exactly as it says to.
Use as few products as you can in the beginning and make sure
they're all salicylate free. Be kind to yourself. Be patient. Try to
take one day at a time, one hour at a time.

—*Cris R., Michigan*

We hear a lot of complaints from patients taking guaifenesin
who lament the loss of their "natural" products. How can they
possibly give up items like jojoba oil face masks, almond oil
skin creams, or cleansers with aloe, witch hazel, arnica, or saw
palmetto? Many have simply been brainwashed by advertising
campaigns that have convinced them that if it is from a plant, it
is "natural" and so it's safer and better. There's just no evidence
that this is the case.

Minerals come from Mother Earth and are also natural.
Animal oils such as emu, lanolin, or cashmere oils have shown
beneficial effects on our own animal skin. And the fact is that
many people have started to be leery of ingredients, no matter
what the source, with unknown actions on the body. For example, those with a family history of breast cancer often decide to
use mineral salt deodorants to avoid aluminum. The bottom
line is that plants contain many compounds, some good and
some not so good for you.

Please remember that the FDA doesn't regulate cosmetic
claims or ingredients, including the use of words such as *pure*
and *natural*. *Natural* on a label can designate something partly
human-made combined with a natural ingredient. It could just
as surely indicate an ingredient synthetically extracted from

plants using some very potent chemicals through a wholly unnatural process. Many "all-natural" toothpastes contain sodium laurel sulfate—a chemical implicated in canker sores. What is natural about sodium laurel sulfate that comes from a chemical factory?

It's also important to remember that when plant extracts are used, preservatives must also be added to maintain freshness. These chemicals are often potent allergens and topical irritants. Skin creams containing cucumber extract have a shelf life of several years. How long can a cucumber last in its natural state, even in the refrigerator? Many dermatologists share this information with patients and suggest those with allergies and sensitivities use simple fragrance-free products such as Cetaphil Cleanser or CeraVie creams.

There aren't very many actual moisturizers and humectants, ingredients that seal moisture into the skin. The workhorse ingredients in most products boil down to a very few chemicals whose names you'll see repeated over and over again on labels. Basic soothing ingredients are such things as mineral oil, glycerine, cyclomethicone, dimethicone, and petrolatum. All are laboratory-made and are mainstays in almost every skin cream no matter what else has been added. The most effective moisture-holding agents are glycerine, ceramide, lecithin, hyaluronic acid, sodium hyaluronate, sodium PCA, collagen, elastin, amino acids, cholesterol, glucose, sucrose, fructose, glycogen, and phospholipids—and none is the name of a plant. There are only three ingredients that protect the skin from photoaging and skin cancer: avobenzone, titanium dioxide, and zinc oxide.

Cosmetics companies shovel plant material into ordinary moisturizers and makeup to make them seem more exotic and to command higher prices. While some plant ingredients do the job asked of them, none is essential to maintain or protect skin. In fact, it's not unusual for us to hear patients say that the quality of their skin improved when they stopped using so many compounds. Patients with skin allergies can attest that using products with fewer ingredients seems to be easier on the body.

We can all agree that not every plant is beneficial or particularly desirable. Natural poisons will kill just as effectively as synthetic ones. Tobacco comes from a plant; poison ivy, poison oak, hemlock, oleander, and toadstools are all well-known, potentially lethal toxins. Our bodies are not flower beds, and nature didn't intend for us to indiscriminately lather on or ingest everything in sight.

Paula Begoun first published *Don't Go to the Cosmetics Counter Without Me* in 1991. She regularly updates it, and also publishes a newsletter and maintains an informative website. She reviews literally thousands of products from companies such as Almay, Avon, the Body Shop, Charles of the Ritz, Dior, Estée Lauder, Maybelline, Revlon, and Vaseline Intensive Care. She reminds us that results are what matter; gouging prices and exotic ingredients don't guarantee a better outcome. Although her book doesn't list the ingredients of each scanned product, it provides an overview and evaluates many ingredients in cosmetics, both natural and synthetic, for their efficacy. Her readers get an inside look at how cosmetics are created, manufactured, and marketed. That's interesting and helpful for everyone, not just patients taking guaifenesin. There is no question that we should all be concerned because ingredients in topical products don't require evaluation for safety by the FDA.

The guaifenesin protocol has benefited hugely from the expertise of Dr. Flora Stay, D.D.S. Her company, Cleure, has products for dental needs, skin care, hair, and cosmetics—all of which will always be salicylate-free. Cleure toothpaste and other offerings benefit from her experience and knowledge as a teaching and practicing dentist who has searched for effective, safe ingredients. Her website, www.cleure.com, contains information about her products and fibromyalgia. She is the author of *The Fibromy-algia Dental Handbook*, published in 2005.

Ruthie Molloy of Illuminaré Cosmetics was inspired by her sister's battle with fibromyalgia. She has a liquid mineral makeup line that can be purchased through her website (www.illuminarecosmetics.com) and other beauty sites. Several other smaller manufacturers are listed in the Resources at the end of this book and on our website. As time goes by, we expect more manufacturers to come forward.

We should mention one other resource before we leave the subject: The Marina del Rey Pharmacy (www.fibropharmacy.com) sells many products that have been carefully screened for salicylates. If ordering from more than one company, you can save shipping costs as well as be provided with helpful, understanding service. We know of many who have called in, too sick to think, and just asked Kay to send them one of every-thing essential: deodorant, toothpaste, mouthwash, and soap. Later, when they recovered enough strength to go out, they added lipstick, eye pencil, and sunscreens and travel sizes of their favorite new products!

It is now possible through the above resources to purchase all the products you need without reading a label. For accu-rate information and changes, always check www.fibromyal giatreatment.com.

> I'm finally having some good days again. I discovered that a vita-min with bioflavonoids and vitamin C with rose hips was block-ing my guaifenesin. Last week, I drove four and a half hours to help my daughter, who was ill. It took a lot of energy to care for her baby and her busy two-year-old, cook, grocery shop, and do laundry. I was amazed at how much energy I had and how little I ached. I could not have done it even three months ago.
>
> —*Mary Ellen Stolle, network leader for*
> *The Vulvar Pain Foundation*

Frequently Asked Questions About Salicylates

Which dishwashing liquids are salicylate-free?

Dish soaps are usually okay to use. A few brands may contain aloe or plant oils. (Those found at health food stores most often contain herbs or seed oils.)

I have eliminated all salicylates from my topically applied products and still don't notice any effect from the guaifenesin. What should I do now?

Recheck everything, even your chewing gum and breath mints for mint, peppermint, spearmint, or wintergreen. Search your vitamins and supplements for bioflavonoids, rose hips, or other botanical additions. If you find nothing, raise your dose of guaifenesin by one or two tablets. Within the next ten days, you should feel distinctly worse. If you don't, be even more suspicious about blocking. Ask for help from the online support group at www.fibromyalgiatreatment.com. If you find nothing, your dosage may need further adjustment.

Should I avoid laundry detergents with phosphates?

You do not need to avoid phosphates in anything. Extra phosphates are not a problem. It's impossible to eliminate them from your life, and your body needs a huge amount to form energy. Laundry detergents don't come in direct contact with the skin since they're rinsed out of your clothes before they're worn. So the answer is no.

I'm a gardener. Is there anything I should be careful about?

You should be very careful doing certain gardening chores. Plant saps are readily absorbed through the skin. For this reason, you should wear gloves if a particular job will expose you to plant juices. The thin gloves worn by surgeons are ideal for delicate tasks, while thicker, plastic gloves should be worn for heavier work. Cloth gloves offer no protection. Leather ones can become progressively saturated with salicylates that eventually soak through and become worse than no gloves at all. Plants such as mint, marigold, geranium, and rosemary have higher salicylate contents than others. However, all plants pose the same kind of danger, even if to a lesser degree. There are many new gardening gloves that are not unwieldy and actually support your hands while you garden. Check your local gardening store.

What about smoking?

With everything we know today, it's obvious that you shouldn't smoke, even if you don't have fibromyalgia. For fibromyalgics, there's added concern: More than one study has shown that smokers have more pain and circulatory problems than others.

However, the topic of this chapter is salicylates. We're also concerned about particulate salicylates inhaled through the bronchial lining by smokers, including marijuana users. We don't really know the full impact of smoking, but some observant patients noticed a distinctly faster reversal at the same guaifenesin dosage only when they quit smoking. We do know from experiments that tobacco plant leaves contain methyl salicylate. They're certainly treated, and dried, but those maneuvers alone would not destroy that chemical. Does the burning or filter change that, and if so, by how much? Obviously, menthol filters create a separate distinct problem.

There's a strong possibility that smoking could make guaifenesin partially or totally ineffective. It might merely depend on the crop's potency, but we tell patients to be as pure as possible and avoid any substance they can't safely validate, and this includes smoking. Obviously, smokeless tobacco doesn't burn or destroy its salicylate content.

Take the easy way in the protocol. By this I mean, don't play around with your dosage, don't use products with salicylates, and try to think positively about the future. Don't let vanity keep you from giving up certain products that interfere with your guaifenesin. If makeup is absolutely necessary in your life, use only what is approved. BE DILIGENT! I can't say this enough. Ultimately you are the one who is going to put yourself into remission. All the information you need is on the website and in the book. You have to have a mind-set that you want to be well. I am extremely SERIOUS. YOU CAN DO IT. You HAVE to do it if you want a good life. It will take time. Just because we live in an instant satisfaction society doesn't mean you can rush your remission by changing the rules. GO FOR IT with all your moxie. Step up to the plate and declare yourself a person who is going to conquer fibromyalgia.

—Nora D., Georgia

Chapter Five

Patient Vindication

I'm now seventy years old and doing great. The fibro pain has been gone for so long but I haven't forgotten how hard it was. If you will do the protocol exactly as Dr. St. Amand teaches, you will be like me...PAIN FREE, FUNCTIONING, ENJOYING LIFE, and hopefully helping guide other fibro patients through the protocol. I now ride my adult tricycle and wear my goofy hat to keep the sun off my face. I'm known in my town as "The Fibromyalgia Lady" and, after all these years, still get calls from desperate men and women who have been diagnosed. I always guide them to "the book."

—*Nora D., Georgia*

OUR THEORY OF fibromyalgia and our protocol have been frequent sources of derision. The initial responses were blatant and attacking. The tone was usually contemptuous with the attached questions: "Where's the proof? Where's the double-blind study?" Though much improved by the protocol, patients would wilt when confronted by their skeptical medical provider. There have also been more elegant, subdued appeals from some of our colleagues, particularly rheumatologists, for definitive studies. Patients have raised little more than emotional defenses because they've lacked supportive, scientific data. Yet we had results.

For years, we've maintained that a double-blind study would not be possible. To refresh your memory, "double-blind" means that patient-subjects don't know if they're on a real medication under testing or on a fake, the placebo. The "double" refers to the fact that none of the participating, research physicians knows which is which. Records are kept secret and identified in computer logs using classified numbers. A matching name is known only to a designated overseer who's entrusted to keep everything well hidden from scrutiny. When the project is completed, codes are broken and statistically analyzed to determine the efficacy of the medication over the placebo.

Attacks continued on our theory, no matter how many thousands of patients provided supportive, though anecdotal data. Medicine ignores "anecdotal" evidence no matter the volume of words and voices raised in support. We, too, decry unsubstantiated claims, but we've nurtured our entire protocol by listening to our patients. We've also gleaned much scientific data in isolated clips from a variety of journals in the past fifty years. Such cumulative information solidified our thinking: Something new did indeed exist under the sun. We were given another boost when the *Lancet*, a prestigious British journal (equal to our *New England Journal of Medicine*), published a letter to the editor. The July 9–15, 2005, issue had this quote emblazoned on its cover: "If everything has to be double-blinded, randomized, and evidence-based, where does that leave new ideas?" That was a spear-like thrust into the realm of medical academia. It fed our resolve and gave us further impetus to keep seeking unassailable, technical defenses for our simple method of treatment.

This chapter is one reason, among a few, for writing a third edition of this book. It presents another opportunity to thank our many patients, not only those who volunteer for our multiplying studies, but also others who've stood proudly in support. They and their cohorts not only inured themselves against derogatory remarks, but also encouraged us while we were guiding them back to health. Our scientific reports are confirming some nuances of the illness as taught us by many, many ailing patients. We can now address some of the alleged weaknesses of our fifty-year-old theory and provide you with some solidly vindicating findings. We're excited because our new, "evidence-based" motifs will empower you to sortie from your defensive positions into a gracious attack mode. What follows should nudge some skeptics to think again because it's difficult to refute the evidence.

Our one attempt at a double-blind study failed in 1995 in that both patients and controls improved overall during the year they were followed. This study failed largely because of our ignorance regarding salicylates. At the time all the researchers (ourselves included) were unaware of the impact of topical salicylates. The speed with which the skin and inner membranes assimilate this compound still amazes us. Procedural errors were also made when it came to excluding hypoglycemic individuals, which skewed the wellness questionnaires. We continue to refute the study's results.

It is our belief that no successful double-blind study will be forthcoming. Guaifenesin is now readily available over the counter. However willing to help, fibromyalgics would hardly continue in a study if they could not see improvement. Remember that only half the patients in a double-blind are given an active medication; the other half receive a placebo, or sugar pill. The placebo group would continue to suffer for a year or more, the time that would be required to harvest interpretable effects. We recognized that likelihood immediately after the negative study was concluded. We knew we needed genetic and/or biochemical research to expose the disturbed, but currently occult physiology that rendered a person fibromyalgic. We're quite excited to introduce you to what our ongoing research is unveiling. Now, how about a little *evidence-based, new-idea* science that needs no double-blinding?

During the past six years, Claudia and I have participated as researchers in studies that have produced two published papers. Two more have just been submitted. Many of you are already aware of the work we've been doing with the world-renowned Beckman Research Institute at City of Hope. Their scientists have melded some of our observations with invigorating data. We've been on an emotional high ever since their teams began searching for genetic mutations and defective biochemistry in our patients. Their dual disciplines blend perfectly to blaze a well-marked trail that will make it easier for others to follow.

The first team was under the direction of John E. Shively, Ph.D. He tested blood from ninety-two of our fibromyalgic patients, sixty-nine family members, and seventy-seven controls (nonfibromyalgics). His team measured twenty-five cytokines or chemokines. Those are tiny proteins that are generated in many tissues throughout the body. They have multiple functions and, in combination with other compounds, greatly affect metabolism, induce immune reactions, and may perversely attack, or protect, the body.

Our highly technical paper was published on June 5, 2008, in the *Journal of Experimental Biology and Medicine* (lead author: Zhifang Zhang, Ph.D.).[1] Twenty-three cytokine/chemokines were elevated in our patient subjects. Another abnormal one has surfaced since the paper was published. Four main cytokines stand out somewhat glaringly. Those of you without foreknowledge in chemistry and immunology may struggle a bit, but may still enjoy reading the paper.

Many of the disturbed cytokines and chemokines are highly inflammatory, as technically advanced readers realize. Yet there is no inflammation in tissues affected by fibromyalgia. That's probably why standard blood tests are consistently normal in such patients. We interpret the findings to show that a mulch of those little errant proteins, in combination, neutralize one another. That seems likely since multiple biopsies from swollen places in fibromyalgia have shown no inflammatory cells. Our coauthors did not address this issue or our interpretation, but we've certainly discussed it.

Please pay attention to the sheer number of the abnormal proteins. If your head doesn't swim just a little, let's make that happen. The preceding paragraph is an indictment of all those who told you, "It's all in your head." You were never a crazy, malingering, lazy, incompetent, or neurotic hypochondriac! Your blood does reflect the bad stuff going on in your body. We're not sure how those many cytokines interplay with thousands of other compounds surging through your genetically unique self. They can wreak havoc as they interface with hormones and other chemical messengers racing to estranged encounters. Intriguing, each of them has a function, at times favorable, but destructive when in the wrong company. It seems that combinations are what count in fibromyalgia.

Now for the clincher: On guaifenesin, ten (10) of the chemo/cytokines dropped lower, some to normal or even below. Five stayed about the same. Eight went up even higher as patients were improving on our protocol. Savor this for a moment. Not only has this one paper shown distinct defects in our chemistry, but it also shows the favorable changes from using guaifenesin. We can now safely dismiss the common criticism that "it's good only for mucus." Congratulations to all of us, especially to you and our fellow sufferers.

But we're not done yet. We've also been working with the genetics department at the same institute. Dr. Shively blended his team with another gifted group led by Dr. Steve Sommer, now replaced by Dr. Theodore Krontiris, both geneticists. Our first paper on the genetics of fibromyalgia was published in the online journal *PloS One* in December 2009.[2] One common and three rare mutations were found in 15 percent of 100 patients ("probands") and 200 of their parents (300 total people). That combination of test subjects provides "trios" and permits reliable genetic screening. Since that publication, another gene has surfaced that affects another 15 percent of our patients: A total of 30 percent of our fibromyalgics have shown mutations. A paper is in preparation as we write.

Is it getting obvious? Since several genes are involved in fibromyalgia, by pure chance, many patients will have various combinations, some dominant, some recessive. Elevated cytokines might waylay messengers sent out to do the bidding of those genes. Then, add such things as injury, surgery, infections, indolence, obesity, or other illnesses into the mix. Complicated? You bet it is. We're even skipping over the involvement of strange little proteins known as micro- and silencing RNAs. Those of you with this disease have always known there wouldn't be a simple answer.

The latter study is ongoing, and even as we write, nearly 300 patient-parent combinations are being recruited. Enough new gene aberrations should exist among them to expand on the earlier findings. The more we can locate, the more likely we'll develop a simple, diagnostic blood test unique to fibromyalgia. We're certainly getting closer.

Let's try to simplify what we've just written. Think of a guitar player when trying to understand genes (DNA), message carriers (RNA), chemokines, and hormones. He sets the music in his brain, sends out nerve messages to the waiting finger. A gene is like a finger plucking a string. RNAs are like emanations caused by vibrations that spread tones throughout the room. However, obstructive barriers exist everywhere: walls, curtains, open windows, and breezes. Sound waves get deflected, muffled, or echoed depending on where the listener is seated. The sound obstructors are like micro- and silencing RNAs and their companion chemo/cytokines. They're directed to certain positions along the way or to the keenest acoustic site. They can muffle, stifle, and alter the melodic message by inserting a flat or a sharp. That would artistically change what is picked up by receivers in targets within hearing distance. The brain knows that its musical score will be mitigated and differently interpreted by each member of the tissue audience. The renovated sound mix is usually harmonious, but not when disease moves barrier-proteins around and adversely impacts the original composition. That's where we aim our treatment: Alter the cytokines, chemokines, hormones, and nerve impulses to better synchronize their effects with their target organs.

Chapter Six

Hypoglycemia, Fibroglycemia, and Carbohydrate Intolerance

The doctor determined that I was hypoglycemic...and he also explained that hypoglycemia and fibromyalgia often go hand in hand. There was a name for what I had, an actual medical term! And there were also websites with information I could read. I was less than thrilled when he told me about the diet I would be on...Sugar was a no-no, as was caffeine...I gulped as he rattled off the list of the carbohydrates I should avoid, including the "Big Five" that figured heavily in my diet: pasta (my Italian heart literally broke in two), rice, potatoes, bananas, and corn...The doctor handed me a list of the permissible and said "Good luck."

This diagnosis meant that a morning might come when I could open my eyes and actually feel good to be alive, without fear of pain. Now four months later, I am pleased to say that I've experienced many such mornings...I have more energy, I sleep better, and I'm in a better mood. Friends, family members, and coworkers all say they've seen a change in me...Six months ago I would not have thought such a change was possible. But thanks to my own stubbornness...and the dedication of my current doctor, I have finally found relief. I guess what my doctor and I have in common is that we refused to give up the search for answers and we chose to ignore people who said there were none. For us both, perseverance has definitely paid off.

—*Michelle Fisher, California*

In 1964, I was treating a podiatrist who suffered from fibromyalgia. Luckily for me, she had many scientific interests and studied a great deal. At one of her checkups, she brought me a pamphlet describing a host of symptoms that it attributed to low blood sugar. As an endocrinologist, I was certainly familiar with severe hypoglycemia, the kind that made patients display severe systemic symptoms, even passing out, because of a sudden excess surge of the hormone insulin, which they were using to control their diabetes. There are a few other quite rare conditions that cause the same catastrophe.

Hypoglycemia—From the Greek, meaning "low [hypo], sugar [glyc] in the blood [emia]." The accepted medical criterion for this condition is a blood sugar reading falling below 50 milligrams per deciliter (mg/dl).

As I read through the gauntlet of listed symptoms, I realized that if the information was even 50 percent accurate, I had been missing the chance to help a lot of sick people. The brochure listed fatigue, irritability, nervousness, depression, insomnia, headaches, impaired memory and concentration, anxieties, dizziness, blurred vision, leg cramps, sugar craving, flushing, nausea, gas, bloating, and constipation alternating with diarrhea as the most common symptoms. We soon realized those were the chronic effects, which we now segregate from the more dramatic ones we recognize as the acute symptoms of hypoglycemia. The latter pounce quite suddenly: shaking tremors, clamminess or sweating, palpitations, faintness or syncope, confusion, and panic attacks. Of course, these are the easiest ones to spot.

Using gout medications the preceding five years, I had been

fairly successful in resolving fibromyalgia in the majority of patients. But there was a subset of people who weren't doing as well. Though they complained less about former pains and even though I noted improvement by palpating regression of lumps and bumps, they were not getting any perfectly normal days. Something was different about this group and their nonresolving miseries. With a few pertinent facts provided by the brochure, however, the picture was now complete. Enter hypoglycemia.

Suddenly the questions posed by the partially responsive patients were resolved. It became clear that not one but two totally remediable diseases accounted for their multiple complaints. As I gained experience, it became progressively easier for me to separate the two and attack them simultaneously as well as to realize the volume of patients who were affected. Luckily, the treatment for hypoglycemia was already well known and highly effective. No medication is necessary or even useful. Resolution simply requires eating the proper diet. Patients were deeply relieved to learn that neither illness leaves residual damage. Our mutual frustration vanished as we medically purged fibromyalgia and the diet corrected hypoglycemia.

I had just begun to hope that I would finally be able to live without the pain from fibromyalgia. The guaifenesin treatment from Dr. St. Amand gave back my energy and mobility. It was all the more difficult, then, to be disabled by headaches. I was aware that my health was not good, so I ate a vegetarian diet and followed the food pyramid recommendations closely; I ate a diet rich in carbohydrates and low in fat, and the worse I felt, the more carefully I followed these recommendations. Despite this, I was always hungry and faint, and my headaches were steadily worsening.

Claudia showed me the diet recommended for hypoglycemia and offered me the hope that by following this regimen

I could control my headaches. I would have tried anything; I had nothing to lose. In fact, I had a lot to lose: pain, fatigue, and even excess weight. From one day to the next my headaches all but vanished; during the first few weeks my migraines diminished to one or two a week and I had no other headaches, either mild or severe. The improvement was so immediate and so unmistakable that I had no difficulty whatsoever following the diet, even though it was just before Christmas and I was surrounded by sweets.

—*Cynthia C., Michigan*

As my education and enlightenment progressed, I became more familiar with patients who had hypoglycemia as a stand-alone illness as well as those who suffered from simultaneous fibromyalgia. At the time, I was a spokesman for the Los Angeles County Medical Association. NBC News wanted to present a segment on hypoglycemia, which was at that time becoming the new fad in medicine. Because I was an endocrinologist, I was interviewed and asked to discuss the condition on camera. I was featured along with physicians who were full-time, professorial staff members from two UCLA campuses.

The story was shown on three consecutive evenings as five-minute, serialized segments during the prime-time newscast. Then, owing to overwhelming viewer response, the program was shown a few more times in the following months. The Los Angeles County Medical Association, UCLA, and Harbor General Hospital were bombarded with phone calls. Since I was the only interviewed physician in private practice, inquiries were funneled to my office. I was inundated with calls from people with hypoglycemia, as well as the as-yet-unnamed fibromyalgia. Combinations of those two were no longer puzzling to me, but the spectrum of symptoms made patients with other conditions quizzical, and they, too, sought help. Many of those were justified in their suspicions and had been either mislabeled as neurotic or had a properly diagnosed illness with the added onus of fibromyalgia and/or hypoglycemia. My patient base grew rapidly to include not only people from our area, but also from other parts of California, soon the entire country, and eventually from all over the world. The sheer number of these has provided us with a huge database. That's the information we're now sharing with you.

To give you insight into hypoglycemia, you should understand the biochemical sequence that follows eating carbohydrates (sugars and starches). Ancient humans did not find food in overabundance. Lean days far outnumbered their days of plenty. In fact, they often went a day or two without any food at all. When they found sustenance, they devoured it on the spot. Rarely were all of the calories in this delightful repast needed for immediate use. Storage capabilities were necessary to provide energy on the less bountiful days that were sure to follow. In more modern times, however, our storage facilities are kept near overflow because calories are so readily available. Every meal provides excess that isn't needed for immediate combustion.

Enter insulin—the only hormone that directs excess food (energy fuel) into storage and attends to the work of conservation even before a meal is completed. It's like an insurance policy that guarantees against starvation, and it's the powerful hormone that kept our ancestors alive in times of famine. It directs cells to store not only glucose, but also fat and amino acids, the building blocks of protein. Insulin sends these stores to the body's energy warehouses, primarily fat cells, but also muscle cells. The liver converts nearly all carbohydrates to the simple sugar glucose. It also jumps to obey insulin's prodding and keeps a bit for itself in a storage form called glycogen. A goodly amount is also dispersed especially to the brain and muscles.

When all of the above are satiated, the remaining glucose

> **Insulin**—A hormone produced by the islets of the pancreas that is released in whatever amounts are needed to clear excess glucose from the bloodstream. It promotes the absorption of glucose into the liver and muscles, where it is stored as glycogen. It also facilitates storage of amino acids and fats, and is known, therefore, as the storage hormone. Without insulin, a person cannot gain weight.

is converted into fatty acids. Those get combined with something called glycerol in a structure we recognize as body fat, or triglyceride. The liver packages these minuscule fat droplets for transport to all tissues, mainly to the storage depots in fat cells. These little packets are what coalesce into the fat accumulations that are situated where we can pinch far more than we like on ourselves. Fat is nothing more than surplus energy maintained in the form of triglycerides. Our mouths and insulin—the caveman's lifesaving alliance—have become, in today's world of superabundance, enemies that make us fat and ensure we stay that way.

> **Triglyceride**—One of three "blood fats" that are known as lipids. Triglyceride is the principal constituent of body fat. It is manufactured in the liver largely from the sugar and starches that you eat.

Some individuals are unable to process carbohydrates without adverse consequences. We often use the term *hypoglycemia*, low blood sugar, to denote a whole disease. More accurately, this is a metabolic error that is really a syndrome, a cluster of symptoms that keep popping up at the same time. The condition could profit by more descriptive nomenclature, but we're accustomed to using that word and it's easily recognizable—most people have at least heard of it. Patients with this illness suffer a distressing insulin-related conflagration that's regularly ignited by eating certain carbohydrates. (See table 6.1.)

Table 6.1
Hypoglycemia Syndrome*

	Male	Percentage Male	Female	Percentage Female
Total number of patients	637		6,201	
Fibromyalgia (FM) only	254	40	1,562	25
FM and sugar craving	290	45	2,974	48
FM and hypoglycemia	93	15	1,665	27
Number of lean patients	520	82	4,283	69
Fibromyalgia only	223	43	1,260	29
FM and sugar craving	232	45	1,865	44
FM and hypoglycemia	65	12	1,158	27
Number of overweight patients	117	18	1,918	31
Fibromyalgia only	31	26	302	16
FM and sugar craving	58	50	1,109	58
FM and hypoglycemia	28	24	507	26

This table was compiled from a total of 6,838 consecutive patients. Diabetics were excluded. A majority of hypoglycemic patients had at least one diabetic parent.

HYPOGLYCEMIA

Chronic Symptoms

- Fatigue, insomnia
- Nervousness, depression, irritability
- Dizziness, faintness
- Blurring of vision
- Ringing ears
- Gas, abdominal cramps, diarrhea
- Numbness/tingling of hands, feet, face
- Flushing/sweating
- Foot/leg cramps
- Bitemporal or frontal headaches
- Impaired memory and concentration

Acute Symptoms

- Heart pounding
- Palpitations or heart irregularities
- Panic attacks
- Nightmares and severe sleep disturbances
- Faintness or syncope
- Acute anxiety
- Hand or inner shaking/tremor
- Sweating
- Frontal headache or pressure

Figure 6.1

There are two ways to produce low blood sugar. The most obvious is by an excess of insulin, but it can also be induced by delayed or inadequate hormonal responses that should have applied the brakes to a rapidly falling glucose. The latter are known as counterregulatory hormones because they normally stop the overexuberant attacks of insulin. All kinds of possibilities exist, because a little too much of this or too little of that creates a whole spectrum of stresses. Combinations of various defects viciously strain a variety of cells.

There are four important counterregulatory hormones, but adrenaline (epinephrine) is the ultimate weapon, and the final safety net. If either insulin or adrenaline is released in delayed, inadequate, or excessive amounts, the other must decrease or increase its output to avoid hypoglycemia. They dance together, but at opposite ends of the ballroom. (See figure 6.1.)

So, you've got the picture. Insulin drives blood sugar down, and adrenaline pushes it up. It's normally quite harmonious. As sugar drops below certain levels, hormones such as glucagon, growth hormone, and cortisol work in unison with smooth orchestration. Normally, we're not aware of the metabolic sounds made by these instruments. In hypoglycemia, however, alarming drops in blood sugar alter the key and discordant notes are sounded. In the overture, sugars and heavy starches are consumed, and this strikes familiar notes in the pancreas. It plays stridently and fast with inappropriate releases of insulin. This threat sets up a chemical counterpoint that, like a loud trumpet blast, awakens the dozing adrenal glands; they respond with a stupendous release of adrenaline. That's when affected individuals first realize that the customary fine-tuning is errant. One or the other hormone gains the upper hand at different moments, and that makes for unusual syncopation. (See figure 6.2.)

Hypoglycemia's acute symptoms, which are triggered by adrenaline, are truly frightening and generally last from twenty to thirty minutes. They most often strike three to four hours

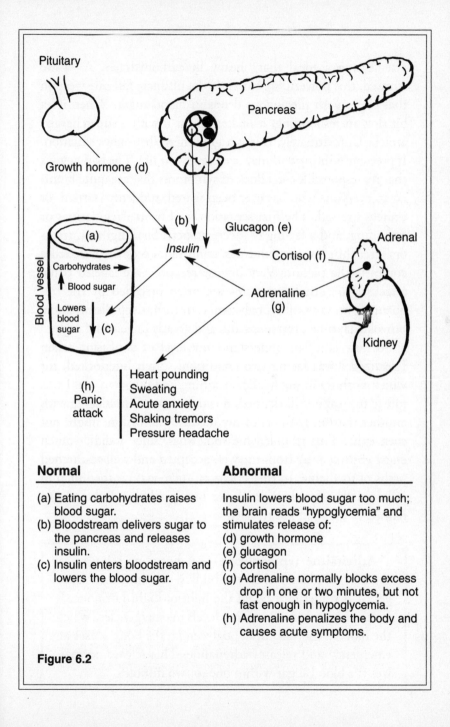

Pituitary

Pancreas

Growth hormone (d)

(b)

Glucagon (e)

Insulin

Adrenal

Cortisol (f)

(a)

Carbohydrates →

↑ Blood sugar

Adrenaline (g)

Lowers
blood
sugar (c)

Kidney

Blood vessel

(h)
Panic
attack

Heart pounding
Sweating
Acute anxiety
Shaking tremors
Pressure headache

Normal	**Abnormal**
(a) Eating carbohydrates raises blood sugar.	Insulin lowers blood sugar too much; the brain reads "hypoglycemia" and stimulates release of:
(b) Bloodstream delivers sugar to the pancreas and releases insulin.	(d) growth hormone
	(e) glucagon
(c) Insulin enters bloodstream and lowers the blood sugar.	(f) cortisol
	(g) Adrenaline normally blocks excess drop in one or two minutes, but not fast enough in hypoglycemia.
	(h) Adrenaline penalizes the body and causes acute symptoms.

Figure 6.2

after eating a meal that's heavy in carbohydrates. As we've stressed, this powerful hormone is the ultimate fail-safe weapon that copes with precipitous drops in blood sugar. When it's a bit slow in responding, it makes up for it with a supercharged attack. Unfortunately, this is a good-news/bad-news situation. It prevents fainting and may even save your life. The bad news is that it's responsible for a flock of symptoms that are quite familiar to everyone who has ever been scared, suddenly startled, or acutely stressed. The first sensation is of heart irregularities or pounding, and a feeling of severe anxiety. Shaking hand tremors, drenching sweats, faintness, and frontal pressure headaches complete the picture. Very intense reactions are labeled panic attacks. Nocturnal symptoms are often preceded by the frequent nightmares of hypoglycemia. In turn, sleep disturbances provoke daytime drowsiness and add greatly to general fatigue.

So now you can understand my level of confusion when I realized I was facing two conditions, often interlocked, for which nothing in my medical training had prepared me. I was forced to treat one ill-defined, misunderstood illness along with another that, in the eyes of my medical profession, might not even exist. This troubled me somewhat, since I didn't much enjoy veering away from the well-accepted and well-researched paths of medicine. In this situation, there was no road map to follow; I therefore had no choice but to take, as Robert Frost named it, the road less traveled.

Adrenaline (epinephrine)—A hormone released by the adrenal glands when the body senses imminent danger. It is sometimes called the fight-or-flight hormone. It is designed to increase energy levels in emergencies. When the blood sugar falls in hypoglycemia, the body senses an emergency and releases adrenaline. This release normalizes the blood sugar within one to two minutes.

> **Endocrine system**—This system is made up of glands that produce hormones (chemicals necessary to regulate the body's functions). They regulate or stimulate metabolism, growth, and sexual development and function, as well as maintain the body in a state of balance (known as homeostasis).

Since patients kept referring others, I was collecting an assortment of conditions I wasn't yet fully adept at handling. I had to look somewhere other than the bibles of accepted textbooks for effective treatments. It's spine-tingling in any field of work to come face-to-face with something exciting and entirely new. It was a little intimidating to find that a nameless disease was actually common, and equally astounding to realize that an existing medication could resolve the condition. I had been taught that results are what count. I remember one of my teachers during grand rounds who said emphatically: "Don't just stand there—do something!" I think this was his interpretation of the Hippocratic oath, which could be paraphrased as: "Get the patient well as best you can, but above all, do no harm." What to do seemed simple, safe, and straightforward. I would offer a diet to erase hypoglycemia, prescribe a medication to control rheumatism—or as it's now known, fibromyalgia—sit back, and enjoy my success. It was never to be: Disagreements and arguments in this field persist even though the opposing voices are getting softer.

THE DIAGNOSIS OF HYPOGLYCEMIA

The glucose tolerance test [is]...the worst torture in a lab that can be done to anyone, especially a hypoglycemic. You arrive following a twelve-hour fast and then, while you are half-asleep, a needle is stuck into your arm and blood is drawn. Then you are given a drink called a GLU-Cola, which is basically a cola with half a bottle of Karo syrup poured into it. You have to drink this down fairly quickly without gagging, and then in an hour another needle is stuck in your arm, and blood is drawn again. They do this ten times during the next five hours. In between needle sticks you sit in a chair in a freezing sterile lab...and you can't walk around because it will cause you to release adrenaline and lower your blood sugar. And you can't eat anything, and you haven't eaten in seventeen hours by the end of the test. Somewhere around the fourth hour you feel like you are going to die, dizzy, sweating, sick, and then you feel like you are going to pass out. Just when you fall asleep, they wake you up to stick you again. When you finally get home, you are horribly sick, and you stay dull-witted and dazed for several days.

—*C.C., California*

The five-hour glucose tolerance test is a standard tool for confirming the diagnosis of hypoglycemia. Patients are given a measured amount of sugar to drink, and blood is periodically drawn to test their response to this glucose load. The former party line was always that, if during the course of the test, a blood sugar reading falls below the magic number of 50 milligrams per deciliter (mg/dl), the diagnosis is confirmed. In my earlier days, we subjected every patient with suggestive symptoms to the rigors of this test. To our surprise, many results revealed nothing but normal levels at any hour. Despite this, the poor patients complained bitterly about a flock of hypoglycemic symptoms they had suffered during and after the experience. Knowing that a spurt of adrenaline can raise blood sugar in one or two minutes, we retaliated by drawing blood more often—every half hour—hoping that added specimens would catch at least one low reading. This worked a little better, but was still far from satisfactory. We quickly learned that adverse symptoms were frequently not synchronous with the rigidly timed blood sampling. In other words, not everyone's blood sugar dropped at exactly the same time after drinking the sugar solution. It was obvious that technicians couldn't insert needles to draw blood fast enough to overcome the rapid effects of adrenaline. No matter how hard lab personnel tried, we all too often missed the glucose nadirs. The hormone was persistently faster than we were.

Finally, because glucose testing failed to confirm our diagnosis about 50 percent of the time, we decided to try a different approach. You can never say we didn't go down trying! We had patients drink the same measured amount of glucose, but omitted blood sampling. Now subjects simply recorded their symptoms during the subsequent five hours. Most of them experienced all of the classic, acute symptoms of hypoglycemia at different hours into the test. Others fell asleep, overcome by severe fatigue. Looking at countless diaries, it dawned on me that patients were simply writing down the very same symptoms they had already related in my office—symptoms that had alerted me to order the test in the first place. So why did we need to subject them to the ordeal and the expense? Why make them drink the horrible stuff? Why not just listen attentively to patient complaints, skip unnecessary testing, and simply accept as diagnostic the symptoms they had so eloquently described on their initial visit?

I decided to use the test only if patients were suffering fainting spells or had an abnormally low fasting blood sugar. Either of those two factors should prompt physicians to consider the possibility of an insulin-producing pancreatic tumor. Our new system paid off. It saved patients five hours of testing, multiple needle sticks, a miserable morning, and the sick days that were sure to follow the sugar cocktail. After all, do you really need a blood sugar reading of below 50 mg/dl to tell you what you already know—eating a lot of sugar or starch makes you feel lousy?

In 1994, Drs. Genter and Ipp published some interesting findings that gave us yet another reason to abandon testing.[1] They conducted a simple and elegant experiment that explained why some patients with symptoms don't register the previously considered mandatory drop of blood sugar below 50 mg/dl. These two doctors ordered five-hour glucose tolerance tests on twenty young, healthy subjects who had no symptoms whatsoever of hypoglycemia. A catheter was placed in a vein so that blood could be sampled every ten minutes without repeated needle sticks. Samples were measured for the amounts of various counterregulatory hormones and the timing of their release following the ingestion of the sugar load.

Surprisingly, during the test about half of the subjects developed varying degrees of the acute symptoms, such as tremors, sweating, heart pounding, anxiety, or pressure headaches. Some had only a few of these effects, but others had all of them. As expected, the battery of tests identified adrenaline release as the cause of these sensations. Very strangely, however, these responses were induced with sugar levels quite in the normal range. The lowest was at 58 mg/dl of blood, but most had levels in the 60s, 70s, and one even at 81! This flew in the face of the accepted definition of hypoglycemia: the magic number 50. This study and a later corroborating paper from France strongly suggest, at least to me, that we each have a set point for blood sugar. If it drops below our own predetermined, ever-changing level, the brain says we've got trouble, and promptly triggers hormonal and nerve impulses to prevent us from passing out.

The problem remains that many physicians are unaware of these studies and persist in ordering fasting blood sugars and tolerance tests when a patient complains of obvious symptoms of hypoglycemia. Normal tests fool physicians into thinking their patients don't have carbohydrate problems. Using purely symptoms for diagnosis, it doesn't much matter what sugar level triggers them. The term *hypoglycemia* should be retained for patients whose blood sugar actually drops below 50 mg/dl. We should accept something that more accurately describes the group we're discussing. The simple designation *carbohydrate intolerance syndrome* wins our vote. Regardless of sugar levels or what name we use, all patients with this symptom complex respond equally well to the same dietary restrictions.

I have now been on the HG diet for over four years and it is still the most important day-to-day thing I do to keep well. Every time I fall off the diet, I suffer in various ways, including getting very anxious and emotional and having trouble thinking straight. So I get a sharp reminder every time about why I bother with the diet! It is worth tackling this issue as a blood sugar problem: It will become clear in a few days whether you are on the right track.

Take a good hard look at what you are eating and when. Do the diet as written, including watching out for the foods and ingredients on the "strictly avoid" list. Make sure you have satisfying balanced meals. Have a snack with protein and fat in between meals and make sure you never go too long without food. Make sure you carry something HG-legal with you. Wherever possible, have food cooked from scratch.

I realize this is an issue in social settings where people are sharing food, but you can make it work. People don't expect diabetics to eat any old thing and it is just as important for your health to be careful.

Mary, New Zealand

Once I had a better understanding of carbohydrate intolerance, I was much better able to discern the overlapping symptoms of fibromyalgia. (See figure 6.3.)

Unless you or your doctor can recognize the distinctive complaints that help separate the two diseases, the second diagnosis might easily be missed. The two diseases share many symptoms: fatigue, irritability, nervousness, depression, insomnia, flushing, and impaired memory and concentration. Anxieties are also common to both conditions, as are frontal or bitemporal headaches, dizziness, faintness, and weakness. Each can produce blurred vision, nasal congestion, ringing in the ears (tinnitus), numbness, and tingling of the hands, feet, or face. In addition, nausea, excessive gas, abdominal cramps, and constipation or diarrhea are frequent. Many complain of leg or foot cramps. When hypoglycemia is the cause of these chronic symptoms, they're experienced even in the presence of a normal blood sugar. That's because of the extensive endocrine and metabolic imbalances brought about by months of insulin-induced stress. (Refer to the Technical Appendix to review the involvement of various endocrine glands.) Even though guaifenesin will correct fibromyalgia, the similarity of symptoms makes it easy to miss the diagnosis of hypoglycemia. Both perplexed patient and physician will think they're seeing only a partial recovery.

There's a certain stiffness of muscles in hypoglycemia, but not the deeper pains induced by the lumps and bumps of fibromyalgia. Much confusion can be avoided by simply using our hands to map swollen areas. This type of examination makes it possible to separate the two illnesses with considerable accuracy. Lumps, bumps, and spastic tissue easily identify fibromyalgia. Fortunately, we also have the acute symptoms of carbohydrate intolerance to dependably point to blood sugar disturbances. These statements are important.

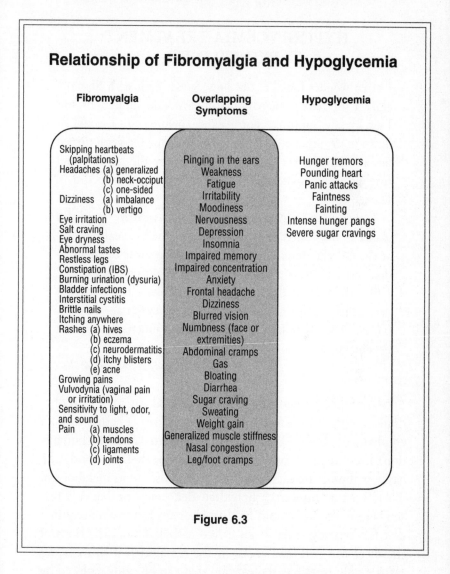

Relationship of Fibromyalgia and Hypoglycemia

Fibromyalgia	Overlapping Symptoms	Hypoglycemia
Skipping heartbeats (palpitations) Headaches (a) generalized (b) neck-occiput (c) one-sided Dizziness (a) imbalance (b) vertigo Eye irritation Salt craving Eye dryness Abnormal tastes Restless legs Constipation (IBS) Burning urination (dysuria) Bladder infections Interstitial cystitis Brittle nails Itching anywhere Rashes (a) hives (b) eczema (c) neurodermatitis (d) itchy blisters (e) acne Growing pains Vulvodynia (vaginal pain or irritation) Sensitivity to light, odor, and sound Pain (a) muscles (b) tendons (c) ligaments (d) joints	Ringing in the ears Weakness Fatigue Irritability Moodiness Nervousness Depression Insomnia Impaired memory Impaired concentration Anxiety Frontal headache Dizziness Blurred vision Numbness (face or extremities) Abdominal cramps Gas Bloating Diarrhea Sugar craving Sweating Weight gain Generalized muscle stiffness Nasal congestion Leg/foot cramps	Hunger tremors Pounding heart Panic attacks Faintness Fainting Intense hunger pangs Severe sugar cravings

Figure 6.3

Either disease standing alone requires its own simple approach. A two-pronged attack demands dual and simultaneous treatment.

HYPOGLYCEMIA TREATMENT:
PROPER DIET

I often wonder how life can be so good, even with fibromyalgia. I still have some pain, I still have some limitations, but I am greatly improved. For instance, before guai, I would sit down in my office chair in front of the computer, get it turned on, and have to get right back up because the burning and tingling in my spine was so bad. That has not happened in years.

I grieve my losses on occasion, such as casting a wistful glance at the dessert menu or passing by the ice cream section at the grocery store. If I weigh that grief against the tremendous grief of years past, however, it is slight by comparison. I find the idea of thinking of my diet like a bank account very helpful. Proteins, fats, and low-carb veggies are deposits, but carbs are withdrawals. Spending too much, my account becomes overdrawn.

—*Jody D., North Carolina*

Many affected people ask if they should eat more carbohydrates, especially during bouts of hypoglycemia. The answer is an emphatic no! In fact, quite the opposite is true. Actually humans don't need sugars or heavy starches from the diet. The body can easily manufacture each and every type it uses in its metabolism. There exist no cases of carbohydrate deficiency for that very reason. However, we should be very clear up front: The required diet for hypoglycemia is not a zero-carbohydrate diet. Both of the diets you will read about in the remainder of this chapter restrict only certain carbohydrates that can be easily replaced by cousin foods—there are many acceptable candidates.

Sugars and some starches start raising the blood sugar within five minutes of consumption. Proteins, and to a lesser extent fats, can provide substrates that the liver can convert to glucose, albeit with a fifteen-to-twenty-minute delay. Not only that organ but also the kidneys easily convert certain amino acids into glucose. Many people consume carbohydrates in the belief that they'll become superenergized. If some of them aren't adversely affected by eating carbohydrates, we salute their remarkable metabolisms. It's true that healthy people compensate for rises in glucose with perfectly regulated bursts of insulin. In all honesty, however, they, too, probably admit to the late-morning, late-afternoon yawns and fatigue following carbohydrate indulgences. What rises must fall, and insulin action substantiates that axiom. Hypoglycemics have an unfortunate and exaggerated response: Their insulin surges incur overzealous carbohydrate control and induce the symptoms under discussion.

Hypoglycemia can be controlled only with a perfect diet, one that eliminates all of the dangerous carbohydrates. As we previously stated, there's no need to add anything; it's what you remove that guarantees recovery. Patients must not eat table sugar, corn syrup, honey, sucrose, glucose, dextrose, or maltose. Lactose (milk sugar) and the significant fructose in fruit can be consumed in rather limited amounts: Only one piece of fruit should be eaten in a four-hour period. All heavy starches must be avoided, including potatoes, rice, and pasta. Eliminate caffeine because it prolongs systemic effects of insulin. It also paradoxically slows entry of glucose into parts of the brain. Caffeine also helps insulin evoke or block responses to hypoglycemia, resulting in an undesirable hormonal combination that blunts release of the expected, salutary countersurge that normally brakes a rapid drop in cerebral glucose. The liver extracts quick energy from alcohol but, in just a few hours, stumbles badly from its effects and temporarily loses the ability to convert stored food residues to glucose. So sorry, but despite everything else we're stealing from your diet, no alcohol. But take heart: For many of you, these dietary restrictions aren't forever.

The elimination of sugars (simple carbohydrates) as well as heavy starches (complex carbohydrates) is mandatory because they push the body into release of so much insulin. Avoid that response, and hypoglycemia will not occur. It's really that simple. In time, each of the affected endocrine glands will recover. In my experience, healing begins with a display of somewhat more energy somewhere between the fourth to fifth day after starting the diet. Some patients feel more fatigue during the first few days as they change their basic energy fuels from carbohydrates to protein and fat. During this initial period, they may also experience headaches from both caffeine and carbohydrate withdrawal. The energy surge that eventually appears may be delayed for those who have been ill for a very long time. Total elimination of sugar and starch may seem like a monumental challenge, but using diligence and willpower, success is rewardingly awesome.

> I have been able to cautiously—and occasionally incautiously—reintroduce a few carbohydrates into my life, learning what my tolerance level is. But I am not tempted to add many; I have my life back, and compared to that, sweets and starches are a truly insignificant sacrifice.
>
> —*Cynthia C., Michigan*

Let's now look at the specific foods that must be completely eliminated if you are to overcome and maintain control of hypoglycemia.

Forbidden Foods List for Hypoglycemics: Foods to Strictly Avoid

Sugar in any form, including soft drinks
Caffeine from any source, including many soft drinks
Fruit juices and dried fruits
Baked beans

Black-eyed peas (cowpeas)
Garbanzo beans (chickpeas)
Refried beans
Lima beans
Lentils
Potatoes
Corn
Bananas
Barley
Rice
Pasta of any kind
Burritos (flour tortillas)
Tamales
Sweets of any kind
Dextrose, maltose, sucrose, glucose, fructose, honey, corn
    syrup, corn sugar (high-fructose corn syrup), molasses,
    cane or brown rice syrup, and starch (caloric sweeteners and
    starches), agave.

Our diet for hypoglycemia is divided into two parts: "strict" and "liberal." Both control hypoglycemia equally well. The strict diet was devised for anyone who needs to lose weight; the liberal diet was designed to maintain weight and still offset hypoglycemia. Take note: The above list, "Foods to Strictly Avoid," is applicable and, in fact, mandatory for both diets. You can't ignore that list in the beginning. Just a little cheat will certainly do you in!

DR. ST. AMAND'S STRICT DIET FOR HYPOGLYCEMIA AND WEIGHT REDUCTION

You can eat freely the foods listed below except for the few items given a quantity limit. You can eat whenever you're hungry—there is no need to starve yourself or eat on any specific schedule. If you don't see something on this list, you simply can't have it. Always check packaged and canned products by carefully studying the list of ingredients. Learn to read labels carefully every time you buy a product. Manufacturers may make changes without warning. Do your homework and don't kid yourself. The very foods that caused you to gain weight are the ones you must give up to lose it. If this appeal to your common sense doesn't succeed, go to the liberal diet. You'll remain heavy but you'll at least control hypoglycemia.

Meats

All meats are allowed, except cold cuts that contain sugar. (Check labels carefully. Low-fat or nonfat and turkey cold cuts usually have added dextrose or corn syrup. Bacon and ham are acceptable, although they do list sugar on the labels. This bit cooks off and is not a problem. Hams that are heavily coated should be washed free of sugar.)

All fowl and game, fish, and shellfish are allowed in unlimited quantities.

Dairy Products

Butter and margarine
Cottage and ricotta cheeses (1/2 cup limit)
Any natural cheese (cheese you slice yourself)
Cream (heavy and sour)
Eggs

Fruits

Avocado (limit 1/2 per day)
Cantaloupe (limit 1/4 per day)
Fresh coconut

Lime or lemon juice (limit 2 teaspoons per day), for
   flavoring
Strawberries (limit 6–8 per day)

Vegetables

Asparagus
Bean sprouts
Broccoli
Brussels sprouts
Cabbage
Cauliflower
Celery
Chard
Chicory
Chinese cabbage (limit 1 cup
   per day)
Chives
Cucumber
Daikon (long, white radish)
Eggplant
Endive
Escarole
Greens (mustard, beet)
Jicama
Kale
Leeks
Lettuce
Mushrooms

Okra
Olives
Parsley
Peppers (red, green, yellow)
Pickles (dill, sour, limit
   1 per day)
Pimiento
Radicchio
Radish
Rhubarb
Salad greens
Sauerkraut
Scallions (green onion)
Snow peas
Spinach
String beans (green or
   yellow)
Summer squash (crookneck,
   yellow, and green)
Tomatoes
Water chestnuts
Watercress
Zucchini

Nuts (limit 12 per day)

Almonds
Brazil nuts

Butternuts
Hazelnuts (filberts)

Hickory nuts
Macadamia nuts
Pecans
Pistachios

Sunflower seeds (small handful)
Walnuts

Desserts

Low-carbohydrate products including sugar-free chocolate
  with sucralose (Splenda) and sugar-free Jell-O
Custard (made with cream and artificial sweetener)
Cheesecake (no-crust or nut crust with cream cheese, sour
  cream, and artificial sweeteners)
Mousses made with whipping cream and sugar-free syrups or
  flavored protein powders

Beverages

Artificially sweetened drink mixes like Crystal Light, Country
  Time, etc.
Club soda, zero-carbohydrate flavored soda waters
Decaffeinated coffee
Mineral or bottled water
Weak or decaffeinated tea
Caffeine-free diet sodas
Cocoa, sugar- and caffeine-free
Bourbon, cognac, gin, rum, scotch, vodka, dry wine (after two
  months on a perfect diet, most hypoglycemics can tolerate a
  bit of alcohol)

Condiments and Spices

All spices including seeds (fresh or dried), all imitation
  flavorings, and horseradish

Sugar-free sauces such as hollandaise, mayonnaise, mustard, ketchup, soy sauce, Worcestershire sauce
Sugar-free salad dressings
Oil and vinegar (all types)

Miscellaneous

All fats
Caviar
Tofu and soy protein products that contain no forbidden sweeteners

> If cholesterol is a problem, avoid cold cuts except sugar-free turkey. Trim all visible fat off meat. Remove the skin from poultry. Broil or grill foods instead of frying. Avoid full-fat cheese, heavy cream, solid margarine, hollandaise sauce, and macadamia nuts. Use egg whites or Egg Beaters instead of whole eggs. Use liquid margarine only. Nuts should be dry roasted only. Use canola or olive oil.

DR. ST. AMAND'S LIBERAL DIET FOR HYPOGLYCEMIA AND WEIGHT MAINTENANCE

(Add these foods to the strict diet)

Fruits (limit: 1 piece of fruit every four hours; no fruit juices or dried fruit)

Apples	Blackberries (1/2 cup
Apricots	limit)

Blueberries (1/2 cup limit)
Boysenberries
Casaba melon (1 wedge limit)
Grapefruit
Honeydew melon (1 wedge limit)
Lemons
Limes
Nectarines
Oranges
Papaya
Peaches
Pears
Plums
Raspberries
Strawberries
Tangerines
Tomato juice (unsweetened)
V8 juice

Vegetables

Artichokes
Beets
Carrots
Onions
Peas
Pumpkin
Squash, winter (such as acorn, butternut, fresh pumpkin, spaghetti, etc.)
Turnips

Nuts (no limit)

Cashews
Peanuts
Soy nuts

Dairy Products

Whole, nonfat, low-fat milk and buttermilk
Yogurt, unsweetened or made with noncaloric sweeteners

Dessert

Sugarless diet pudding (1/2 cup a day limit)

Breads

Three slices a day of sugar-free white, whole wheat,
  sourdough, or light rye. No more than two slices at
  one time or three servings a day of sugar-free flat bread
  (no more than two servings at a time). Low-carb
  tortillas—two is one serving. Corn tortillas—two are
  a serving.

Other Food Items

Carob powder
Flour, gluten or soy only
Gravy made with gluten or soy flour only
Wheat germ
Puffed rice, shredded wheat, or other sugar-free cereals
Popped popcorn (1 cup limit)
2 tacos or 2 enchiladas (2 corn tortillas only)

Most of the questions we are asked about the diet stem
from confusion regarding the built-in nature of various carbohydrates. Many people have difficulty understanding why
they can't eat a tiny bit of potato instead of the daily allow-
ance of sugar-free bread permitted on the liberal diet. Most
of those individuals have repeatedly tried calorie-restrictive
diets. The number of calories contained in foods are simply
added up, and if the total sum is kept low enough, weight loss
should begin without regard for the dietary mix. So carbohydrate substitution, gram for gram, would seem logical. Wrong!
That type of math won't cope with our problem since not
all carbohydrates are created equal. Since a calorie is a measure of heat, a portion of meat can be equal to a very different amount of candy. Note that a pound of feathers is larger

in size than a pound of lead, but the weight's the same. A carbohydrate-restrictive diet adds up very differently: A gram of dextrose is not equal to a gram of lactose relative to the insulin response.

The glycemic index (GI) ranks foods on how they affect blood sugar levels in comparison with straight glucose. It's mainly used to evaluate the metabolism of carbohydrates. Protein and fat don't induce much rise in blood sugar unless eaten with carbohydrates. Initially based on glucose with a number 100, the United States more commonly uses white bread as 100. (To convert to the white-bread scale, multiply by 0.7.) We'll stick with the original since white breads differ in the amount of insufflated air and the creative styles of different bakers. Tables exist to permit food comparisons by the rise in blood sugar or by the level of insulin they induce. As examples, potato, a bunch of glucoses strung together, is assigned the GI of 98; on the other hand, fruits contain fructose, which is quickly shunted to the liver, doesn't raise the blood sugar to the same extent, and releases far less insulin; peaches have a glycemic index of 26. Perhaps you can now appreciate that, though fructose and glucose are both carbohydrates, we can't substitute their effects on GI ounce for ounce (gram for gram). In general, you'll find that foods with a high GI are excluded from the hypoglycemia diet; lower-numbered ones can be consumed in moderation, the lowest in unlimited quantities. Please note, the glycemic index is not a perfect system. Expert studies have shown that this system is quite fallible. Individual constituents are not eaten by themselves and our foods exist in multiple combinations with others. A good example of this is the carrot, which we allow on our liberal diet despite its fairly high glycemic index. Its fiber content makes the difference.

When we first designed these diets, we had to rely on our

patients as test subjects since the glycemic index didn't yet exist. Any food that induced symptoms of hypoglycemia in even one patient was relegated to the forbidden list. We gradually boiled it down to the roux, the sticky residue that's the foundation for our diet listings. Nearing fifty years later, the diets still work without much revision. If you try to use recipes and foods from other low-carbohydrate diets, beware if you're hypoglycemic. Most of those were primarily devised for weight reduction and don't fit our requirements.

In our experience, about two months of perfect dieting are needed to wipe out all the symptoms attributable to carbohydrate intolerance. Consider the dietary process as if you were building a checking account. First, you must make deposits. If you're well disciplined, you can rebuild energy reserves to the highest level allowed by your genetic makeup. Only when your account is full should you begin experimenting with other carbohydrates, and begin making withdrawals on your balance.

Twenty Common Foods and Their Glycemic Index[2]

Food	Index	Food	Index
Fructose	25	Bananas	62
Yogurt	32	Brown rice	66
Milk	34	White bread	69
Tomatoes	38	White rice	72
Apples	39	Wheat bread	72
Pasta	45–50	Cornflakes	80
Peas	53	Honey	87
Sucrose	59	Carrots	92
Sweet corn	59	Baked potato (russet)	98
Corn	59	Glucose	100

You may never be able to indulge in wanton spending. You should be cautious in the beginning. Uncontrolled spending, or too much cheating, produces sequential debits. You may have to push away from the banquet table now and then and take time to replenish your reserves. A negative balance will put you right back into hypoglycemia. If you permit that to happen, brace yourself for the fury of renewed adrenaline surges and panic attacks. Once you've followed the diet for a while, your body is resensitized and its hormonal emissions synchronize, but resume disharmony if you excessively challenge the system. If that happens, there's no choice but to go back and restart the process of restoration. It's far better to heed whatever early warning signals you're given; tighten up on your diet and avoid disaster. That's the key to damage control.

It's in your best interest to become an A student by being observant. Learn to recognize the very first symptoms that follow dietary indiscretions. Enervating fatigue often leads the way, but frontal, pressure-type headaches are almost as likely. A few setbacks from hit-and-miss dieting will develop an instinct when to retreat. Mental or physical stress, the premenstrual week, and injuries render you especially vulnerable. They'll continue to sap your reserves, but if you're careful, you'll avoid fully subjugating deficits. You'll be far less fragile if you can anticipate before major symptoms resurface. In time, you'll properly ration meal contents to match energy expenditures.

Physicians or dietitians can't predict if you'll need permanent dietary restrictions. In a majority, a certain amount of leeway develops as fibromyalgia improves. Recall that illness causes much of your body to work day and night, thereby expending huge quantities of energy. When the overworked, contracted tissues relax, you may be rewarded by being able to eat almost indiscriminately. Unfortunately, genetics plays a part: Some patients will never be able to eat much carbohydrate. A family history of diabetes is sufficient warning that you were born with a genetically vulnerable pancreas. In that case, lifelong adherence to a low-carbohydrate diet would be safest.

> I got on the liberal hypoglycemia diet and have dramatically improved since then. I feel clear-headed with very little muscle pain on most days...If I cheat on my diet more than once or twice a week, I pay with nervousness, fatigue, and pain. I had serious withdrawal from refined carbohydrates. It felt like an addiction to me. I now look at foods as nourishment, not a reward or something to soothe me.
>
> —*Heather, Texas*

FIBROMYALGIA + HYPOGLYCEMIA = FIBROGLYCEMIA

Our statistics on nearly six thousand consecutive patients with fibromyalgia are telling. Twenty-nine percent of our females and 15 percent of our males have concurrent hypoglycemia. Most of our patients begin having low–blood sugar attacks after the onset of fibromyalgia. Many fibromyalgics feel worse depending on the amount of carbohydrate they ingest at one time. They don't get hypoglycemic or severe pain, but become generally more fatigued and stiff after eating starches or sugar.

We wanted a single name to cover patients who have both conditions. We've chosen *fibroglycemia*. So, you might ask, what is the reason that this combination is so common in our patients? Let's review a bit. We addressed our mapping system for making the diagnosis of fibromyalgia (see chapter 2). Our hands can easily identify the swollen areas of the body as contracted portions of muscles, ligaments, and tendons. Such areas are puffed up mainly because of accumulated intracellular fluid under high pressure, but they're also working tissues, as demonstrated by their spastic, constricted state. These tightened segments are steadily pulling on bones, joints, or adjacent structures twenty-four hours a day without respite. Though the effort is low grade, these sinews eventually fatigue and begin hurting just as expected from a never-ending workout. For every lump and bump we draw on our maps, there are many other affected areas too deeply hidden for us to feel. They're invisible accomplices that also contribute to the exhaustion. People who exercise stop when they get too much pain and fatigue. Fibromyalgics don't enjoy that luxury: They can never stop their muscles from working.

Remember that the currency of energy for all cells is ATP. Eighty-five to 90 percent of the food we eat is converted into this substance. Every bodily function demands huge supplies of this chemical. We can't even think without using large amounts of ATP for brain activity. Ounce for ounce, the central nervous system—especially the brain—uses more than any other tissue. Fingernail and hair growth, digestion, fat deposition, breathing, urinating, fighting infections, or healing tissue trauma all utilize ATP. The bulk of production and consumption occurs through muscle activity. As overworked tissues fatigue, they use nerves to signal the need for more fuel. The brain receives the message and immediately thinks: I'm tired. Give me a candy bar. When ATP production is normal, energy should be available within five minutes of eating such carbohydrates. That's no longer true in fibromyalgia. No amount of eating will totally satisfy the steady or sudden demand for energy.

Most fibromyalgics fall victim to carbohydrate cravings throughout the day in an unconscious attempt to create energy. Those sugars and starches are quickly digested and converted to glucose. Unfortunately, the carbohydrate-craving fibromyalgics quickly saturate their systems with glucose molecules, which force the pancreas to release large amounts of insulin.

Such surges rapidly lower the blood sugar by driving it mainly into muscles, but also into fat cells, liver, brain, and most other hungry areas of the body. These repeated insulin surges eventually cause hypoglycemia in genetically susceptible individuals. Both the chronic and the acute symptoms of that condition are added to those of fibromyalgia. There you have it: fibroglycemia!

These are the sickest of our patients. For them, dietary modification isn't merely a good idea, it's mandatory. They face a huge metabolic chore. They must eat themselves out of hypoglycemia while simultaneously accepting the increased symptoms of fibromyalgia reversal. There can be no compromise for this group. They would continue to feel terrible on a freewheeling diet even when guaifenesin had purged much of the fibromyalgic debris from their tissues. Fibroglycemics must either choose to eat correctly or choose to remain sick!

Over the years, my blood sugar has been slowly climbing as my weight rose, and now I am prediabetic. I am in a serious battle to lose weight, lower my blood sugar and my cholesterol, and not cross over the line into diabetes. I lost a lot of weight years ago on the strict HG diet, then coasted for a long time on the liberal diet, fell off the wagon a couple of times, and gained back what I'd lost, and now here I am today, trying not to become diabetic. It's not a symptom of fibromyalgia, but carb intolerance very often goes along with it, and can ultimately become diabetes. I thought it wouldn't happen to me.

Outcomes like this are what motivate us to keep harping on controlling your blood sugar and getting as much exercise as you can handle. As for me, I'm not giving up. I'm wearing a pedometer, and eating from the strict HG diet. Spring is coming to Minnesota, and cleaning up my yard and gardening will give me more opportunity for exercise.

—*Anne, Minnesota*

Obesity sometimes offers some protection against hypoglyce-mia, but only in males. That's a Trojan horse reenactment. Once fat is overexpressed in the system, chubby cells are gradually provoking a more serious disturbance. The larger a cell gets, the more resistant it becomes to further storage attempts by insulin. It's much more difficult to prod obese cells into opening their transport tunnels when they consider themselves already over-stuffed. As a result, fewer amino acids (building blocks for pro-tein) and fatty acids can be inserted into the usual warehouses. The pancreas, ever mindful of the waste-not-want-not principle, presumes its message is not being received. Rather than waste the digested food residues, the pancreatic islets instead increase their output of insulin. That's like hitting deafened fat and muscle cells with a hormonal two-by-four. Reawakened by this louder shouting, they dutifully respond, and storage resumes. Most structures of the body are willing to accept a bit more fatty acid and that's what insulin orders be done.

Overweight becomes heavier on the way to frank obesity. Now the bulging fat cells refuse to be fatter and fight back by becoming profoundly perverse in following insulin's instruc-tions. The step beyond simple insulin resistance (as this meta-bolic state is called) is type II, or adult-onset, diabetes. Cells that are unresponsive to insulin don't absorb glucose as read-ily as they once did. At this point, the blood sugar no longer drops abruptly; eventually, it doesn't even bother to stoop a little. This is the way obesity sometimes corrects hypoglycemia and dupes patients into thinking they've outgrown their sugar problem. But there's a heavy price to pay down the line. The health ravages of insulin resistance are many, and those of dia-betes several times worse. There's a special subset of individuals who have family histories of diabetes in parents and grandpar-ents. They are born with insulin resistance and will invite the same fate for themselves unless they heed our warnings about carbohydrates. We won't explore those hazards any further.

Nevertheless, we're adamant in warning you that neither low nor high blood sugar is healthy. We refer interested readers to our book *What Your Doctor May* Not *Tell You About Fibromyalgia Fatigue.*

Many patients crave sugar but are not yet hypoglycemic. For those of you who like statistics, here are some numbers. Not counting hypoglycemics, 43 percent of our lean and 57 percent of our obese fibromyalgic women crave carbohydrates; men don't fare much better: 44 and 48 percent, respectively. For all patients combined, including hypoglycemics, the lip-smacking demand for sugars can be rounded out to 75 percent incidence. Just like the other patients with blood sugar fluctuations, they suffer all of the aches, pains, and fatigue but aren't punished by the sudden adrenaline surges of fibroglycemia. During perverse situations, they can be pushed into that category by heavy sugar bingeing, alcohol abuse, emotional stress, infections, and even the trauma of an accident, extensive dental work, or surgery. Women are especially susceptible during the premenstrual week. It's as though they're teetering on the edge waiting for a nudge over the precipice.

Though no diet is necessary for people with fibromyalgia, those who regularly yield to their cravings could consider it. Sticking to a low-carbohydrate diet for one or two months might well provide surprises. Considerable energy and cognitive improvements are the rewards. Some encouragement is exhilarating while waiting for guaifenesin-induced improvements to begin. Even noncravers get some of those benefits. It's great just to get rid of some of the fibrofog, getting better sleep, and avoiding the drowsiness that regularly follows carbohydrate meals. It's certainly worth a month-long experiment. A prime function of insulin is to drive glucose into cells. Especially in tissues such as fat and muscle, it has to tag a phosphate onto it. That's how glucose is prevented from escaping back out of their cells. It's a great way to lock in a substrate for quick energy needs. Insulin also signals certain kidney cells to reabsorb phosphate that was just filtered from the blood and into the urine. By sucking it back into the bloodstream, more phosphate ions are made available for glucose trapping. Muscles are especially cooperative and some are more obedient to insulin than others. They snap to attention and soak up big phosphate loads, more than their fair share. You'll recall our theory suggests that phosphate excess is what eventually slams the brakes on energy formation. The chemistry of fibromyalgia, hypoglycemia, and the combination disease, fibroglycemia, is quite complex. But in simple terms, if you've got a few warped genes, and yield uncontrollably to carbohydrate craving, your cells will get a heavy phosphate dosing.

As if the picture weren't bleak enough, let's paint it worse! When insulin and glucose appear in fluids bathing the outside of cells, they insist on other visitors besides phosphates. Not too strangely, bloated fat cells and, especially insulin-resistant ones, make oppressive, militant demands. Together, they further subjugate cells into luring calcium into their enclaves and overzealously welcome all such guests. Though we should consider phosphate the prime villain, calcium is a steadfast accomplice. It unrelentingly goads already exhausted cells into further exertions. The low-carbohydrate diet thwarts the propensity for excess calcium and phosphate from insinuating themselves into mischievous places. It does that by thwarting excessive insulin extrusions.

As you'd surmise, fibroglycemia patients have the same salvaging dietary response as do those purely hypoglycemic. Please follow our earlier advice: Adhere to the strict diet if you're overweight and to the liberal diet if you're happily trim. Remember, both versions of the diet similarly prevent excessive swings in blood sugar. The added benefit of the strict one is weight reduction. It doesn't correct carbohydrate-induced hypoglycemia any better or any faster.

I stopped all my medications cold turkey and went on the hypoglycemia diet. I started guaifenesin and went through some bad cycles. I fell off my diet and suffered for that. But slowly things have gotten much better. I'm down twenty-five pounds in weight, my mind is clearing, my muscle spasms have cleared, and I can sleep. I am not perfectly well but I can make it through the day without having to lie down for most of it. The most important thing is that I now have a life.

—*Gwen, California*

When we begin treating fibroglycemia, we don't wait for the dietary benefits to kick in before starting guaifenesin. These people are very sick so we can't think of any reason for delay. Once the hypoglycemia part of the combined disease clears (usually within two months), patients can judiciously add more carbohydrates. We discussed how to do that earlier in this chapter. Since people are genetically different, they each have to find their ultimate dietary limitations. There's a spectrum of possibilities ranging from permanent restrictions to none whatsoever.

There are no current modalities other than proper diet and guaifenesin treatment to reverse the mix of fibromyalgia and hypoglycemia. It's mandatory, but it takes plenty of discipline to avoid any source of salicylate while adhering to the required diet. Success in chronic conditions depends greatly on the tandem efforts of individuals and their physicians. The patient is the primary player in this recovery game. Though the demands are great, the appearance of the first good hours and days makes it all worthwhile. It's highly exhilarating when contrasted with the preceding years of disabling symptoms. Euphoria is the reward.

From the abyss of terrible to the heights of wonderful isn't such a long climb. We're offering you, the patient, a ladder. You'll have to climb it rung by rung or else you'll not likely even stay where you are, but continue the descent into your personal hell. Those of us who've recovered urge you to resurface and join us in living.

LIVING LOW-CARB: THE FIBROGLYCEMIA AND HYPOGLYCEMIA DIET

Since I have begun treatment with guaifenesin for my fibromyalgia, my carbohydrate cravings have lessened and it is really not so hard to follow the hypoglycemia diet. I would have expected it otherwise—that with the worsening of symptoms, my carb cravings would have become intolerable. But that is not what I have experienced.

—*L.N., Massachusetts*

Down to Specifics

Since the first edition of this book, low-carbohydrate dieting has become very popular. Where choices were once rare, there are now hundreds of them. Products are better labeled and fast-food joints, even fancy restaurants, not only accommodate but actually court low-carb dieters. There are ample cookbooks, low-carb grocery stores, websites, and bakeries that compete for the market. "Low-carb" is now an established way of eating.

Most people begin their new diet reluctantly and timidly, quite afraid of making mistakes. That's the way it should be. Earlier in the chapter, we stressed that a certain reverence must be applied to the required restrictions. Errors are costly, and early on, gains are easily erased. Unlike the sequences necessary to determine guaifenesin dosages for fibromyalgia, the low-carbohydrate diet can be presented in black and white. Your predecessors have done all the work. This you can have and that you can't. Be dedicated and accurate. Don't even consider cheating or getting creative for the first two months.

For most people, breakfast is the most difficult meal. Yet there are plenty of choices. By habit, we tend to define only certain items as being "breakfast foods." But really, it's all the same to your digestive tract. Even if you don't want to consider anything out of the usual, just look around you. On both the strict and liberal diets, eggs can be prepared any style: fried, boiled, or scrambled. Omelets are a bit more work but can be made with any of the usual additions—cheese, bell peppers, sour cream, tomatoes, avocado, and sprinkled herbs. You can eat any kind of meat such as breakfast steaks or pork chops and even sugar-cured bacon, since frying burns off that bit of carbohydrate. (Watch out for sausages, though: Most mulch in some kind of sugar.) Hams frequently have honey or other sweeteners that should be washed off.

Breakfast drinks can be made with unsweetened protein powders, egg, or soy. There are even ready-made choices, including sugar-free Instant Breakfast! Toss in strawberries unless you want to spare your quota for later in the day if you're on the strict diet. Clever thinking creates other possibilities—say, making a smoothie using fruit, tofu, milk, and sugar-free syrups. There's nothing wrong with a scoop of cottage cheese, a slice of cantaloupe, and an added piece of sugar-free flat bread if you're on the liberal diet. Smoked salmon and cream cheeses aren't bad choices, either. Egg custards are particularly refreshing, especially on warm, summer days. They can be made in batches using heavy cream, eggs, vanilla extract, and sugar substitutes. The liberal diet permits you to spread unsugared peanut butter on toast made with sugar-free bread. A tiny spoonful of sugar-free jelly is a nice addition. On the liberal diet, unsweetened cereal or oatmeal with sugar-free sweetener is allowed. On both diets, you can find recipes for acceptable quiches, or breakfast casseroles. Yep! We keep repeating this, and we're still not done: Your diet should be *sugar-free*.

Lunch on the strict diet could include vegetables with or

without meat. Deviled eggs make wonderful snacks; they're safe if made with sugar-free mayonnaise and aren't stuffed with sweet relish. Liberal dieters might well get by with sandwiches that use the thinner types of sugar-free breads, tortillas, wraps, or flat breads. When I wanted to lose a few pounds, I used two cabbage leaves as my "bread." Large lettuce leaves can be used to form wraps. A bit stickier, but slices of roast beef or cheese can substitute. Composition salads are great with added bits of beef, chicken, shell- or other fish, cheese, egg, sour cream, and avocado. Taco salads can be made with low-carb tortillas and bean-free chili on the liberal diet. Inspire yourself by creating your own versions, including variations on the traditional Cobb or Caesar salads, as long as you keep dressings sugar-free. You can always eat hamburgers and cheeseburgers with a fork after tossing out the bun.

Just by custom, we usually conjure a different vision for the components of our evening meal—we're usually less interested in eggs and sandwiches. We also tend to prepare our food somewhat differently, using a lot more grilling, broiling, and baking. Fish is less often eaten at lunch but is something we can add to our dinner menu. Vegetables may be marinated, stir-fried, roasted, baked, or grilled along with meats or separately using the same oils and sauces. Steamed vegetables with cheese and nuts are delicious. On the strict diet, it doesn't take much imagination to use al dente cauliflower, daikon cubes, or chunks of summer squash as replacements for potatoes in certain recipes. Celery root or cauliflower can be cooked and whipped into faux mashed potatoes with butter, sour cream, and a little garlic or bleu cheese. Artichoke appetizers dress well with butter or sugar-free mayonnaise, sauces, and shrimp. Slip in curry or hot paprika. Batter is easily made from eggs and crushed pork rinds to coat meat such as chicken on the strict diet. Nut flours make delicious piecrusts or coatings for chicken or fish on the liberal diet. Your taste buds might like the dramatic change offered by blackened meats. You could stuff large mushroom caps or green peppers with spinach, cheese, or bits of anything you dream up. Spareribs made with sugar-free barbecue sauce or meat loaves that have been stuffed with cheese or topped with sugar-free ketchup make a nice change. Stir-fry shrimp with bell peppers, mushrooms, and scallions; lace scampi with extra butter, garlic, and a few gourmet herbs to avoid menu ennui. Chopped cauliflower or shredded lettuce can serve as a replacement for rice.

There's a world of flavors just waiting for your creativity. There are no restrictions on spices; mustard and chili powders; sugar-free sauces; Liquid Smoke; horseradish or garlic paste; or piquant Thai dressings. These ingredients add great zest to whatever you're preparing. The liberal diet certainly provides more variety, but somewhat restricts the amount you can eat. Use unusual items such as spaghetti squash or zucchini ribbons to fake pasta dishes. Toss with any of your favorite (sugar-free) sauces or serve it simply with butter and Parmesan cheese. You gourmet people are still permitted favorite escargot preparations and caviars. Several desserts work in nicely on either diet. Whip up egg custards, sugar-free cheesecakes (nut flour shell) on the liberal side, and sugar-free Jell-Os. There are plenty of other delicious concoctions, even ice creams, now being made with artificial sweeteners such as sucralose (Splenda). Mousse can be easily made with whipping cream and a flavored protein powder. Would you perhaps consider floating sugar-free ice cream or whipping cream on top of a diet root beer? One patient melted sucralose-sweetened chocolate bars in her microwave oven and poured them on her strawberries.

Eating out is getting safer as more restaurants are responding to the growing demand for low-carbohydrate fare. Most readily accommodate their clientele and substitute vegetables in place of rice or potato. Cottage cheese or sliced tomatoes provide suitable options. Fibroglycemics should bring decaffeinated coffee in packets, order a pot of hot water, and make their own brew because a stressed waiter might mix up coffeepots and serve you the real thing. The main courses are usually as safe as what you would have eaten at home. Ask the waiter if the Caesar or bleu cheese dressings are sugar-free. If not, use oil and vinegar with or without a squeeze of lemon juice or a little mustard. Occasionally, restaurants have flavored olive oil sitting on the table or at least honor your request for some. In Mexican restaurants you can order various fajitas, ropas viejas, machaca, or even the chiles rellenos if they're only lightly floured. Italian restaurants usually offer veal or chicken piccata, bistec, osso bucco, and assorted seafoods including scampi and calamari. Satisfy your tastes but choose restaurants with cooperative chefs who'll tell you what's in their sauces.

Our book *What Your Doctor May* Not *Tell You About Fibromyalgia Fatigue* also contains many suggestions. We've added some of these and other helpful references to the Resources at the back of the book. The website www.fibromyalgiatreatment .com has recipe pages that also contain many recommendations for snacks. Included is a complete Thanksgiving Day dinner, all low-carb (liberal diet), including faux yams and pumpkin pie or mousse.

It's not within the scope of this book to adequately discuss the merits of fats versus carbohydrates as fuel sources. The battle is finally disengaging: Heavy carbohydrates are more often implicated as dietary villains and certain fats as okay guys! Though the hormone cortisol can store belly (visceral) fat, only one hormone can store lipids in all fat cells, and that's insulin. It's predominantly released in response to carbohydrates as we've already discussed; fats beg for insignificant amounts and proteins only a bit more unless they're eaten along with carbohydrates. Our strict diet permits weight reduction for three main reasons:

1. It avoids heavy insulin outputs.
2. Protein digestion and storage require more caloric expenditures than that particular food contains.
3. In the absence of surplus carbohydrates, metabolism must burn fat for energy. Fats are loosely divided into two categories: cis and trans fats. Many products now show on the label which one(s) they contain. It's easy to remember which are the good ones with the phrase "I love my SISter," which reminds you that trans are the bad ones. There aren't many concerns about unsaturated fats from olive oil, vegetable oils, and liquid margarines. Most popular weight reduction diets are simply variations on the original theme. Well-executed studies are accumulating that back the safety of low-carbohydrate diets and contradict the notion that it's the fat in the Western diet that's making you obese; our diet is indeed healthy; put the blame where it belongs: Look to the carbohydrates and their buddy insulin. Most are killers and their weapon is insulin.

Several large issues were discussed, including my lack of progress with weight loss on Weight Watchers and the zooming rise of my triglycerides on my last four workups at my internist's office. Funny thing is, my rheumatologist said the same thing that Dr. St. Amand said, "You know what you have to do on both issues." Back to the strict diet it was. I asked Dr. St. Amand if I went back on the strict [diet], would it affect my labs being done three days later and he wasn't too sure I'd see any improvement that fast. I'm here to say my triglycerides went down from 299 to 169, my cholesterol dropped from 184 to 162, and even a couple of my liver tests improved significantly. My appetite is greatly reduced and it takes much less food to satisfy me. Guess I am carb sensitive…duh!"

—*Marsha, California*

We are all witnesses to the explosion of obesity and adult-onset diabetes two generations of high-carb eating has fostered. Medical doctors such as Richard Bernstein and the late Robert Atkins have made this point and have eloquently defended their positions.[3] What has been handed down is not safe eating: The incidence of obesity is escalating as are diabetes, high blood pressure, and insulin resistance. Heart disease and hardening of the arteries are the sequels. Weight reduction is easily and comfortably achieved with sufficiently low carbohydrate intake. Effected in time, that offsets the risks. Those who've been unsuccessfully trying to lose by shunning fats instead of carbohydrates have been seriously duped. What you've been eating is what's made you fat, hypoglycemic, or diabetic. In deference to my colleagues, I'm not your doctor and can't impose my recommendations over those of your personal physician. But if you have a weight problem, you owe it to yourself to do some research and ask hard questions. Although my patients don't always follow my advice, they'll certainly continue hearing from me on this subject.

I've been on the low-carbohydrate diet for more than forty-five years. I confine myself to the strict diet during the week. It prevents late morning and afternoon energy depletion. It also drops my weight one or two pounds below my desired level. By the weekend, I go into my liberal mode, but I confine my cheating to eating pizza, bread, or rarely rice. My eating style keeps me contented—though it might not do so for you. Each of you may eventually develop your own ritualistic system of dieting and cheating. But first, you must get out of your hypoglycemia funk. In that process, if you need to, why not take your weight down to a healthier level? After you've reached your goal, allow yourself only enough cheats to keep you on friendly terms with your bathroom scale.

I have to say that when I stop and take stock, I am amazed at what I can do now. When I started the diet and guaifenesin,

I never dreamed it was possible to get my life back this way. I only hoped I would get at least a little better. I never dreamed I would have this much energy. I never dreamed I could get strong. I never dreamed I could be there to care for my parents in the end. There was a time I had nightmares that they would die and I could not get to them.

—Gretchen, South Carolina

Chapter Seven

The Protocol

Last winter, I was ready to apply for Social Security disability payments. I only dared to drive my car one or two miles on a "good day." I hadn't had a social life for three years. My credit rating was ruined because I was so exhausted I would let bills pile up for months, then try to catch up with them all at once. Nights were torture. I woke up every hour to hour and a half all night long. I had irritable bowel, irritable bladder, and restless legs. In the mornings, my joints ached so much that at times I was forced to get down on my hands and knees and crawl from the bedroom to the bathroom to the kitchen...

By March, I'd decided I was willing to try guaifenesin. Maybe it wasn't for the faint of heart, but neither was the quality of the life I was living. For the next several weeks I felt miserable most of the time and then, suddenly, I had two days of total reprieve from FMS. Not just "good" days—extraordinary, amazing days. Then I started into the next cycle. I've had all my old symptoms return in full force. Tomorrow will be two months on guaifenesin, and according to the protocol, I should have reversed one year of symptoms of FMS by now. I can honestly say that I feel better than I did a year ago, and I certainly bounce back from exertion much faster than I used to. So, this isn't easy; it isn't fun; but it works. Follow the protocol to the absolute letter, be ruthless in getting rid of products and foods that aren't good for you, and go for it!

—*Anne, Minnesota*

I$_T$'s TIME TO take a closer look at our protocol. We're going to lay out each step carefully. We've tried to write this chapter as clearly and concisely as we could. We'll skip over some explanations that we've already detailed in previous pages or will subsequently outline. Please digest what we say and don't allow yourself seemingly harmless deviations from what is a proven path. Some ten thousand patients have scouted the way: Take advantage of the trail they've blazed. You're about to benefit from both their successes and their mistakes. Please, do it exactly our way.

FIND A DOCTOR WHO'LL MAKE
THE DIAGNOSIS

Obvious as it sounds, first make sure you have fibromyalgia. That sounds silly, but it's important to rule out more dangerous or potentially lethal conditions. If you haven't been diagnosed, pointedly ask your doctor or consultant about the disease. Ask if he or she understands and believes in fibromyalgia; even at this stage, some don't. Don't be shy: Even tell the secretary who makes appointments that you suspect what you have, but you'd like expert confirmation. You get the wrong vibes? Choose another doctor. Fibromyalgia is difficult enough as it is. Without an ally it's just too stressful.

If you need help finding a doctor, there are several things you can try. First, ask your friends. If one of them has a doctor he or she describes as an open-minded good listener, start there. Most rheumatologists, internists, and family practitioners are familiar with the entity though a few still pooh-pooh it or too closely adhere to the "party line." You might try calling a local fibromyalgia support group, the local chapter of the Arthritis Foundation, or any group that keeps lists of doctors sympathetic to fibromyalgia or chronic pain. Online you can locate practitioners through websites such as the National Fibromyalgia and Chronic Pain Association or our own www.fibromyalgiatreatment.com.

General practitioners or internists are perfectly qualified to help you precisely because they're generalists and not super-specialists. They're less likely to squeeze most of your symptoms into the smaller-size container of their limited specialty. This is not the time for preconceived notions that will force you to fail on yet another course of worthless treatment. Any physician or other licensed health practitioner might be able to guide you, especially now, since guaifenesin is readily available without a prescription.

Face-to-face with a doctor, what should you expect? If you've not had recent blood tests, he or she will likely order some. A basic workup will survey your body for adverse conditions since many diseases have symptoms in common. Some tests are altered by recent food or drink, so give fasting samples. Normally included will be a blood count looking for anemia, infection, or inflammation; a chemistry panel will check organ function, lipid abnormalities, diabetes, and the chemical composition of your plasma. Warnings: A normal blood sugar does not exclude hypoglycemia. A substantially low fasting glucose demands further investigation, possibly by an endocrinologist.

It's true that 85 percent of fibromyalgics are women. Equally so, 5 to 10 percent of women develop thyroid dysfunction, mostly low (hypothyroidism). Expect the two illnesses to overlap, just by chance. It's also a fact that each condition will make the other worse. They're not otherwise linked, though they cause a mutual intensification of symptoms—as you'd surmise from the superimposition of any second disease. The ultrasensitive test, TSH (thyroid-stimulating hormone), is mandatory since it's outstandingly accurate for detecting thyroid glandular dysfunction and will help separate the two conditions. Unfortunately, there remains much misinformation about this test. Very few illnesses fail to share symptoms with several other diseases. Some areas of the country are rampant for Lyme disease. Extensive foreign travel might have exposed you to diseases such as hepatitis or parasites.

If you have many aches and pains, your doctor will probably include an arthritis panel to help uncover the presence of lupus or rheumatoid arthritis. If you're over fifty, a woman, and have a particular distribution of pain, testing should be expanded to include the CRP and the ESR (erythrocyte sedimentation rate). If they're markedly elevated, the diagnosis of polymyalgia rheumatica will be considered. Though it's not related to fibromyalgia, like other adverse conditions it will certainly intensify symptoms. Polymyalgia reaches emergency status because of the threats it poses, including blindness and strokes.

At your initial appointment, bring your doctor a list of all of your medications and supplements. This is no time for trying to avoid a professional opinion on the merit of such combinations. Include any over-the-counter products you take, even now and then. Certain herbs and nonprescription items can seriously affect liver enzymes and kidney function. That's why your honesty coupled with appropriate blood tests could well expose problems while they're still minor and correctible. In short, there's nothing ever gained by playing games with your doctor.

We remind you that there are as yet no distinguishing tests for fibromyalgia. The work being ordered on your blood is to reassure you and your physician that something more urgent does not exist coexpressed with fibromyalgia. When such entities are excluded, you and your doctor will feel far safer and can get on with this protocol clearly focused on the problem at hand.

The diagnosis of fibromyalgia is properly made in two parts. The doctor begins by taking a detailed medical history that includes a full systems review. Since fibromyalgia causes fatigue, pain, depression, irritable bowel syndrome, irritable bladder, numbness, leg cramps, headaches, palpitations, and a host of

other diverse symptoms, your doctor will explore them, sometimes in detail. Many doctors use check sheets for baselines
that itemize symptoms and, later, to track changes. Refresh
your memory ahead of time so you can help your professional
establish a chronology of your complaints, including onset and
progression. This sequencing will also provide you a rough
guide as to when and in which order you should expect the
reversal of your symptoms.

After your doctor is satisfied that your complaints and medical history suggest fibromyalgia, an examination will surely
follow. He or she may not feel comfortable "mapping" as we
do, but at the very least should do a hands-on search for the
so-called tender points (see the description on page 28). We
think physicians should also feel places where you hurt even
if they're not included in those predetermined zones. Finally,
armed with normal blood tests, a sympathetic ear, and tender-
point or mapping results, both of you should feel secure with
your diagnosis.

ADDRESS THE CARBOHYDRATE-INTOLERANCE/HYPOGLYCEMIA FACTOR

Assuming you've been officially diagnosed with fibromyalgia,
you may have another important item to discuss with your doctor. As we explained in the previous chapter, there's no totally
reliable blood test for hypoglycemia. Your experience is really
sufficient. You're very well aware of what happens when you eat
foods high in sugar, or potatoes, rice, pasta, and other wrong
carbohydrates. As much as you'd like to deny it, you've actually done the best test in existence, over and over again. You
ate and you suffered. Tell that to your doctor. Very few will
accept a verdict that's based purely on the symptoms you feel.
The chances are that he or she may not agree with you, but on
your own, you can easily modify your own diet as outlined in

this book. We've described how you do that, so take your own symptom inventory and trust what you feel.

Ideally, what you and your physician should look for is what follows. Remember how symptoms cluster into two fairly separate batches, the chronic and the acute? To review: The latter are the scary ones and typically strike two to four hours after eating, often during the night. They're sudden in onset and sometimes violent enough to be labeled "panic attacks." Hand or inner shaking, sweating or clamminess, headache, heart flip-flopping or pounding, anxiety, irritability, weakness, dizziness, faintness, or occasional passing out are the rest of the litany. These unwelcome complaints may not all appear at once or as intensely in everyone. If eating makes them go away, but they recur when you're hungry, hypoglycemia is the likely culprit.

The chronic symptoms are more generalized. They're with you most of the time no matter what the blood or brain sugar levels. They don't materialize because of any drastic fall in circulating sugar or surges of counterregulatory hormones. They're mainly due to metabolic fatigue from so many fluctuations. Headaches are frontal, suggesting sinus problems, or disposed like a contracting rubber crown, wrapped circumferentially around the head. Fatigue, irritability, nervousness, flushing, impaired memory and concentration, tight muscles, abdominal pain, bloating, excess gas, and diarrhea are part of the not-too-pretty chronic picture. This symptom complex isn't helped by eating, unlike the acute ones. Treatment requires the longer and more determined dietary effort.

If you're hypoglycemic, you have no choice but to follow our dietary advice. We discussed carbohydrate intolerance in chapter 6, but it bears repeating. Give the diet a try and see how it makes you feel. Reread chapter 6 and make a couple of copies of the diet. When you're first getting acquainted with its variations, keep one in your wallet or on your smartphone and another taped to your refrigerator door. It might be best to slip one into your desk at work or even your car. Before you eat anything, make sure it's on the approved list. You can't afford mistakes. You should follow the diet perfectly for two months before you begin experimenting with off-list foods. Our diet is one of the few that will dependably control hypoglycemia.

If you're heavy, you belong on the strict diet. Proper behavior will provide striking rewards: You reduce weight and simultaneously battle hypoglycemia. Carbohydrate craving starts to ease in about ten to twelve days, and that makes it easier to stay the course. You may not get all of the goodies you previously enjoyed, but at least you can eat all you want and not go hungry. Once you've shed the surplus baggage, you're free to add everything on the liberal diet.

Normal-weight hypoglycemics can enjoy the liberal diet since it restores control just as quickly as the strict diet. We've told you that most fibromyalgics feel better on carbohydrate restriction using either diet. There's an inspiring boost in energy beginning about the fourth or fifth day, the brain fog lifts appreciably, and soon, the irritable bowel eases greatly. This applies to almost all fibromyalgics even if they're not carbohydrate intolerant or hypoglycemic.

If you're underweight, you may have some difficulty maintaining your weight even on the liberal program. Eat more volume of the foods on that diet as best you tolerate if your scale starts dipping into lower numbers. It's tough to correct hypoglycemia and not lose weight. Nevertheless, concentrate on fruits, nuts, dairy products, sugar-free grains, and the higher-carb vegetables listed on the liberal diet. Even for the slim and trim folks, dieting is still necessary for a couple of months. Hopefully, you'll sneak in more of the forbidden starches later and regain any lost weight.

I have been on the guai protocol for almost four years and have been following the HG diet. At the time I started the diet, my pain and fatigue were extreme. My level of whole body pain averaged 7 to 8 out of 10 every day, with no reprieve. I never experienced any good days or even good hours. I had never thought of myself as having typical HG symptoms, but I was hoping the diet would help my fatigue. Instead it helped my pain. I now have very little whole body pain, between 0 (most days) and 2. I am sleeping better, which I attribute to being diligent about the diet. Too much carb = restless night.

—*Carol, Canada*

Plan and brace yourself for your first visit to the grocery store. You'll need more shopping time to move at a snail's pace as you pause to read labels. Until you get the hang of the diet, give yourself the luxury of leisure study. In fact, let's do it really right! Carry a magnifying glass and a copy of the diet. Focus attentively on the "Foods to Strictly Avoid" listings. "Low-carb" on the label isn't enough. "Sugar-free" isn't always accurate, either, because it may only mean no added table sugar. Lactose-free milk sounds like a good idea until you read the ingredients and realize it's sweetened with corn syrup. Did you remember to avoid caffeine?

You may feel more tired and irritable for the first several days after you start ditching carbohydrates. You've been together for a long time, and they don't let you easily break the connection. It takes about one week before you glimpse a few rewards. Some of your symptoms begin to ease, and a bit of energy pops out through the snowed-under feeling. Within six to eight weeks, assuming you haven't cheated, you'll get most of the benefits the diet can provide.

MAP YOUR LUMPS AND BUMPS

"Mapping" is our coinage for our manual examination of a patient. We look for lesions: the swollen tissues of fibromyalgia (spastic muscles, tendons, ligaments, and some joints). We draw our findings on a printed caricature of the body. We depict the size, shape, and location of each and shade it according to the degree of hardness. The first such is our baseline for future maps that we'll compare for progress under treatment.

If your physician doesn't feel confident using this novel technique, you have a few alternatives. Ask for a referral to a physical therapist, chiropractor, or licensed massage therapist whom your doctor considers adept. Copies of your first and subsequent maps can be sent to the medical office for professional monitoring of your progress. Preferably, you'll visit someone who is at least somewhat familiar with fibromyalgia. It takes good hands to feel the lumps and bumps. Show that person a copy of one of our body-map illustrations.

The examiner should use the pads of the fingers as though smoothing out tissue wrinkles, not digging into them, thereby creating ripples of flesh. We draw the size and location of lesions as we find them and press a bit harder or lighten up on the pen to illustrate the hardness of each lump. It's not mandatory for examiners to use our exact system. Variations can be introduced as long as the same examination is conducted on all subsequent evaluations. Would-be mapmakers should only record objective evidence to illustrate nothing but the swellings they palpate. They mustn't be swayed by subjective expressions of tenderness since dominant pain sites change from day to day and obscure others. Because of that, impressing locations of pain on the map is unacceptable and would totally invalidate comparisons. Our method of mapping is on a DVD that is sold at www.fibromyalgiatreatment.com.

In the unlikely event your doctor has no suggestions for potential mapmakers, ask friends for someone they've used. Hospitals and orthopedists usually have a staff of physiotherapists or can refer you. Most chiropractors now know the diagnosis and will either willingly do the job, or use a massage therapist on their staff. Local fibromyalgia support groups maintain lists of capable people. You can also post your needs and ask for help on the online Guai Support Group, which you can join via www.fibromyalgiatreatment.com. It was created to help solve these and many other problems.

Go to your first appointment with a blank copy of the body map and give it to the professional who will do the examination. You can get it from this book, but it might be better to download it from the website so it's full sized. This way, the experienced or novice mapper can quickly scan what you want done and make a reasonably similar search of your body. Do your best to obtain copies of this and sequential records.

The first map is very important and should be created before you begin guaifenesin. It's the baseline that provides a startling reminder of what you were and helps substantiate progress when comparing subsequent maps. If you've already medicated yourself before being mapped, you've lost some detail, but it's still beneficial to ensure favorable progression.

All of the professionals we mentioned are quite accomplished in palpating muscles and tendons. They know the feel of tissues and have to make only minor adjustments in their techniques to accurately sense the lumps and bumps of fibromyalgia. We happily allow anyone to copy the caricature we use for mapping purposes.

Now we really need your attention. Be you patient or practitioner, here is an extremely valuable clue—probably the most significant one in this book. Read this paragraph over and over again until you've mastered it. If I had to choose only one muscle to make the diagnosis of fibromyalgia, I would immediately select the left thigh, the quadriceps muscle. The name tips you off that it's a four-part muscle. The outside portion is called the vastus lateralis; the front is the rectus femoris. Patients should be checked lying in the supine position. A trained examiner will easily feel spasm (and may evoke considerable tenderness) in 100 percent of adult patients in these sites. We've found this so in more than six thousand consecutive, untreated males and females. Equally fascinating, both of the structures clear completely within the first three weeks on an adequate guaifenesin dosage without salicylate blockade. The front of the right thigh is also affected, but usually shows only two or three swollen lumps. However, the back of the right thigh (hamstring muscle) is usually involved as a long, tight band, but not so the posterior left. The differences between the two sides are indeed striking.

The left lateralis (side) segment is often the tenderest of all of the involved muscles of fibromyalgia; its spastic portion is quite long, smooth, and only occasionally felt in separated bundles. The left rectus (front) is not as even and its affected areas are made up of four to seven separate, spastic bundles. They feel firmer, undulated, and progressively tenderer going from the top down to just above the knee. We're giving you a major shortcut: The diagnosis is readily confirmed by just examining the thighs, and since their lesions all disappear within three weeks, the guaifenesin dosage is quickly established. This confirms that reversal is under way even though there are potential pitfalls down the road and some dosage adjustments may be necessary.

Take the lead with doctors—even if you can interest them in only a minimal examination, plead that they feel the left thigh. Preach a bit if you must, but get them to palpate those muscle bundles, confirm the diagnosis, and secure the dosage. If those sites clear within the first month, the dosage should also be correct for the rest of the body. Unfortunately, once those are wiped out, what can the doctor monitor for future progress unless he or she has done a more thorough mapping? We do a diligent, body-wide search, on every patient on every single visit. We rely on our examinations to chart progress and also for early detection of salicylate blocking. Do your best to get

Patient: _____   Date: _____

—FATIGUE	—OCCIPITAL HEADACHES	—DYSURIA
—IRRITABILITY	—DIZZINESS	—PUNGENT URINE
—NERVOUSNESS	—FAINTNESS	—BLADDER INFECTIONS
—DEPRESSION	—BLURRING VISION	—WEIGHT CHANGES
—INSOMNIA	—IRRITATED EYES	—BRITTLE NAILS
—IMPAIRED MEMORY	—NASAL CONGESTION	—ITCHING
—IMPAIRED CONCENTRATION	—ABNORMAL TASTES	—RASHES
—ANXIETY	—RINGING EARS	—HIVES
—SUGAR CRAVINGS	—NUMBNESS	—NEURODERMATITIS
—SALT CRAVINGS	—RESTLESS LEGS	—GROWING PAINS
—SWEATING	—LEG CRAMPS	—VULVODYNIA
—HUNGER TREMORS	—GAS	—PAINS
—PALPITATIONS	—BLOATING	
—PANIC ATTACK	—CONSTIPATION	
—FRONTAL HEADACHES	—DIARRHEA	**Figure 7.1**

yourself detailed, but thigh checking provides you assuaging information. You can make do without remapping unless you get worse down the line on the protocol.

If someone other than your doctor maps you, ask for copies to insert into your personal medical files. Your mapmaker can focus on the preceding sketches, hopefully spot improvement, and sequentially palpate for even minor changes. It's highly encouraging for everyone involved to look at serial drawings that visually document clearing. Barring permanent tissue injury, most of those graphic lumps and bumps should become just unpleasant memories. (Figure 7.1 shows a blank map.)

ELIMINATE ALL SOURCES OF SALICYLATES

Learn how to check for salicylates on your own. Stay 100 percent salicylate-free. Don't try to gamble with the protocol's rules. You will lose! "If in doubt . . . leave it out!" Make sure you are on your correct dose and then "ride out the storm." Follow the diet if you need it. Exercise when you can. Don't look for instant success, but instead, enjoy the small improvements that occur as time goes on. The last piece of advice I will share is for you to "live your life to the fullest now." Don't wait to get better. Life is too short. Try to find the joy in your day!

—*Cheryl K., Canada*

Here comes our very deliberate redundancy. Before you begin the protocol, you have one last crucial task. If you don't accomplish it successfully, forget ever starting. Do the thorough search for salicylates in your medications and everything that goes on your skin. We provided extensive material in chapter 4 to guide you. Sorry, no shortcuts—you must check everything! Too many physicians allow or even suggest that patients try guaifenesin and then tell them little or nothing about salicylates. We've repeatedly seen minuscule amounts introduced in the wrong places stop all progress dead in its tracks. Blockade from this unfriendly chemical is the overwhelming number one reason for failure. If you're going to ignore this warning, don't waste your time reading the rest of this book.

Get a big garbage bag and gather up everything in your home or office that you plan to use on your body. Set aside undisturbed time. Magnifying glass in hand, have a dictionary and the Quick Check in this book handy, and do your homework. Type on packaging can be exasperatingly tiny, which is possibly deliberate! You should end up with three piles: products you can keep using, some you must toss out or bequeath to a grateful recipient, and stuff that requires deeper investigation. Those with incomplete descriptions such as "and other ingredients," or products that list only the active ingredients, must be researched or simply dumped in the giveaway pile. Use no product in which you can't identify every ingredient. If you want to rescue any of these, you'll have to get on the Internet, go back to the store and look for more complete listings, or perish the thought, call the manufacturer. Don't rely entirely on the person at the other end of the phone to check for you, who may insist such and such product doesn't have salicylates. Too often you've reached a customer service representative who has no idea that all plants pose problems. Always get a list of ingredients.

Check all medications be they prescription or nonprescription, such as pain relievers, wart removers, first-aid creams, dandruff shampoos, and skin treatments, anything applied topically. That includes nasal sprays, patches, eye drops, suppositories, over-the-counter or prescription preparations such as cortisone, acne lotions, and other dermatologic creams. Vitamins and supplements should invite your scrutiny. Don't forget what you're looking for: any plant name and the bioflavonoids quercetin, hesperiden, and rutin. Pharmacists compound topical hormones such as estrogen, progesterone, DHEA, which are fine, but you must check the cream base, which may contain a plant oil or extract. When you see the word *flavor* on a label, you need to make sure it doesn't contain mint or menthol.

Off we go to your bathroom. Here you'll find mouthwashes, toothpastes, soaps, shampoos, conditioners, razors, shaving creams, deodorants, nasal sprays, lotions, toners, masks, ointments, suppositories, and acne medications—all need to be scrutinized. Creams for relief of muscular pain usually contain menthol or methyl salicylate—the identical substance that flavors both artificial and natural mint. If you've ever used one, recall how your skin tingles immediately after application. That's how fast salicylate is sucked into your body through skin. It's appreciably faster through the thin membranes of your mouth if you use minted (peppermint, spearmint, wintergreen) mouthwashes, gums, toothpastes, and other dental hygiene products.

Your beautiful garden is all abloom with natural salicylates. Remember: All plants make salicylate; it is part of their immune system. Come in contact only with their intact surfaces. When their saps or juices are absorbed by your skin you will block your guaifenesin. Year after year we go on summer alert since we know a bunch of our patients will begin working in the garden. Be sure the gloves you wear are waterproof so you don't absorb salicylates through them—cotton gloves and light leather become saturated easily. Luckily there are many wonderful gardening gloves available in local stores, even some that will help support sore or arthritic hands. You can also locate these easily online. Your biggest task will be to keep the gloves handy where you can find them easily and not forget to put them on.

BEGIN TAKING GUAIFENESIN

As we stated earlier, guaifenesin is no longer a prescription drug. You can get it in various strengths: 200, 300, 400, 600, and

1,200 mg tablets. We've mostly worked with the longer-acting 600 mg forms, but any kind will do if you take the right amount of a quality product properly spaced for near continuous action.

Long-acting guaifenesin, by definition, has sustained twelve-hour action. We instruct patients to take it twice a day. Short-acting tablets or some encapsulated powders are effective for four or five hours. They're more rapidly absorbed, stimulate the kidneys faster, and quickly fade away. They're often ineffective when they solo without added longer-acting stuff. High-dosage patients do better by using short and long in combination. The patented release system in the 600 mg tablet, Mucinex, is a fast- and slow-release formulation. It's also the most expensive.

Some short-acting tablets or powders come in poorly sealed capsules or are sold in bulk. Patients stuff their own gelatin capsules as a do-it-yourself money-saving scheme. We've seen too many failures in this home-based production. We think malfunction is due to repeated opening of the container and exposure to air: potency wanes with time. Manufactured medications are produced and stored in climate-controlled laboratories; they're retailed as soon as feasible. Once pressed into tablets or sealed in capsules, the contents are well preserved for even more years than stated on labels. Tablets are only as good as the powder from which they were pressed; buy faster-moving stock from a reputable manufacturer.

It's difficult for us to recommend one company over another and ignore perfectly good manufacturers. Some formulas contain fillers problematic for hypoglycemics, such as maltodextrin; lactose may be bothersome for a few who are extremely intolerant to that sugar; and dyes and saccharin, which our chemically sensitive patients need to avoid. Our website, www .fibromyalgiatreatment.com, monitors products we've successfully used and lists the formulations as well as their inactive ingredients. Since our repeated mapping documents progress, we can accurately confirm a drug's efficacy for fibromyalgia.

FIND YOUR DOSE

My first cycle lasted twelve days. The second one lasted eleven days. And so it went, slowly, slowly getting better. If I had to make a graph of the first several years, it wouldn't be a smooth straight line going upward. It would be more like a staircase. Every winter I felt worse, but not quite as bad as the previous winter. Every summer was a little bit better than the summer before.

—Ann, Minnesota

Please be systematic and stay at dosages for the times we specify. Stick with our outline until your basic need is confirmed. Trust us—though it's tempting to bounce the medication up and down according to how you feel or you think you should feel, don't do it! Otherwise, you'll only succeed in confusing yourself and whoever is trying to help.

There are always uninformed persons who'll dash in with brash suggestions. That often includes patients who've attained alleged expertise though they've only treated their first case, their own! Ignore anything contrary to the following paragraphs. We're going to spell it out as we've learned from the past several thousand patients. In the early reversal period, mapping provides a perfect directional signal. If you're uncertain about the skill of your mapper or are in solo flight winging it alone, follow our suggested flight path to assure a healthy landing. Using the guidance of our website support group, you can avoid the guessing game. Freely consult member-experts who know the protocol and enforce it as written.

Once on guaifenesin, focus your semi-addled, fibromyalgic brain on daily messages. This is not a board meeting: You don't need to keep elaborate minutes. Scribble on a calendar or daily log pad just a couple of words—enough to jog your memory when you need to look back. It's tempting to create 1 to 10 ratings for each symptom, especially pain. That's okay in the beginning, but over time it's difficult to equate today's knee pain with the severity of last year's headache. Fatigue is still fatigue, but is it now less? Once you've experienced runs of several good weeks, amnesia gleefully sets in: Who wants to remember how bad was bad? During treatment, worse days may become better than the good days were before you started treatment. Keep notations simple: For instance, bad, good, lousy, horrible, same, or so-so. Other possible entries might read: "headache half day," "neck very sore," "more energy A.M.," "back better," or "shoulder stopped hurting." Soon, you'll decipher favorable patterns etched by your jottings. Summarize your notations, and on your next visit, make a brief presentation to the medical guide, who can incorporate your observations in determining progress.

Only one brand of guaifenesin (Mucinex) may currently claim to be "long acting." The original company, Adams (sold to Reckitt Benckiser), proved that the 500 mg blue portion of their tablet worked for at least twelve hours. The Federal Drug Administration has mandated that any company promoting guaifenesin as long acting must provide similar evidence. Unfortunately, the blue dye in Mucinex upsets some of our patients. The tablet also has a 100 mg white layer that is fast or short acting. Cutting that tablet in half would, therefore, provide 250 mg of long-acting and 50 mg of short-acting drug. This splitting could cause some powdering and a scant loss of dosage, and the combination poses a problem for patients initiating treatment. Fast-acting guaifenesin alone may initiate reversal too abruptly, especially in patients with unusual sensitivity to drugs. Such intensity is highly impacting on individuals with low pain thresholds. Since people absorb drugs at different rates, we usually begin with 300 mg tablets or capsules that work long enough for our purposes. We like to use preparations that work somewhat longer than a short-acting tablet even though they may have a less determinate duration of action. Those are "compounded" drugs and can only be sold by prescription. At least such allows us better, tailor-making dosages. We can thereby avoid the heavy assault of short-acting guaifenesin. With a less heavy hand, we begin at low dosages, then increase later if we must according to our needs rather than using preset formulations. Since the drug has no known toxicity, we have the luxury of moving slowly upward until we begin and sustain reversal.

Hold your beginning dosage for just one week. If you become distinctly worse, you've likely found your correct personal level. That small amount is sufficient for only 20 percent of patients. Please remember, nearly all of you will get recognizably worse when you meet your basic needs. If you're already tired, you may become exhausted; if you ache, you'll hurt more. Symptoms that were mild or barely noticeable may suddenly demand your attention. Briefly, symptoms reverse much faster than they set in, so you could sense some entirely new ones. What was gentle could now be harsh; what was soft, hard. Never doubt that there are underlying problems lurking in deep areas below your level of past perception. The speed of tissue clearing often accelerates above subliminal, and symptoms become more and more intense.

If you're not worse during this first week, double up to 600 mg twice a day, for a daily total of 1,200 mg of longer-acting tablets or capsules. Currently, all tablets lower than 600 mg are short acting so you'll have to spread doses into three or four well-spaced intervals to obtain round-the-clock effects. If increased dosage proves effective, you'll notice an exacerbation of symptoms within three to ten days. Most readers will find these new amounts sufficient: 80 percent of patients begin reversing at this level. You should hold here for a full month before further challenging yourself. Then, if you're unchanged, you're one of the less fortunate 20 percent who need more, or you're blocking, or you're lucky and don't hurt more while reversing.

Where do you go from there? If you're sure you're not blocking, raise the dosage to 1,800 mg per day. (That's Dr. St. Amand's dosage: 600 mg in the morning and 1,200 at night. Claudia's is higher.) You don't have to split the tablet or try to remember a midday dose. You've now reached an amount that offers a 91 percent success rate. Some patients improve faster by adding short-acting to the longer-acting medication, e.g. 200 mg, 400 mg, or 600 mg twice daily taken at the same time. If you keep to 1,800 mg a day for another month and get neither worse nor better days—suspect blocking. Because success rates are so high at 1,800 mg, it's time for a thorough, repeat search. We ask our patients to "bag their groceries" and bring us all their topicals and supplements for staff inspection. We can offer faraway people only the online support group to guide them through the maze. In our office we have the luxury of individualizing dosages for our slower responders.

If the anticipated worsening of symptoms doesn't appear and the next map shows no change for the better, we again raise the dosage with two options. We could pump in an extra 600 mg to 1,800 mg of the more prolonged, gentler-acting tablets or capsules as we offered in the previous paragraph. We could alternatively add faster, short-acting guaifenesin. Short acting is available in most pharmacies as 400 mg tablets. When we attach such to the daily dosage, we begin with only one-half tablet (200 mg) twice daily to be taken with the longer-working product. If we still need more down the line, we can keep adding 200 mg in monthly increments up to patient tolerance or hold at any satisfactory level of map clearing. Because of its two layers of varying action, such moves are difficult with Mucinex; patients must do some basic math and extrapolate the amounts of fast or long that implement the desired dosage.

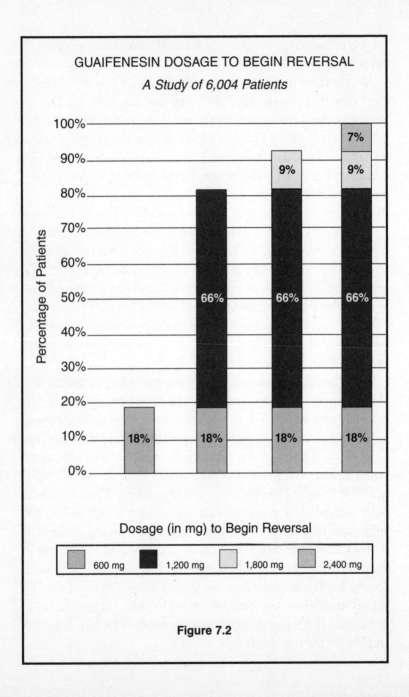

GUAIFENESIN DOSAGE TO BEGIN REVERSAL

A Study of 6,004 Patients

Percentage of Patients

Dosage (in mg) to Begin Reversal

600 mg   1,200 mg   1,800 mg   2,400 mg

Figure 7.2

The majority of people find their cycling dosage with relative ease. They get worse and they get better. They forge ahead, whether slowly or quickly, and soon determine the direction of their recovery. By now you've guessed that it's not so simple for everyone. A small number of patients, possibly 5 percent, get barely perceptible symptomatic increase during treatment. They erroneously think they have to get hammered with pain when they reach healing levels. For those lucky people, it's not so. If mapping is not available, this group may unwittingly keep raising their dosages by unnecessary amounts in a quest for dramatic reversal symptoms. There's no real downside to this error (except expense), and those who push the dosage do get well at accelerated rates. We should also mention that a significant number of patients get better for a few days after beginning guaifenesin and start to cycle later than most. That's why we hold patients at specified dosages for a designated time. Until we find a blood test for fibromyalgia, mapping is the best method we have to determine patient status. We highly recommend that examination for anyone who can find talented hands. (See figure 7.2.)

REMAPPING WHILE ON GUAIFENESIN

Remapping is best done by the same person who did the initial exam using the same technique to ensure that an exact comparison can be made. Certain tissues clear fastest and the lumps and bumps will disappear first in these areas. Even when considerable improvement has been achieved, remapping remains important because lesser remnants make percentage changes difficult to quantify. This especially applies to the delayed retreat of tendons and ligaments. Those structures have marginal blood supplies and only reluctantly release their accumulated debris. The trained mapper will detect subtleties that others could easily miss.

During our office revisits, we query our patients about their observations good or bad. We remap them at every visit. We hide previous maps and refer to them only after completing the new one. This is the best and most objective procedure we can suggest to monitor activity. Lumps and bumps should get progressively smaller, softer, or more mobile. Larger lesions such as those at the hips, tops of shoulders, and shoulder blade areas may split into two or more smaller bumps. Once you're sure of dosages and reversal rates, you and your mapping professional should agree on the frequency of examinations—whatever scheduling makes you both comfortable.

Don't overlook an important fact: Until late in the reversal game, mapping adroitly detects blocking by some source of salicylate. New lesions are obvious on a deteriorating map. Blocked patients are finally alerted when they get sufficiently worse, something that mapping will sooner determine. The earlier people report setbacks, the quicker we can help recheck products or adjust dosages. We've effectively used our system for many years. Thanks to astute teacher-patients, we can identify most occult sources of salicylate. (Figure 7.3 shows maps of a patient before and after starting treatment.)

Patients usually ask how long they should continue taking guaifenesin. Once symptoms are gone, some are tempted to stop. There's a simple answer: The genetic defects that cause the illness are unchanged by medication, so stop the drug and symptoms will resume. The illness probably won't reappear all at once or overnight, but come it will! In time, a better medication will surely be discovered. But for now, rather dependably, the dosage that reversed you may be what you'll need into the distant future.

If you increased your medication just to speed up the reversal, lowering your intake to the originally effective dosage is proper. But if you try dropping too far, below your therapeutic level, brace yourself for the gradual return of your complaints.

These maps show results in a 39-year-old woman who has been on guaifenesin 600 mg bid. She was initially seen and mapped on November 7, 1995, but did not begin treatment until May 14, 1996. The results you see, therefore, are the effect of medication over a span of 10 months (from May 14, 1996, to March 11, 1997).

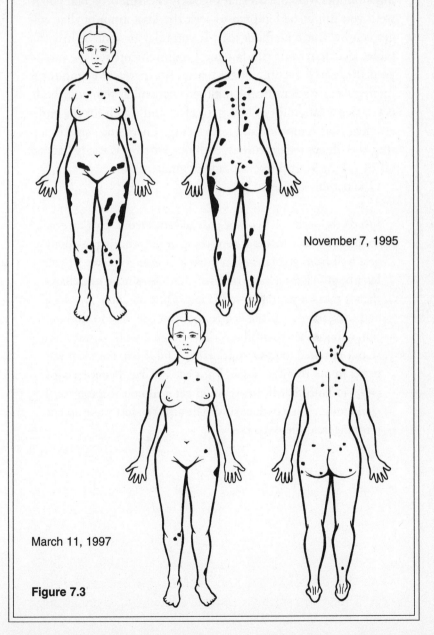

November 7, 1995

March 11, 1997

Figure 7.3

There's no harm experimenting if you want to, since the reversing amounts were not all that precisely measured. When you're well, you might be tempted to seek the least amount that will get you by. But remember this: If you take just one eighth of a tablet less than your fundamental requirements for the rest of your life, you'll eventually get worse. An ineffective amount is ineffective! Be scientifically inclined; remember that your body is your only laboratory, so remain alert and watch for the earliest clues that symptoms are resurfacing. There's no sense in letting the illness regain full ascendancy when it is easily headed off by taking your proper dosage of guaifenesin.

One patient advises:

Just do the protocol. Let time pass and stick it out. Don't worry so much about whether it is working or not working. Nobody gets well from guaifenesin in a week or even a month. If you have been sick for a long time, which it seems most of us have, then it takes time to get well. Time. Quit watching the clock and live each day to the degree that you can. Try to think of something other than illness. Let the guai work. I was constantly tempted to raise [my dosage]. Did I? No. For me it was better to not think so much. I just tried to live. I concentrated and had faith that if others could get well on this protocol, I could too...It is a path of stealth health. You just wake up one morning, and there you are.

—*Gloria, Florida*

Part II

‿❧‿

Distinguishing the Many Faces of Fibromyalgia

Part I of this book provided a sweeping overview of fibromyalgia. We've given you some of the historical background and experiences that led to our current method of treatment. We touched upon the medications we used in the early years, and explained how we found guaifenesin. We went through the details of the theory behind our approach, explained what we think goes wrong in fibromyalgia, and told you how you can fix it. We hope that in the process we gave you a solid explanation for your symptoms and validated the reason for all of your complaints.

Now we're going to delve into a little more detail. We want to focus on your symptoms, explore the causes, and give you some ideas about how to handle them. In the process, we will cluster them together to structure syndromes simply for convenience and easy reference. We're aware that this creates an artificial set of divisions and suggests a series of different diseases. Please don't be led astray. All you feel is related and fundamentally interconnected. We ask that you keep this in mind when reading through this part. We've also included quotes from other patients who've shared their experiences at various stages of reversal. As you'd expect, we've included mostly favorable statements, but believe us, they're the norm and not the exceptions.

I suppose that progress reports COULD be seen as "too good to be true," especially when one is in pain with untreated fibro or painful early-days-on-guai cycling.

I personally read them preguai as inspirational and possibly a teeny bit exaggerated, but basically true. Now, at 6+ years on guai, I can tell you that they are indeed TRUE, and not exaggerated. If anything, most understate how far they've come because they're afraid to paint too rosy of a picture to the remaining fibro-skeptics.

—Millie, Illinois

Chapter Eight

The Brain Symptoms

Chronic Fatigue and Fibrofog

I thought I was developing Alzheimer's at a young age due to the mental fogginess of fibro. I've never taken narcotics or any medication that affects mental function, but I once stopped at a red light as if it were a stop sign and proceeded through the intersection. People were honking, tires were squealing on the pavement, and my youngest daughter screamed at me that I was gonna get us killed. Luckily, we escaped this incident without injury or even a scratch to my SUV. She asked me why I did it and I honestly didn't have an answer. I had also experienced very short-lived disorientation. Once while driving, for a split second, I had no recollection of how I had gotten to where I was or why I was even behind the wheel driving. Once I identified familiar landmarks, I regained my memory of where I was going and why. It was such a scary experience, that I wondered if I should be driving at all.

—*Deb B., South Dakota*

THE CEREBRAL CYCLES of fibromyalgia entered medical literature somewhat late in the game. You'll recall that descriptions of the older disease, fibrositis, made no mention of brain involvement. When this term was replaced with the name *fibromyalgia,* problems with gray matter were still overlooked in the official description of the illness. Fairly rapidly, however, academic researchers began connecting the physical pains and brain aberrations as facets of one disease. About that time, a few psychiatrists bravely took a defiant counterstance against their colleagues and flatly stated that the mental disturbances were not psychologically based. In 1996, when Devin Starlanyl wrote her landmark book, *Fibromyalgia and Chronic Myofascial Pain Syndrome: A Survival Manual,* she unhesitatingly described the toll the disease had taken on her energy and cognitive abilities.

The overall change in medical attitude was very refreshing for patients who had been repeatedly embarrassed by past it's-all-in-your-head verdicts. Yet it did nothing to help them understand the illness or to offer relief of symptoms. One author summed it up: "Fibromyalgia was often considered to be a manifestation of hysteria and was equated with psychogenic rheumatism in the 1950s and '60s. However, with recent controlled studies it became evident that patients with this syndrome had uniform, stable and reproducible symptoms and signs rather than the bizarre and changeable symptoms of hysteria."[1]

Ten years ago, I was ready to let my husband divorce me and keep the kids (I simply could not take care of them) so that I could move into my parents' basement and just suffer alone. I was in daily severe pain. It began to get much, much worse in my thirties. I could barely function day to day. Pain meds did mostly nothing but make me sleepy or nauseated; maybe took the edge off, but I still couldn't function. My brain fog was so bad that I couldn't plan dinner, or get myself to the doctor when the pain was at its worst. All I could do was to practically crawl to a hot shower in the morning, get the kids fed and off to school, and then I would do basically nothing for the rest of the day. A trip to the store for groceries would exhaust me. I could not socialize. I was in too much pain.

—*Millie, Illinois*

CHRONIC FATIGUE SYNDROME— FIBROFATIGUE

It is a huge store and you have to walk a couple of miles to just get around to everything. When I got to the back of the store, I saw a lady sitting down in a chair that was on display. She had a grocery cart full of groceries, and her husband and son (about ten years old) were standing beside her waiting for her. I heard them ask her, what can they do, what does she need. They looked helpless. She reminded me of ME before I started guai. I can remember getting to the back of the store with my grocery cart and thinking, "How am I going to make it back up front?" I was trying not to stare at her. But I couldn't help but look at her and wonder if she had FMS. It didn't look like a medical emergency (something that would require a 911 call). She just looked like someone who had made it to the back of the store and didn't know HOW she would make it back up front. I could see the look of helplessness on her family's faces. I felt so sorry for them.

I can't get her off my mind. I remember how I used to feel on Saturdays, the day that I had to get everything done, the laundry, the shopping, the cleaning, etc., etc. I wasn't able to do any of it. I used to spend most of the day in bed. I would cry and cry and feel so hopeless.

—*Jan, Kentucky*

Fifty years ago when I began working with the disease now named fibromyalgia, I was struck by how many people had the same symptoms. Often enough to keep me on my toes, however, there was considerable individual variability. We speak in medicine of the "chief complaint," which is the single worst symptom that brings a patient to us. Many complained bitterly about the intense, widespread pain they were experiencing. Others launched into a series of descriptive words trying to make me grasp how severe was their continuous and numbing fatigue. Yet most of the time, there was that inexorable duet, both pain and exhaustion. In the end, it didn't much matter which of their complaints brought these people to my office; when I examined them, they all had the same widely scattered, easily palpable lumps and bumps in muscles, tendons, and ligaments. All I had to do was connect those physical findings together with the roster of symptoms patients provided to finally convince me this was a single, bad disease!

Table 8.1
Central Nervous System

	Male	Percentage Male	Female	Percentage Female
Number of patients	596		3,444	
Fatigue	560	94	3,348	97
Irritability	503	84	3,038	88
Nervousness	404	68	2,616	76
Depression	441	74	2,917	85
Insomnia	484	81	3,070	89
Impaired concentration	465	78	3,010	87
Impaired memory	477	80	3,097	90
Anxiety	422	71	2,627	76

Nowadays medical literature abounds with well-detailed studies of both fibromyalgia and chronic fatigue syndrome.

Many physicians believe they are the same illness. We've treated more than ten thousand patients in these categories, and we can assertively say that we've never seen a case of pure chronic fatigue syndrome. Notwithstanding the variations in history, body mapping reliably ties complaints to physical changes and amply satisfies the criteria of fibromyalgia. Fatigue is the dominant complaint of people with high pain thresholds. Carefully questioned, they relate the symptoms of irritable bowel, bladder or vulvar pain, and musculoskeletal complaints, however minor they may seem. The worst map we ever created was of a woman who swore she had no pain at all, only mild stiffness. Later she admitted that she had dental work and delivered babies without anesthesia. While most patients have a combination of hurting and fatigue, they can lie at opposite ends of the bell-shaped curve and experience very little else.

Most patients suffer daytime drowsiness, which is nevertheless accompanied by nocturnal sleeplessness. Even in healthy people, insomnia results in impaired mental function. Fibromyalgics may or may not get to sleep easily, but most of them awaken frequently throughout the night. That's even more likely to happen during more intense pain cycles. There just aren't enough comfortable spots left on the mattress so the brain orders an intermittent roll from side to side seeking a better position. Once awakened by such exercise, how can one find a comfortable spot and get back to sleep? When these symptoms occur on sequential nights, patients are sorely tempted to increase their dosage of sleeping medications. Adding hangover effects to an already exhausted body and brain further hinders next-day mental clarity. Sleep deprivation isn't the fundamental cause of fibromyalgia, but it certainly doesn't help.

Exhaustion has always been a major problem for me. I've been in the habit of taking some form of natural energy boosters (ginseng, guarana, etc.) for at least the past ten years. Since I'm on guaifenesin, I can't do that anymore, so I'm now having a very hard time making it through each day. Sometimes I think I feel good, and then go to the grocery store, and after five minutes feel like I have walked five miles. Sometimes I have to rest my head on my desk or my hands, and take a little "nap" at work. I have a high tolerance for pain, but also for medications. My body just laughs at OTC stuff. I even have to take double what most people do for prescription drugs, so I mostly just have to deal with the pain on my own, unless it is so bad I can't walk, write, etc. I think exhaustion is a big part of FMS, and that we all have to endure it. For me it is always there, even when the pain isn't.

Progress report—a few months later:

As an update, I am so much better it's unreal. I'm on 600 mg/day of guaifenesin now, am working 40 (or more) hours a week, and even take the stairs at work! I still have a bad day now and then (one or two a month), but my progress is so amazing, my doctor has started other patients he has with fibromyalgia on the protocol, which he named after me because I was his first patient to try it. Between the guai and changing all my medications around (I finally got off Prozac after ten years!), I've lost the bluish color in my hands, I don't sweat all the time now, and overall, I feel pretty normal. My doctor says he's amazed at the difference from when I walked into his office last April.

—*Sherry, Georgia*

The omnipresent fatigue of fibromyalgia is scary enough, but it becomes terrifying during flare-ups when concentration and memory vanish. Together they create the perfect profile of the early stages of Alzheimer's disease. To say the least, it's a bit difficult to combat this trio, especially when you add to them irritability, nervousness, depression, apathy, and surges of anxiety.

If you can indulge yourself with a nap, you can improve a bit, but an intended short doze might easily extend into lifelessness for several hours, which makes it even more difficult to sleep at night. Exhaustion puts you to sleep on the couch despite the blaring TV. Unfortunately, that wreaks further havoc with your internal clock. You almost hate going to bed early since you know you'll be just as tired in the morning and you'll face the pains of your nightly muscular thrashing.

The good news is that guaifenesin will reverse the fatigue and insomnia of fibromyalgia. They will yield to the same cyclic purging as the rest of your body. Eventually, fewer and fewer days of exhaustion will hound you; the positive rewards are startling. There will be energy to fit your lifestyle and enough left over for your social enjoyment. At first these will appear as isolated hours, half days, and then single days. A glimmer of hope of what lies ahead is enough to keep most people on the protocol. If you are like the rest of us, you will never forget your first energized day.

In the meantime, what can you do about the combination of fatigue and poor sleep patterns that plague fibromyalgics? So prevalent were these that, at one time, they were thought of as the malfunctions that induced the disease. There are pharmaceuticals to help you, of course, and those will be discussed later, in chapter 15. But the problem with this solution is that sleeping medications make you tired and diminish mental clarity. Should you use them every night? No, but you may have to anyhow. Are they acceptable occasionally when you absolutely need them? Yes. But that doesn't solve the every-night problem.

The first thing that helps sleep is exercise. Getting some during the day will ease stiffness, increase the right kind of fatigue, and even help clear your mind. Endorphin release will cause drowsy, pleasurable feelings, and exercise promotes that. So will pleasant thoughts and peaceful meditation, funny movies, or enjoyable activities. Do anything you can to relax your muscles and mind—mild stretching to beautiful music, for example, done early in the evening might help considerably. Comfortable mattresses, dark rooms, and fewer distractions are also helpful. Some people derive a great deal of help from sound machines at night. They muffle outside noise and can make the bedroom more peaceful.

FRUSTRATIONS OF FIBROFOG

These bad periods creep up. You think you're handling everything and then the pain starts to increase and suddenly you are in a panic... When the pain starts, I think I can still continue doing what I have been doing. What creeps up on me is the brain confusion. I get so frustrated trying to sort out the simplest things, until I give up and then I get depressed.

How do I handle it? Recognizing it for what it is comes first. Then I just have to let go of everything I don't have to do, and keep things very simple, rest a lot, baby myself. Get a massage, physical therapy, pool therapy for pain, or take whatever medications help.

It is interesting for me to watch this cycle towards depression and see how it is based on brain dysfunction and expectations. The mood swings go with the cycling, too... You can't expect too much of yourself when you don't feel well. Your brain is just trying to tell you that.

—*L.N., Massachusetts*

Physicians who treat fibromyalgia regularly hear, "I can stand pain, but I need a brain." Someone other than us aptly coined the term *fibrofog*. The term connotes a deep overcast full of heavy toxins that prevent brain-body interactions. Equally disconcerting, it renders patients partially unresponsive to the rest of the world. So bad is short-term memory that it's not uncommon for patients to forget something while it's being told. Sense of place and direction are sadly disrupted. How many of us have lost the way home and suddenly found ourselves in a strange location? You forget what you're doing midtask or what you're saying midsentence. Reasoning and deduction may range from difficult to impossible; math becomes a challenge even with a calculator in hand. Patients read without seeing the words— and why bother anyhow if they can't absorb the material, follow a plot, or remember the characters? Words stumble out of the mouth in strange sequences as though letters were glued together. They're frequently misspelled or look that way even when correctly written. Patients attempt to use dictionaries for assistance, but during bad fibrofog, there's no conception of letter sequences or recall of the alphabet. Names are interchanged and children become each other; floor may become desk.

Put yourself in the shoes of family members who are forced to play hide-and-seek with various items. Where in blazes are the car keys? For that matter, where's the car? Where did you leave your purse or did you donate it to some charity? Are the groceries out there fermenting in the trunk? The corollary: Patients can't see what they're looking at directly. What's the point of looking for something when you know it won't be there? Patients forget to pay bills, honor appointments, and meet friends; some have even left their kids stranded at school waiting for the delinquent parental chauffeur. Inability to count on your own brain is demoralizing and doesn't do much for irritability, nervousness, anxiety, and sense of isolation. Go through just a few such experiences and you'll understand why we won't even bother to define fibrofrustration.

During brain cycles, it's common especially for female patients to experience oversensitivity to sounds, lights, odors, and other external stimuli. Women already have more highly tuned senses; now the intensity gets kicked up an octave. Ordinary TV sounds may cause severe discomfort; fluorescent lighting can be intolerable, and even expensive perfume can cause nausea. Not too surprisingly, those may also induce headaches. Such symptom combinations have erroneously led some doctors to look for strange allergies or chemical sensitivities. Many patients go though extensive testing in an attempt to uncover unusual responses to the environment. Patients are quick to tell us, "It's not the chemical I touch; it's the odor that gets me." In our experience, as patients improve, these symptoms usually recede along with all of the other expressions of a totally upset metabolism.

It's up to you, the patient, to learn skills for coping with fibrofog. Understanding its nature and fundamental cause certainly helps anxiety and, in turn, fibrofrustration. With reversal, temporary cycles of cognitive impairment become more bearable. In the meantime, certain tricks soften the blow. They'll help erase the fear of forgetting important items when you well know you can't rely on your memory.

• Practice being methodical, so that it becomes second nature. Convince yourself to put things in the same place every time. For example, car keys should have their own peg by the door. If you work at always putting them there, eventually you'll do it automatically. Mailbox keys, glasses, unpaid bills, mail needing responses, shopping lists should all have special, designated places. No matter how exhausted you are, each time you have one of those things in hand, go to the predetermined site to hang or file it.

• Post a big calendar in a prominent place—say, on your refrigerator—preferably close to the phone if you make appointments on a landline. Write down every appointment the minute you make it. Every morning and every night, check what's written there. Do it at two specific times: just before you go to bed and when you have your breakfast. If you're afraid you'll forget something during the day, hang a note where you're sure to see it. You can also enter the information into your computer or smartphone and set it to notify you. Having it on a written calendar as well is important if you forget to charge your batteries or don't check your electronic gadgets regularly.

• Make a list of what you have to do. Then train yourself to check it routinely several times a day. Do it on a small pad you can carry with you or on your phone or tablet computer. When you awaken, scrutinize it carefully. Each time you complete a task, cross it off immediately—if you wait, you won't remember having done the chore. Never leave the house without checking that bunch of to-dos. Before you head out, make sure you have a list of which errands you have in mind. Don't trust yourself with the master list—you'll surely misplace it.

• If you use a landline, keep a pad and a pen near the phone and leave them there. Don't walk off with them. When you take a message, write it down right now! When the fog is exceptionally bad, cradle the phone (poor neck!) and make notes as you're talking. If things are really bad, scribble the name of the person to whom you're speaking. Keep notes concise and meaningful enough so that you'll actually grasp what you were trying to recall.

• Post notes somewhere and everywhere. Even if you carry a tablet or smartphone, they will only help you if they are switched on or you are looking at them. Many patients tell us they can't imagine what they did before Post-its! We've heard of people who hang notes reminding them to turn off lights, lock doors, water plants, remember shopping items, and even to pick up their kids at school! Make sure you carry a copy of children's schedules, including when they need to be at extra curricular activities. Buy one of those small clipboards that attach to dashboards so that you can write memos when sitting in your car, but not while driving.

• Make lists to take to appointments. When meeting with a teacher, boss, repairman, or client, prepare notes of pertinent topics. Prior to a doctor's appointment, itemize your questions and concerns before you leave home. We usually allocate enough time per patient, but we get frustrated when we try to walk out of the examining room and get stopped a few times with an "Oh, Doctor, I forgot…" Jot down pithy phrases to remind you of the answers you've just been given. Do the same for meetings at your children's schools or when making dates with family and friends. When discussing business matters, such as with your insurance company, get the name of the person with whom you spoke. These rituals might save you embarrassing, repeat phoning and the frustration of trying to find the right person to refresh your faulty memory.

• When you're suffering from intense fibrofog, limit your driving. At the most, run one errand at a time and save the more complicated tasks for a better day. Turn off the radio while driving and concentrate on the bigger task at hand. It's not polite, but apologize and ask your children or other passengers to keep as quiet as possible. If noisy children confuse or distract you, pull over and firmly review your current status. It's easy to miss a freeway exit so use local roads for shorter excursions. Never talk on the phone while driving: We all know that even so-called normal people don't perform that duet too well!

• At home and at work, decrease sensory inputs as much as possible. Many patients find they absolutely can't function well with even minor distractions. For good, fibromyalgic reasons, they lose the ability to tune them out or relegate them to the background. Turn off music while you're working. During bad cycles, even soothing sounds can put you into overload after a while. Close the door to filter outside noise from a room where you're working: It's a small luxury to concentrate in silence.

• Start working on projects early. Some take you twice longer than normal to perform. Don't fight it. On adverse days, your ability to absorb information has gone to La-La Land. If the task seems insurmountable at the moment, give it up and try later. Sometimes you'll have no alternative but to take a break and dry that clammy little sweat that signals frustration.

MOOD SWINGS (FIBROFLUX)

There are days like today when I feel as if my ears could explode. Every single noise is so intensified. I have to walk around with either ear plugs or fingers in my ears. My husband just does not get it. It takes every bit of energy I have to go about the day without going into a nervous breakdown.

—*Tracy, Washington*

Some horrifying facets of brain cycling are the sweeping mood swings. For the most part, patients are acutely aware of them but feel powerless to exercise control. Anger, frustration, fear, depression, and self-pity can attack with great intensity then disappear in a matter of minutes. Unfortunately, their negative effects linger. How do you retract some of the horrible things you've just said? How will your spouse, friends, or family members retract what they said in response? Female patients often cry buckets with minimal upsets; both sexes can become uncontrollably angry at the slightest provocation.

Try to recognize what your seesawing moods are like during times when the teeter-totter is level. During an outburst, you may grasp how irrational you're being, but you're neither able to stop nor admit how wrong you are. On a calmer day, chat with your spouse and children. Tell them you're sorry for your outbursts and beg them to ignore the past and, unfortunately, any future displays. As a modest excuse, remind them that you're sick and your brain is involved in the illness. Stress that you're firming up a plan for getting well. Not a bad idea to affirm the same message to everyone else in your life. So confess your past and pre-regret your future.

Pause when you start feeling superemotional. Try meditation plus warm showers or baths: Both can soothe your daily stresses. Imbue yourself with the old strategy of counting to ten before reacting; take a walk. Sneaking away from a problem before it fully surfaces isn't always feasible. But practice the technique and it might save you confrontations, the ones wherein you always lose. When you know the situation is getting out of hand, say to your inner self, "I'll stop now and deal with this later." You'll calm down.

Recognize that cognitive impairment and emotional overreaction are abnormal normals of fibromyalgia. They're experienced to some degree by all who suffer its ravages. It's okay to be patient and understanding of self, but not altogether forgiving. Give yourself an inside slap and apologize for your angry outbursts and overreactions to minor provocations. You know why those happen, but it's not equally apparent to the person at whom you direct your dragon fire. Laugh when your fibrofog causes you to do something slapstick. Laughter is therapeutic and closes the gap between people.

> She started going off on illnesses, saying the more you talk about illness, the worse you make it, and if you don't talk about it, then you can get better. So I took it she meant she was tired of listening to me talk about my fibro. It really hurt my feelings.
>
> When I talk about it, I don't feel so alone. I wish I could be positive—and think my illness away. I told her people who don't have chronic illnesses don't understand. I'd like to see someone stick a knife in her leg and leave it there for years and have her not talk about it or think about it, hoping it will go away.
>
> —*Wendy, Kansas*

Chapter Nine

Musculoskeletal Syndrome

I am feeling trapped by this new world of pain right now. I feel pain in my hands, arms, feet, ankles, and back. I feel my resistance to pain is especially low and that I feel especially beaten by it. I think to get control of the pain, I need to get control of the stress and grief. The medications I have been on are just not working for this low point. I feel in a metaphorical sense that the pain is a prison. It makes the stress worse and the stress makes the pain worse.

—Camilla, Michigan

MUSCLES, TENDONS, AND ligaments combine to keep us erect as bipeds, motor us to our destinations, and not least of all, help us raise food, prepare it, and carry it to our tables. They're also involved in the digestion and elimination of nutrients, and even play a role in reproduction. They're the largest structures of the body and outweigh the skeleton. They're constantly supporting, pulling, yanking—and in fibromyalgia they hurt! Muscles and their cohorts, tendons and ligaments, are dedicated to physical work. They never get the downtime and the relative rest enjoyed by bladders, stomachs, and fingernails. These hardest-working tissues are often first to be affected by fibromyalgia.

Table 9.1
Musculoskeletal System

	Male	Percentage Male	Female	Percentage Female
Number of patients	596		3,444	
Numbness	417	70	2,781	80
Restless legs	371	62	2,283	66
Leg cramps	349	58	2,438	70
Pain	595	99	3,421	99
Growing Pains	259	43	1,581	46

You may not know that there are different types of muscles. They have somewhat different physiology and, therefore, are affected differently by fibromyalgia. Oddly enough, they get involved in a rather predictable sequence though not always exactly true. Both statements are correct. We'll present some supportive evidence in chapter 14, "Pediatric Fibromyalgia," and we provide even more detail in our book *What Your Doctor May* Not *Tell You About Fibromyalgia Fatigue.* Let's do a superficial summary here anyway.

There are two fundamental types of muscle fiber and subgroups that we'll ignore. Most animals, including humans, have red (type I) and white (type II) meat. The colored strands are particularly germane to our discussion since they're the ones most distressed by fibromyalgia. Unlike chickens, our muscles are not constructed with one-color fibers to the exclusion of the other. Oddly, fiber distribution on the left side of the body is different from the right. The same muscle on the alternate side may have more type I or II. The differences in composition alter function. Stranger still, handedness makes little difference from one side to the other. We learned this as we said in the previous paragraph, because some muscles are consistently affected much sooner on a particular side of the body. We'll shortly explore this disarray, but let's dwell a bit on fiber types.

In this discussion, we'll largely ignore white meat. Its fibers are designed for speed and short-lived action. They don't have sufficient energy for a long haul, but they're great for sprints. Fibromyalgia barely glances at them and brushes them with only a light stroke: It fixates on far better prospects. Red meat is that color because it has a much richer blood supply. It contains far more mitochondria since red needs to make energy for sustained action. As you'll recall, these little powerhouses convert foodstuff to energy, the protein ATP. Type I fibers are hardworking muscle components with many functions that ensure survival. They are literally our strongest supporters, the hold-you-up and balance muscles. Workaholics, they turn us from side to side and shuffle our arms and legs from uncomfortable to comfortable positions all night long.

Aerobic workouts, running, and distance walking actually develop red fibers. Anaerobic, resistance exercises such as weight lifting produce mainly white fibers. You can see why pain and fatigue are so prominent in fibromyalgia. It's a disease with red overtones, right smack in the heart of our most productive energy factories. Selected muscles are the first to suffer from ATP deficiencies and, for safety reasons, fret around in a partially contracted state. Calcium promotes this sort of hibernation trance because it can't escape from the precise site where it was assigned to duty. It just goads muscles into continuous working. We've surely got a problem with pump failure—it's supposed to eject from inside cells. That's the only way they can finally relax. Guess the problem? Fibromyalgics don't have enough ATP (energy) to work the pumps.

We already had an extensive outline depicting what percentage of the time any given muscle, left or right, was involved by the time we see an untreated patient. We extracted data from body maps of 200 adult females. Our compilation was averaged by including recent-onset as well as advanced patients to produce a midcourse look at fibromyalgia. When we applied the same technique to the children's group, our findings on the 187 maps was truly revealing: We had a few two-year-olds, with the rest scattered up to our cutoff age, sixteen. We learned not only which muscles would be first affected at discovery, but also the pecking order of sequential involvement. That was of great help in transposing expectations for what we would always palpate in adults.

The left side of the neck, tops of shoulders, and inter–shoulder blade muscles are swollen in 96 percent of the kids; 84 percent on the right. Better still, the inside and outside elbows had our bumps in all the children we examined. Those are good areas to begin a search for fibromyalgic muscles. They're where muscles attach (called entheses), the best telltale signs in tots even for kids without many other defective sites. The older they get, the more muscles, tendons, and ligaments will develop swollen segments. Those lumps are similarly present in adults and are the earliest arrivals in longest residence. There are lots of other places where adults display their fibromyalgia. Though repetitious, let's disclose those post-adolescent, not well-disguised locations.

The most rewarding, diagnostic muscle group in anyone past age fifteen or sixteen is the left thigh, the quadriceps muscle. It's involved in 100 percent of adults of both the front and the outside. The lateral part, the vastus lateralis, is distinctly tender even using only moderate digital pressure. The less sensitive front of the thigh, the rectus femoris, is regularly affected likewise. It's not a long-structured smooth band like the outer thigh, but is made up of sequential, separate bundles. Since the left quadriceps is always involved, it should be the finger target for all untreated patients. It's not only diagnostic of fibromyalgia, better yet, it totally clears within three weeks on guaifenesin.

Assuming that the history fits snugly with fibromyalgia, can a would-be mapper ignore checking anywhere but at the muscles we've just delineated? That notion offers a tempting shortcut, but since under treatment the thigh clears within three weeks or so, what's left for follow-up exam? The answer is simple: More extensive mapping is required to collect a larger variety of other swollen places. The more thorough the discovery effort, the more tissue will be available for future monitoring. Sequential mapping can then assure ongoing recovery as lumps keep vanishing in concert with patient symptoms.

We can't ignore the body's many ropy connectors. There are two main types. Tendons blend with partner muscles, and hook on to bones at the other end. Ligaments, on the other hand, connect bone to bone. These widely distributed structures are deeply involved in fibromyalgia. They're serious abettors along with affected muscles in causing most of the pains. We urge examiners to roll their fingers over the cord-like structures and feel for unusual hardness and, particularly, for swollen segments. Patients respond during this search by expressing considerable tenderness.

Let's point out just a few places where those members of the musculoskeletal system are usually ignored or misdiagnosed. Pain from the deltoid tendon on the outside of the shoulder, most often the right, is sometimes attributed to the rotator cuff. Inguinal ligaments connect the front part of the hipbone to the pubic bone. The outer portion is almost always swollen, especially in women. It produces pain at anchorage across the lowest part of the abdomen by constantly pulling and irritating where it splays like Saran Wrap across the pubic bone. If doctors fail to put their hands on that ligament and examine it for swelling, they'll erroneously suspect ovarian or bladder problems. The peroneus muscle is on the outside of the lower leg; it begins at the outer knee and goes all the way to the foot. It curls around the ankle and joins another muscle to create a tendon that hooks onto the top of the arch. The right one is much more affected by fibromyalgia than the left. They may both visibly swell just below the outer anklebone and suggest water retention. The sole of the foot is more commonly involved than not. Invariably, doctors say the pain is due to "plantar fasciitis" when it's actually due to a swollen tendon. "Itis" implies inflammation: There isn't any in fibromyalgia. Structural abnormalities and swellings described in this paragraph are easily palpated with just a bit of practice. Simple hands-on efforts can quickly expose the cause of the pain at such locations and save a lot of anguish and investigative costs.

FIBROMYALGIA AND OSTEOARTHRITIS

Seven years ago I barely functioned. I went to work, stopped to pick up fast food on the way home, and went to bed. I called my home my fibro-home because I let everything go. It was a disaster. I missed paying bills and could not clean up the clutter, which kept getting worse. I lost friends because I kept canceling activities. Now I feel twenty years younger than when I started this journey. Much of my medical problems were predicted by Dr. St. Amand in his book. I don't feel any fibro issues, but I do have severe arthritis. So it is better to get on this journey sooner, rather than later. I feel well enough to now begin attacking my weight—to cut the blood pressure and cholesterol issues. This will also dramatically help my arthritis.

—*Gail H., Illinois*

What is generally accepted as fibromyalgia is only the beginning of a long, miserable progression that ultimately leads to osteoarthritis. This isn't the kind that causes crippling deformities, though it can gnarl joints a bit and cause enough joint damage to require knee or hip replacement. Most people accept aches and stiffness as a normal part of growing older, so

osteoarthritis is considered "wear-and-tear arthritis" and natural for the elderly. Don't you believe it!

You recall we tease a lot of history out of patients on our first
meeting. We ask if their parents and grandparents had similar fibromyalgic symptoms or arthritis. If we're lucky, some of
those family members accompany the patient and speak for
themselves. As we check off answers to our long symptom list,
we often see older relatives nod as if they were being quizzed.
Most of the time they eventually verbalize and suddenly
explode with "and now I've got osteoarthritis" (*osteo* is from *os*,
the Latin word for "bone"). They describe X-ray findings that
show spurs and degenerative bone changes that confirm that
diagnosis. They aren't alluding to traumatized joints, but to the
getting-old type.

It's quite striking how body smarts manage to avoid fibromyalgic damage to essential organs. There's no increased cell
death, muscular wasting (atrophy), or nerve damage. Kidneys
perform smoothly with the possible exception of our theoretical, putative metabolic error. The liver remains completely
functional and the heart pumps just fine at metronome pace.
The brain thinks, remembers, and still directs traffic, although
some cognitive function may be erratic in the presence of fibrofog. Cuts still heal, and the immune system remains capable of
fighting disease, though perhaps a little reluctantly. Not so with
the joints. The prevailing medical opinion holds that fibromyalgia is a nonarticular (nonjoint) disease, but we strongly differ. They're frequently involved early in the disease, but it takes
years before damage is perceptible to a radiologist on an X-ray.

As fibromyalgia progresses, something has to give. If I were
a body, here's how I'd think: I'm getting punished with less
energy and I've got to give up some less crucial functions. I
sense the rising levels of phosphate. It's safer to load muscles
with metabolic debris than it is to let it circulate uncontested in
the bloodstream or end up in vital tissues. We have ample data

to underscore that protective stance by the body. It makes sense that stacking the junk into expendable structures can preserve activity in essential areas.

From birth, bones have accepted as much phosphate as their periodic growth status would allow. Once they must refuse more, tendons and ligaments are the next safest places. Even with a little excess mineral, they still perform reasonably well because they're only called upon to perform short contractions. Muscles are next in the reception line and finally step out to share the load. In their distress, they'll collectively flash messages from the ailing periphery to the brain, pleading for relief. The already enfeebled central nervous system can't help, and in turn, it, too, capitulates: Energy, fatigue, and cognition line up the wimp column. Now, most patients seek professional help.

Fibromyalgia is a jerky process in affected tissues before they totally succumb. The system remains somewhat fluid, and there are momentary though often only partial recoveries. Serial failures progressively sap other tissues. Salutary energy comes only in spurts, and in emergencies, some tissues steal energy from others heretofore unaffected. At any given time, 25, 50, or 75 percent of the body may also be struggling. Rest or minimal-load exercise improves percentages, but untreated, it's eventually a losing proposition.

Collectively, fibromyalgic muscles and bones, the largest structures in the body, accept much more than fair shares of the load. Finally, generalized exhaustion taunts the body into finding new reservoirs for the accumulating debris. Joints are attacked and will yield to become the ultimate repositories for calcium, phosphate, and other miscreants. Realistically, joints have an inexhaustible capacity and, once pressed into full service, will continue accepting deposits the rest of the fibromyalgic's life. Tartar-like crystals actually form whereas, in other tissues, calcium and phosphate almost always remain in solution. Even one of these crystals contains an inordinate amount of calcium phosphate compared to the minuscule bit that effectively disturbs metabolism in mobile cells. Fluid from osteoarthritic joints consistently shows every known shape of calcium phosphate crystal. Such microscopic rocks abrade and irritate cartilage, ultimately leading to bony overgrowth, spurs, erosions, and irreparable destruction. Sadly, that's tangible evidence of permanent damage that cannot be reversed by guaifenesin. We make this a compelling argument for early diagnosis and treatment.

The body waits a very long time before resorting to this drastic solution. The scenario concludes a long-fought and gallant attempt at damage control. Because joints have such a huge capacity for accepting the offending ions, essential organs such as the heart, brain, kidneys, and liver are forever spared damage from fibromyalgia. Viewing the progression of our illness in this light, feel blessed that joints are so responsive. It's a good solution for a bad condition and allows you to stay alive, the body's first priority. Osteoarthritis may be uncomfortable and ultimately disabling, but at least takes years to surface. By that time, nature assumes we'll have procreated, raised our young to maturity, and are fully expendable in a biological sense.

Our protocol doesn't offer relief from osteoarthritis other than prevention before it occurs. It does, however, help clear tissues that constantly pull on or in joint surfaces. From the sequence we've outlined, know that damage begins with the first microscopic crystals that start the abrasion in a very lengthy process that defies X-ray detection. Patients relate joint complaints for a number of years before very-delayed validation appears on X-rays. Once damaged, anti-inflammatory and pain medications are the choices until sufficient damage leads to the operating table and joint replacement.

Many medications are given for muscle pain: Analgesics, muscle relaxants, nonsteroidal anti-inflammatories (NSAIDs), antidepressants, and anticonvulsants are the most offered. Heat and ice are local modalities that may help, the choice determined by which works best. Unfortunately, most muscle creams (Tiger Balm, Aspercreme, Bengay, Icy Hot) contain salicylates, but lidocaine (Lidoderm patches) and Voltaren gel do not. The little heat pads that can be applied over painful areas won't block. Gently performed massage and other bodywork can make symptoms manageable. Acupuncture and acupressure offer relief for some. Used in tandem, various modalities blend to mutual benefit. Less reliance on medications avoids escalations in dosages and side effects.

Fibromyalgics have to be prodded into following the one piece of advice consistently given by experts: exercise. It's inexpensive, has no enduring side effects, never fails to show benefits, and even a bit helps. Unfortunately, this lead-in won't fully convince many, but let's try. Even the gentlest type such as stretching can temporarily soothe ailing muscles, tendons, and ligaments. Sustained aerobics, however light, quickens the rebuilding pace for mitochondria, ATP-making power stations we've already discussed. Increased energy production introduces stamina to push ahead even faster. For those with arthritis or severe back pain, water aerobics provide a good reintroduction to exertion. It's buoyant and combines some of the cardiovascular benefits of walking with those of resistance training initiated to overcome the water pressure. Exercise stimulates production of our natural pain-relieving compounds, endorphins, and their receptors.

We think the disease first appears because of faulty ATP production and greatly worsens by becoming sedentary. Inactivity invites willful destruction of a seemingly inexhaustible supply of mitochondria. The body stops feeding what it doesn't use so your power stations are closed down. Indulge your chronically afflicted musculoskeleton and only slowly begin any exercise program. DVDs exist to prompt neophyte workouts. Sneak them in when you're sure of your energy-limited schedule.

Don't demand instant results. Over time, confidence, strength, and energy recharge their own batteries. Fatigue, weakness, and long-gone stamina plague fibromyalgics not only while they're ill, but also when they head down the road to recovery. Deconditioning is the price of inactivity.

There were days that at times turned into a week, when I was cycling so hard I couldn't exercise. Instead of feeling guilty, I gave myself a break. Dr. St. Amand says that after two weeks of no exercise, you pretty much lose what you've accomplished to that point. So I would discipline myself to do something as soon as I could. Many times I had to start over with very light exercise and build up to where I was before the hard cycling began. The secret is not comparing ourselves to the normal people around us that are exercising. Just do it no matter how insignificant it seems. Be patient. You will eventually see results. I have, and it's great!

—*Carol H., Texas*

Chapter Ten

The Irritable Bowel Syndrome

Fibrogut

I was never diagnosed with IBS until we arrived at the FMS and HG [hypoglycemia] diagnosis. Everything was a mystery. I had been plagued all my life with inexplicable stomach and intestinal pains, gas, and bloating, alternating diarrhea and constipation. The most common medical advice was to "relax" and take antacids. I have been on the hypoglycemia diet, alternating between strict and liberal versions, for almost a year. It only took a month for my IBS symptoms to improve once I knew how to diet properly.

—*Gwen, California*

SOME FIBROMYALGICS ARE overwhelmed by their uncomfortable bowel symptoms. Their other problems seem relatively minor annoyances. They go on a quest for relief and aren't too likely to get much. Physicians understandably have a bit of difficulty in assessing problems deeply hidden within the abdomen unless they're given sufficient patient history. We see individuals who poorly describe dull, steady aching in particular locations and wince from tenderness from light digital pressure. That's not much information to suggest what testing might be appropriate. Luckily, proper questioning narrows down the field of possibilities. We're on the very end of the doctor visit spectrum so by the time we see patients, they've been tested and probed myriad times and have taken every over-the-counter medication and herbal supplement available.

When a patient complains of persistent aching or abdominal pain, the primary physician usually does a basic manual examination followed by blood tests. One example, pain in the pit of the stomach and sour belching, will promote a test for the ulcer-causing bacterium, *Helicobacter pylori*. Excess gas, nausea, diarrhea, cramps, or constipation evoke different evaluations. Further testing will likely follow using ultrasound and X-ray.

Nothing abnormal? Off goes the patient to a gastroenterologist. This specialist reviews the lab reports and other findings and confirms everything is functionally normal. Other tests might eliminate the likelihood of celiac disease, a condition we can't adequately discuss here. Let's be thorough since symptoms persist. That segues into an endoscopy of the esophagus, stomach, and upper part of the small intestine followed by the ultimate indignity: a colonoscopy and exoneration of the colon. Our totally tested subject now has a complete, certified list of normal results. It's good to have a result, but you still feel terrible and demand, "What's really wrong?" The final consultation sums it up: "You've got irritable bowel syndrome."

So where does this leave the patient? As comforting as it is to have a name tagged onto a validated ailment and reassurance that it's not deadly, the next step isn't exactly clear. Some suggested solutions are to "eat more fiber; take stool softeners; use prescription medications to reduce gas, diarrhea, and cramping." This might offer temporary relief, but it is only temporary. What is this irritable bowel mess? What's the underlying cause? How can we get rid of it forever?

IBS is one of the overlapping FMS and HG symptoms. I don't think it pays to debate whether it's from FMS alone or HG

Ultrasound—High-frequency sound waves are passed by a transducer through the area of the body to be studied, to make an image of solid organs such as the liver. These waves cannot pass through bones or make images of gas.

Endoscopy—A procedure that is done with a fiber-optic instrument, enabling direct visual examination. A long, narrow tube is inserted through the mouth, down the back of the throat into the esophagus, down into the stomach, and into the duodenum, the first part of the small intestine.

Colonoscopy—Colon probing with a similar but longer endoscope (colonscope) inserted rectally and passed upward. The doctor then withdraws it slowly, as each part of the intestine and rectum is examined. This procedure is usually done in the doctor's office or hospital "GI lab" with the patient mildly sedated. If only the lower portion of the colon is to be examined, a shorter instrument is used for a sigmoidoscopy.

Table 10.1
Irritable Bowel Syndrome

	Male	Percentage Male	Female	Percentage Female
Number of patients	596		3,444	
Nausea	237	39	2,045	59
Excess gas	388	65	2,447	71
Bloating	351	59	2,573	75
Constipation	274	46	2,252	65
Diarrhea	283	47	1,983	58

alone. Where does that get you? And what if you're wrong? If you just do the HG diet perfectly for a couple of weeks, and it helps, that answers your question. If you do the diet perfectly and there is no difference, then it could be just FMS, or it could be a side effect of a medication you're taking.

—*Anne Louise, Minnesota*

Over the years, many other names have been used to describe IBS, including *spastic colon, mucous colitis, toxic gut, leaky bowel syndrome,* and *functional bowel disease.* Most of those alternative terms are inaccurate attempts at designating a cause for the condition. For example, the term *colitis* means "inflammation of the colon." There's rarely such irritation in IBS. We consider them all as synonyms for the same condition. As in the rest of the body, nothing exposes affected systems biochemically or anatomically enough to provide diagnostic proof. There's much upset, but no damage.

As in all other facets of fibromyalgia, women are affected by IBS in greater numbers than men. Expectedly, like other symptoms of the disease, intestinal complaints are usually worse premenstrually. Its clustered symptoms begin at any age, but surprisingly, often in children and young adults. It may appear dramatically as the first symptoms of the disease. Adults often recall recurring bouts during early school years.

Since my teenage years I have had stomach pain and cramping...My general practitioner would say it was "a little gastritis." He would prescribe an antacid and send me home with a pat on the back. I suffered like this for about ten or twelve years...I went to a very eminent gastroenterologist... He pronounced "irritable bowel syndrome." When I asked him what I could do for it, he said, "Nothing. Just stay away from green vegetables."...I also experienced insomnia and some muscle pain since I was a teen. I had no idea they were all

related to FMS. A few years ago, the FMS came on with a ven-
geance, and after seeking a diagnosis for about nine months,
I finally found a doctor who told me I have FMS with gastroesophageal reflux.

—Marie, Nevada

Sixty percent of the fibromyalgics we've seen have IBS. The
complex has so many symptoms that not all patients get all of
them. There could be intermittent difficulty in swallowing,
and acid might reflux back up the esophagus from the stomach. That's so-called heartburn, the burning sensation named
gastroesophageal reflux disease, or *GERD*. Irritation may cause
esophageal spasms and produce chest pain closely mimick-
ing angina or a heart attack. It's more common in overweight
patients and often occurs at night. Waves of nausea sometimes
appear out of nowhere. They can last for hours or for only a few
minutes, often in staccato, repetitive waves. Gas and bloating
are almost regular, but just as high on the patient's list is constipation alternating with diarrhea.

Confronted with IBS symptoms, doctors might order a battery of expensive blood allergy tests and find alleged "multiple
food sensitivities." Skin tests are complementary or alternatives.
Assessments may be correct, but patients often tell us they have
no problem after eating some supposedly offending food. We
suggest a cheaper eating test by simply sequentially using a tiny
amount of one item at a time; in this way the gastrointestinal tract becomes the diagnostician. If sensitivity truly exists,
symptoms should get decidedly worse, and then the patient
knows to stop eating the irritating food. This is the true proof
of sensitivity, because, too often, sensitive skin simply over-
reacts to an injected foreign protein.

Constipation and diarrhea can take turns in rapid shifts. It's
not unusual to have one problem for months or years, then suffer from its inverse. Particularly, recurrent diarrhea may lead

to stool testing for candida (yeast) or parasites. Stool examinations are not for novice technicians. It takes a well-practiced eye to avoid being duped into thinking food residues are cysts or parasites. Cultures are frequent sources of error since yeast is normal in stool specimens. Repeatedly, patients have undergone varieties of herbal purges aimed at the liver or colon in cathartic washouts. Those are usually cleansings for something that was never there. Still others have spent months or years on antifungal (yeast) medications, such as Diflucan (fluconazole) or Mycostatin (nystatin), without experiencing much change in symptoms.

> How does it feel physically? I described it to a friend this way: "Imagine you are just recovering from a bad case of the stomach flu, where you're better but still shaky and not sure how loose your bowels still are. Now imagine you're going to try to carry on a normal life, and pretend you're fine. And imagine every day is like this." It's hard, it's uncomfortable, and the emotional component is hard, too. Cramping, urgency, a feeling of "looseness," burning pain in the lower back, nausea, acid reflux, shakiness, and weak knees. These are all symptoms I associate with IBS.
>
> —*R.A., California*

We know fibromyalgia and undigested carbohydrates combine as preeminent forces to cause IBS. Like other cells anywhere in the body, those of the gastrointestinal tract also suffer energy deprivation. The three smooth muscle layers of the intestinal wall become dysfunctional, just as can skeletal muscle. The small intestine has the assigned task of churning and mixing nutritive elements with digestive juices. Such activity begins the breakdown of fats, protein, and carbohydrates into absorbable components. Alternate contraction and relaxation of the intestinal wall propels raw materials to the next digestive station, where they submit to the action of various hormones and enzymes. The results are minuscule food particles that may now be assimilated and made ready for body-wide distribution. Quite likely, intestinal glands share in the general problem of fibromyalgia and, along with the musculature, become inept for ideal digestive sequences. Nausea, gas, and bloating are disconcerting enough, but the ensuing constipation and diarrhea are more alarming. Like uncontrolled traffic signals, they switch from stop to go in prolonged cycles that greatly interfere with digestion as well as elimination. Imagine the backing-up effect this has on the entire gastrointestinal tract: a serious malfunction that produces all of the symptoms of irritable bowel syndrome.

Food processing is mainly done in the small intestine. Bile and pancreatic exudates massage fats into microscopic, digestible fragments. The colon (or large intestine) lies downstream, all six feet of it, and also serves various functions. Similarly affected in fibromyalgia, its glands and muscles contribute to the irritable bowel syndrome. The main job here is to remove salts and water from the mulch, a process that may take a few days. It sequesters friendly bacterial residents that live in the colon. These organisms use our food residues for their own metabolic use and, in the process, create items for our special needs. As much as 20 percent of ingested carbohydrates reach the large intestine undigested. They're the main feed for certain bacteria that thrive when so abundantly nourished. Unfortunately, they create great amounts of gas as they ferment sugar and starch residues. Gas can cause repetitive cramping and sharp stabs anywhere in the abdomen but mostly when it's whipping through the small intestine. It doesn't linger long in that location since it's quickly propelled forward and expelled into the much larger reception chambers of the colon. There, it encounters forceful contractions of more powerful muscles that shove the now hardening remnants toward the rectum.

Origins of Abdominal Pain

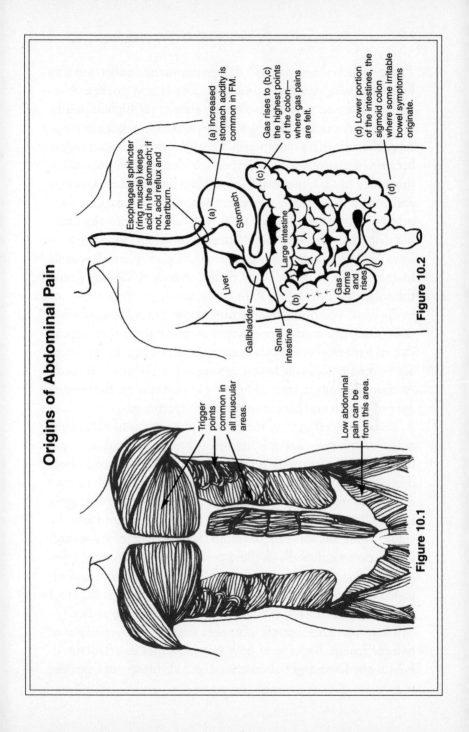

Figure 10.2

Esophageal sphincter (ring muscle) keeps acid in the stomach; if not, acid reflux and heartburn.

(a) Increased stomach acidity is common in FM.

Gas rises to (b,c) the highest points of the colon—where gas pains are felt.

(d) Lower portion of the intestines, the sigmoid colon where some irritable bowel symptoms originate.

Liver

Gallbladder

Small intestine

Large intestine

Stomach

(a)

(c)

(b) Gas forms and rises

(d)

Figure 10.1

Trigger points common in all muscular areas.

Low abdominal pain can be from this area.

The large bowel gets distended from improvised collection sites where gas temporarily accumulates. The largest pockets accumulate in the upper reaches since air rises to the highest points.

Gas produces an amazing variety of sounds, but it's nothing more than air that's temporarily trapped. Forced to accumulate because of constipation, it further dehydrates stools and makes them rock hard. Cemented food residues plug up the rectal area and, like a dam, further interfere with gas elimination. Pressure builds up behind this solid wall, and adds to the existing discomfort of bloating, nausea, and perhaps sour belching (acid reflux). Added pressure also induces painful spasms mainly in the lower left side of the abdomen. Glands lining the colon react to surface damage by making slimy mucus just as the nasal and bronchial membranes do in response to irritation. The purpose of this mucus is to make the colon slippery so that hard stools can slither out without causing further damage to the sigmoid (the lowest segment of the colon) or rectum. At times the longer, stained mucous strings take on the appearance of worms and lead to unnecessary treatments.

The cemented head of the bowel movement is often so hard and slow to exit that it scratches the rectum, causing some bleeding and rectal pain. If encrusted food particles are embedded on the surface, the laceration may be deep enough to produce what we call in medical parlance a rectal fissure. Higher up, small pockets (diverticula) may extrude outward from the colon. Stool contents can push into them, attract infection, and induce diverticulitis. Rock-like stools can also push rectal veins ahead of them like an ocean wave. They may get inflamed, sandpapered, swollen, or clotted, recognizable as hemorrhoids. Stool blood demands testing to eliminate more threatening causes.

There are certain predictable sites where gas accumulates as painful locales because of how our intestines are structured. First is the lower right abdomen, where air blasts out from the small intestine into the colon. Pressure builds in this area, and a bit later gas is propelled to the upper right abdomen near the edge of the liver. Cramps cut across the belly from right to left as gas is squeezed toward the highest place in the bowel, the left upper quadrant. A huge air pocket can form under the thin diaphragm muscle that pushes upward toward the heart. Sharp-stabbing or pressure pains reflected into the front of the chest can mimic a heart attack. You may ask, "Why doesn't gas move along with the forming stools?" The propulsive efforts of the intestinal muscles are a bit like grabbing a long, sausage-like balloon in the middle. The gas squeezes in both directions, but as soon as you let go, it gushes back to the center. The result is repeated pains from the same gas bubble whether it lingers somewhere or rapidly shifts position. (See figures 10.1 and 10.2.)

Often, patients suffering from such gastrointestinal conditions are miserable and yearn for "comfort foods," the easily digested sugars and starches. (Sixty percent of our fibromyalgics crave sweets in a vain attempt to make energy, as we've discussed.) But excessive carbohydrate consumption only makes things worse, promoting genetic tendencies toward hypoglycemia, weight gain, and diabetes. Repetitive releases of insulin force the liver to convert carbohydrate excesses to fat. Obesity is responsible for many health problems beyond the scope of this chapter, but it also adds to gastrointestinal misery. Heartburn and gastroesophageal reflux occur primarily in overweight patients.

Pains arising from the abdominal wall provide diagnostic pitfalls for doctor and patient. The diligent physician completes the normal examination and testing, surveys the results, and ascribes the discomfort to IBS. Internal pain is not quite the same, however: It presents gas-like, as colicky cramping unlike the duller, steady, and hard hurt on the outside surface. The outer abdominal muscles suffer the same as other muscles throughout the body. Unrelenting spasm, a bit more to the right of the pit of the stomach, instigates much unnecessary testing. It's quite easy to identify: Patients lie supine and simply raise their heads off the bed. The doctor palpates both sides of the uppermost abdomen and compares the tension under his fingers. Both sides may be involved, but the right is usually more tender and swollen.

In chapter 9, we discussed diagnostic problems caused by the inguinal ligaments. It bears repeating. Those are parallel, double cords, located on each side of the groin. They originate from the front pelvis and anchor at the pubic bone. They're actually part of the abdominal wall muscles that originate adjacent to the lower ribs and spread downward. In the groin, they curl around each other to create rope-like structures. Those connections are what let you brace and give leverage to do a sit-up. They're almost always involved in fibromyalgia and are easily felt as swollen segments in the outermost parts of the ligaments. They stay tight day and night, exerting a steady pull on the attached abdominal muscles. The pain described in the previous paragraph is the result and may even become a rib-side charley horse. Both the tight ligaments and their muscle cohorts exert an unrelenting drag on the pubic area, yielding the sensation to urinate. However frequently the patient goes to the bathroom, nothing much comes out, but the sensation continues. Physicians don't often palpate the groin ligaments when doing an in-depth, pelvic examination. If you have these complaints, request a full examination before submitting to an ultrasound and invasive searches.

IBS symptoms are usually treated with an assortment of medications. They sometimes help, but with almost equal success, patients get partial relief with over-the-counter products such as antacids, cathartics, and gas-reducing agents. Often, especially when treating themselves, efforts are misdirected and bypass the underlying cause. Because symptoms are confusing and changeable, suspicions arise about yeast and parasites.

Prescriptions are too often added to over-the-counter stuff in a "shotgun" approach. Costs mount with expensive digestive enzymes, cleansing compounds, and even colonics. Adding this fistful of pills to those for sleep, nervousness, depression, and pain helps make their pharmacist's monthly car payments but also invites drug interaction disasters.

Sometimes irritable bowel symptoms are actually side effects of a medication taken for another symptom. Narcotics such as codeine, OxyContin, and morphine and muscle relaxants like Flexeril and Soma cause some degree of constipation in nearly anyone. Antianxiety drugs such as Klonopin and Valium can do it as well. Over-the-counter magnesium is sometimes touted for fibromyalgia, but an excess may cause diarrhea. Constant use of laxatives is habit-forming, and even recovering patients are afraid to stop them and too impatient to wait for resumption of normal function. Losing what little benefit they've obtained from their drugs can't be risked; they fear their whole system will fall apart. This concern is not ill founded: They're barely coping as it is and have no emotional or physical reserves. The following story is typical.

> For the last ten years or so I have been diagnosed with every-thing from colitis to food allergies to systemic Candida infection because I have had so much trouble with diarrhea. Sometimes I would go for days with no bowel function and then out of the blue I'd have diarrhea...I had constant pain-ful intestinal gas that was very embarrassing because I could not control it. I was treated for colitis and then sprue or gluten intolerance. Neither of those treatments helped. Next, an aller-gist diagnosed me with intestinal yeast infections from anti-biotics. He said I had developed food allergies from the yeast and put me on an antifungal drug called nystatin. That helped a little. The next doctor...did a two-year series of European allergy shots and gave me an even stronger drug for the yeast.

[He] had me injecting myself with allergy shots two to three times a week and taking doses and potions of various things by mouth four times a day. My diet was very restricted, and my weight fell from 118 to 98 pounds. The doctor had me on a high-carbohydrate diet in a failed attempt at weight gain.

In desperation and prayer I turned to the Internet and found Dr. St. Amand's information. After comparing his description of hypoglycemia and IBS to my symptoms, I hoped I had found an answer. I dropped Dr. St. Amand and Claudia an e-mail. Dr. St. Amand assured me I was on the right track. Claudia helped me get started on the diet and told me what to do in the stormy early weeks, as my body fought to adjust to the new fuel. She promised after the first six weeks things would settle down. They did. The gas and diarrhea and other symptoms are gone now as long as I stay on the diet…The good news is I can now eat anything on the HG diet and not have diarrhea or gas. I no longer look like a starved waif, having put on 14 pounds as well.

—*Gretchen, South Carolina*

Patients with irritable bowel syndrome often avoid intimate relationships, as do those with vulvodynia or bladder dysfunction. All three of these conditions isolate the individual because of the personal nature of the affected areas. Most people suffer in silence and resist explaining their illness to others because it's so vague, mysterious, and embarrassing. The good news is that websites and support groups exist. A good place to start for basic information is the online support site: www.ibsgroup.org.

TREATMENT FOR IBS

So how do we treat this irritable bowel syndrome? These are the two simplest paragraphs we've written in this entire chapter. Begin by eliminating all sugars and complex carbohydrates.

You'll find the proper diet outlined in chapter 6 and on our website. The diet is the same as for hypoglycemia except that you don't need to avoid caffeine or alcohol unless they upset your system. The diet alone will quickly eliminate 60 to 70 percent of your symptoms. Dietary restrictions will be temporary for most of you. Once you feel better, add one favorite food at a time beginning with anything but sugar, sweets, and the heavier starches, such as potato and pasta. Unsweetened grains, brown rice, and the dairy products, yogurt and sugar-free ice cream, are good places to start your experimentation. Promptly back off if symptoms return, trusting them as reliable indicators that you've added too much, too fast, or too often. This hunt-and-peck system is the only way to learn which foods and in what quantities you can tolerate. The premenstrual week is the riskiest of the month for resurrecting adverse effects. In time, you'll learn what you need to restrict, if anything, on a permanent basis. You'll dependably evolve your own personal program.

Over-the-counter preparations work quite effectively when combined with the diet. Gas-X contains mint oil; use Phazyme instead. Both charcoal and dimethicone products may work quite well for gas and bloating. Calcium carbonate antacids such as Rolaids, Mylanta, and Maalox are good choices for an upset or acidy stomach but use only the fruit flavored. Prilosec, Pepcid (famotidine), Zantac, and other histamine-2 blockers are available in over-the-counter strengths and also counter acidity. Prescription strengths may be needed if the weaker ones prove inadequate. Prelief neutralizes food acids and is a good choice for women who get bladder burning with such. Over-the-counter Imodium helps control cramping and diarrhea during flare-ups.

Fiber and extra fluid intake ease constipation, but titrate up gradually so you won't make things worse. If you add fiber, stick with sugar-free formulations such as those made by Metamucil,

Fiber Choice, Konsyl, or Citrucel. Sugar alcohols such as sorbitol and xylitol are in vogue, but varying from person to person; a few fibroglycemics get worse from an undependable effect on blood sugar. They are also well known for causing diarrhea and gas, especially maltitol. Magnesium is a standalone supplement that should be titrated up gradually for constipation. Calcium on the other hand may squelch diarrhea.

Titrate—to determine the proper amount of medication needed for therapeutic action by gradually and systematically raising the dosage until the desired effect has occurred.

If you're taking antibiotics, add acidophilus, which can help maintain healthy flora in the colon. It's an inexpensive insurance policy against a severe bout of diarrhea.

Rectal pressure from constipation can be relieved quite safely by inserting a glycerin suppository. Hemorrhoids may be treated with topical preparations, but beware of those containing witch hazel or other plant extracts. Over-the-counter anti-inflammatories such as naproxen or ibuprofen may help within a few days. Highly effective for constipation is good old-fashioned exercise. If you get moving, your bowels may follow suit!

There are prescription drugs on the market for IBS symptoms as well. Hopefully, you will not need to use these for long. Some patients actually get relief from diarrhea and some pain when taking tricyclic antidepressants. Unfortunately, side effects of these include dry mouth, fatigue, and weight gain. In June 2002, the FDA approved Zelnorm for IBS patients with constipation, but it was withdrawn in 2007 because of serious side effects. Lotronex (alosetron) is a newer drug aimed at IBS with diarrhea. It has also had problems with the FDA and was off the market for a time but is now allowed as a second line therapy. This means that patients must have failed on all other existing treatments before it will be considered.

> At the end of my first year, my IBS was almost gone. My energy level got better. I was able to stay out of bed when I came home from work in the evening. I was able to get a shower, dry my hair, and put on my makeup without taking several breaks. I was able to go to my grandson's football games and sit on the cold bleachers late at night. Some people never cycle severe pain but have other symptoms instead.
>
> —*Jan H., Kentucky*

Many other medications are currently used by physicians. Older tricyclics are often prescribed because of their relaxing effects on intestinal smooth muscles. Anticholinergic drugs also relax such muscles and ease cramping. Two commonly used for IBS symptoms are Bentyl (Dicyclomine) and Levsin (hyosycanine). Librax has similar benefits, but contains a benzodiazepine that should be withdrawn only with caution as patients can develop a tolerance to it. The newest IBS drug to be approved is Amitizia (lubiprostone), which is approved for adults with constipation. It works by increasing fluid secretion in the small intestine. Side effects include nausea and abdominal pain. Before it is prescribed, patients should try stool softeners such as Miralax or Perdiem. Milder laxatives such as sennocides may also help.

Serotonin-reuptake inhibitors may be helpful because they keep that neurotransmitter at higher, available levels. One study using one of these, Paxil, showed promise. Whereas 26 percent of patients were greatly improved by simply increasing fiber intake, 63 percent fared equally well by taking a small daily dose of that drug. Peri-Colace is both a stimulant and stool softener, a combination directed toward constipation. GERD is sometimes resolved by weight loss, but until that's accomplished, a class of medications called proton pump inhibitors will prove effective. This group includes Protonix, Prevacid, Prilosec, and Nexium. True to their promise, they disable a pumping effect in acid-making cells and potently block production. For diarrhea, standard treatments are over-the-counter Imodium (loperamide) and prescription Lomotil. These may be used whenever a problem occurs and work quickly, within an hour or so.

The remaining treatment format is equally simple. The steps you should follow are clearly defined in chapter 6. Basically, you must find your guaifenesin dosage and eliminate all blocking sources of salicylate—that's your job, and only you can do it! This entire book has been written for one purpose only: purging fibromyalgia and controlling the hypoglycemia that often accompanies it. Long before you picked up this book, many of you already suspected that interconnected symptoms were being erroneously separated to form so-called syndromes. We strongly advocate the use of only one medication and one diet for a sustainable control of all the symptoms of both those conditions.

Warning

Irritable bowel syndrome and fibromyalgia do not cause a high fever or severe pain that is persistent. If you are experiencing these symptoms, with or without nausea, diarrhea, or constipation, see a doctor to rule out more dangerous conditions such as appendicitis or diverticulitis.

As a teen I had the symptoms of what I now recognize as IBS. I never knew there was a name for the things that plagued me. Other kids dreamed of their futures and what they were going to be when they grew up. I found it hard to have those dreams. Sometimes I wondered if I was dying slowly but I never told that to anyone. All I knew was other kids my age weren't sick all the time.

—*Cris, Michigan*

Chapter Eleven

Genitourinary Syndromes

The bladder thing was my most serious symptom and it was guai that allowed me to get off Elmiron, a depressing (literally) medication that controlled the bladder pain. Possibly I would have committed suicide because of bladder pain because it was so bad for years. Within a couple of months on guai I was mostly free. I still have a little blood in my urine sometimes and a tendency to feel bladder irritation but nothing like the intense pain of those years.

—Hannah, California

THE BLADDER, URETHRA, and vaginal tract share in producing some of the most overwhelming symptoms of fibromyalgia. They can induce oppressive feelings that totally overshadow brain, muscular, and intestinal complaints. This intensity leads patients to seek relief from urologists or gynecologists. Unfortunately, while most of these specialists administer local remedies, they fail to recognize the broader picture. In the end, because the underlying disease hasn't been treated, these initially helpful therapies fail. Fibromyalgia is not part of their field of expertise, and patient and physician become increasingly frustrated. Worse still, desperate patients will finally try anything with a ghost of a chance, and all too often succumb to damaging topical applications or destructive surgeries that

Table 11.1

Genitourinary System

	Male	Percentage Male	Female	Percentage Female
Number of patients	596		3,444	
Dysuria	157	26	1,153	33
Pungent urine	216	36	1,596	46
Bladder infections	66	11	2,215	64
Vulvodynia	N/A		1,360	40

fail to live up to promises and, worse, leave scar tissue in their wake.

BLADDER

Fifty percent of female fibromyalgics give a medical history of three or more bladder infections before we first see them. Some tell us they've had fifty or more documented attacks and other repeated episodes of painful urination when no infection could be detected. Bladder infections in males are quite uncommon and therefore require more through investigation.

Routine urinalysis, even in healthy individuals, often shows varieties of amorphous calcium crystals in combination with oxalate, phosphate, or carbonates. You'll recall that the entire body participates in trying to get rid of excessive phosphate. These acid particles are secreted through tears, saliva, sweat, vaginal fluids, and bowel excrements. This output is not negligible except when compared with what's excreted in the urine, which is the major dumping system.

Calcium and phosphate don't crystallize inside cells. The two substances coexist in solution. It's the same effect when you drop salt in water: It immediately enters into solution though the sodium and the chloride are still there. Sufficiently diluted, they won't form particles. Phosphate surges out of the kidneys in a dissolved state, but things change in the bladder. That reservoir holds liquid waste until sufficient volume demands voiding. While waiting in the bladder, phosphate often solidifies in combination with calcium, oxalate, or magnesium. The weight of these microscopic crystals makes them sink to the base of the bladder and at the opening of the urethra. That's similar to sand in a swimming pool that gradually migrates to the deepest area, around the drain. On urination, particles are swept out and, like liquid sandpaper, abrade the delicate lining, the mucosa. If the scraping effect is sufficiently injurious, the integrity of the membrane is compromised and, once broken, allows bacterial penetration. The short female urethra—the tube that drains the contents of the bladder from the body—presents only a small distance for infectious agents to travel from where it exits the body, near the anus. Bacteria from the vagina, rectum, and skin find their way up into the bladder and cause cystitis. Consequently, this is the anatomical reason why women have far more problems with their urinary tracts than men. (See figure 11.1.)

Cystitis—Infection of the bladder. Symptoms include a constant urge to urinate, pain above the pubic bone, burning, searing urine, and, upon urination, producing only a small amount of urine. Antibiotics are commonly prescribed to treat the infection, as well as local analgesics that work on the urinary tract.

Under the same circumstances, intercourse is even more traumatic. Most women know about "honeymoon cystitis," which

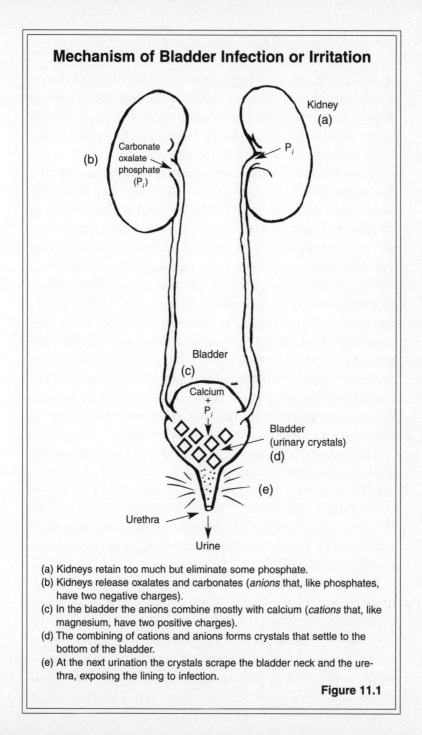

Mechanism of Bladder Infection or Irritation

Kidney (a)

Carbonate
oxalate
phosphate
(P_i)

(b)

P_i

Bladder
(c)

Calcium
+
P_i

Bladder
(urinary crystals)
(d)

(e)

Urethra

Urine

(a) Kidneys retain too much but eliminate some phosphate.
(b) Kidneys release oxalates and carbonates (*anions* that, like phosphates, have two negative charges).
(c) In the bladder the anions combine mostly with calcium (*cations* that, like magnesium, have two positive charges).
(d) The combining of cations and anions forms crystals that settle to the bottom of the bladder.
(e) At the next urination the crystals scrape the bladder neck and the urethra, exposing the lining to infection.

Figure 11.1

occurs during periods of heightened sexual activity. Pooled crystals damage the urethral and bladder walls from friction effects of penile strokes. Even the tougher vaginal lining is treated just as harshly and reacts like the bladder, as we'll discuss later when we get to that portion of the anatomy.

When bladder infections are recurrent, patients are given a low-dose antibiotic for an entire year to achieve complete eradication. Infection is detected by the presence of blood or pus in the urine but it may not be visible to the naked eye. In most cases only a microscopic examination in a laboratory can distinguish them. In the event of severe pain, especially pain accompanied by fever, a physician should be consulted for an accurate diagnosis and treatment. Without urine culture, even veteran patients are fooled into thinking there's infection where none exists. Prolonged use of antibiotics can cause diarrhea, vaginal yeast infection, or bacterial resistance. Urinalysis is certainly cost-effective. Antibiotics such as levofloxacin can stamp out infections in short order, making them popular choices for quick results. Because infections can travel from the bladder up into the kidneys via the ureters, it's important to treat them promptly.

The symptoms of urinary tract irritation commonly occur without infection. Burning urination (dysuria) sometimes appears for only a few hours or days and resolves spontaneously. Patients may have an unbearable urge to urinate with the sensation of a full bladder but voiding produces just a small amount of fluid. It is not uncommon during a cycle to urinate multiple times an hour.

Eventually, repeated cycles of cystitis invite more thorough investigations by urologists. When multiple urinalyses fail to expose infection, they seek to uncover another villain by looking directly into the bladder (cystoscopy). That search almost always proves futile, so the physician resorts to a biopsy of the bladder wall. Frustration mounts if such specimens appear normal under microscopic scrutiny. Sometimes, surface irritations or small clusters of certain white blood cells are found and, though hardly conclusive, at least point to a possible diagnosis.

> All my life I've had recurrent vaginitis. When I had a vaginal culture, it sometimes came back no Candida (I used to wonder if the lab mixed up the cultures) and yet all this irritation and discomfort continued. I used to buy Monistat cream four at a time when they were on sale. My GP even suggested I might be allergic to my own menstrual flow (if you can believe that one) and also said I might be allergic to my husband's sperm (not very helpful). Now, thirteen months on guai this pain is taking a bit of a break. I actually have days when I don't have it at all.
>
> —*Vera Lynne, Canada*

Those minimal and inconsequential findings or no abnormal findings earn a commonly proffered diagnosis of "interstitial cystitis." There is no definitive test for IC, so the diagnosis is largely based on symptoms. These include steady hurting in pelvic, pubic, or lower abdominal areas and an urgency to urinate so strong that patients might void twenty or more times a day. Urine cultures are routinely negative. Rectal pain may be intensified by hard spasms in muscles lying between the vagina and rectum, the perineum. Decreased bladder capacity and painful intercourse are two other common complaints. A succinct description would be: It's like a ninth-month, never-terminating, pregnant-bladder condition. The diagnosis of interstitial cystitis is rarely offered to males and is often misdiagnosed as nonbacterial prostatitis, prostatodynia, or prostalgia. Only about 10 percent of those diagnosed with IC are males. Men may have the same symptoms as women, but add scrotal or penile pain. If you've been diagnosed with IC, you were 10 percent more likely to have had childhood bladder problems.

Cystoscopy—A procedure done in a doctor's office, in which the urinary tract is viewed through a cystoscope inserted through the urethra and up into the bladder. Through this fiberoptic scope, the doctor can examine the lining and structure of these organs. A patient is usually given a local anesthetic or a mild tranquilizer to help with the discomfort.

Affected individuals have joined in support groups all over the world. It's estimated that some 450,000 have interstitial cystitis in the United States, but likely too few have been diagnosed. The average age at diagnosis is forty, about the same as for fibromyalgia. Both of the two large IC organizations, the Interstitial Cystitis Network (www.ichelp.org) and the Interstitial Cystitis Association (www.ica.org), are aware that fibromyalgia coexists in a large percentage of members. They include information about fibromyalgia in their brochures and websites. Group surveys have shown fibromyalgia, irritable bowel syndrome, and vulvodynia as frequent, concurrent conditions. Both the ICA and the ICN give out dietary suggestions and other hints for abating symptoms.

The most common dietary triggers for painful attacks are cranberry juice, coffee, tea, alcohol, citrus, artificial sweeteners, hot peppers, carbonated beverages, tomatoes, and tobacco. Vitamin C is ascorbic acid and, even if buffered, can irritate the bladder, but you can get your vitamins from other sources: half a cup of red bell peppers contains the same amount of vitamin C as an orange.

Pyridium (phenazopyridine HCL) is generic and available

> **Insterstitial cystitis**—A disease defined by the absence
> of a positive test for other bladder conditions, manifested
> by bladder and pelvic pain and the constant urge to uri-
> nate, which produces only a small amount of urine.

both in over-the-counter and prescription strengths. It numbs
the bladder and relieves pain but is designed for only short-term
use as it can build up in the body. Be careful when checking
both over-the-counter and prescription medications for bladder
pain as many of these contain salicylate (by name). Over-the-
counter Cystex and prescription medications such as Prosed,
Urised, Urelle, Uribel, and Utira will all block guaifenesin.

Half a teaspoon of baking soda in six ounces of water three
times a day can help cut the urine's acidity. Prelief (calcium
glycerophosphate) can do the same. Cranberry juice or tablets
are touted as prevention from infections, but the tablets will
block guaifenesin. Juice works as well as the tablets but it can
raise urinary pH and create more pain. D-mannose, the active
ingredient in cranberries, can be purchased as a supplement
and will not.

One oral medication, Elmiron (petosan polysulfate), is
approved for IC. It is believed to provide a protective coating
inside the bladder. It has not performed well in studies but
may help some patients. Other therapies include bladder instillations where various substances are inserted directly into the
bladder. It is worth noting that only one, DMSO, is actually
approved for this type of delivery. Other instillations include
BCG, heparin, lidocaine, Elmiron, and sodium bicarbonate.
Two new compounds, Cystistat (sodium hyaluronate) and
Uracyst (chondroitin), are currently being tested in the United
States and Canada.

Elavil and other tricyclic antidepressants act on smooth

muscle and cut pain perception and can be somewhat useful. Newer antidepressants (SSRIs and SNRIs) have not demonstrated any efficacy in treating IC. Antihistamines including the histamine-2 blockers are often included in a multipronged attack because they work on the mast cells which line the bladder. In IC, these cells are stimulated and release histamines, which cause local pain and irritation. Over-the-counter antihistamines such as Benadryl help sufferers sleep and also provide some assistance in subduing mast cells. Antispasmodics can help subdue frequent urination. Ditropan and Levsin are two of these. Unfortunately their side effects include fatigue and vision changes.

> When you're having an attack, the constant pain…the fear of sex making more pain is debilitating. It weighs down your life, your lightness, destroys spontaneity, makes you standoffish with the man you love because you just don't want to have to explain you're having problems again. That part is bad, but the symptoms that you live with night and day are even worse: never sleeping through a night, having to sleep on the outside of every bed, always worrying whether there will be a bathroom close by, stopping often on car trips, dodging into fast-food places, hoping they won't catch you not buying anything and telling you the rest room is only for customers.
>
> —*C.C., California*

Guaifenesin eventually clears IC complaints, but may initially worsen them like other symptoms of fibromyalgia. After the first few reversal attacks, future bouts become relatively minor and will likely disappear. Fight back early by drinking extra fluid and watching your diet and by using appropriate medications at the first hint of urinary burning. Prelief may be taken daily as a preventative measure, especially when traveling. Car and airplane rides are notorious triggers. It's far easier to abort an early onslaught than to subdue a well-established attack. Exercise, especially stretching, has been helpful in the long term. Take guaifenesin and begin a fitness regime sooner rather than later to help restore you to normal.

VULVAR PAIN

As a senior gynecologist with special training and expertise in vulvar disease, I have been striving to help women with the enigmatic disorder called vulvodynia, and its most common subset, vulvar vestibulitis. In recent years there has been increasing appreciation of other conditions reported as commonly associated with vulvodynia, such as irritable bowel syndrome, fibromyalgia, and interstitial cystitis. In my own practice at Scripps Clinic and Research Foundation, I've discovered that fibromyalgia is at least three times as common in vulvodynia patients as in the general population. I've also noted that vulvodynia tends not to respond to therapy until the underlying fibromyalgia is treated...Dr. St. Amand has done groundbreaking work in the evaluation and treatment of fibromyalgia as opposed to medications that only reduce or help control symptoms. His research, and that of those who follow in his footsteps, will permit fibromyalgia to become merely a painful memory for patients and their spouses. I salute his effort.

—John Willems, M.D., FRCSC, FACOG, head,
Division of Ob-Gyn, Scripps Clinic and
Research Foundation, La Jolla, California

All too many fibromyalgic women develop extreme sensitivity and irritation of the inner vaginal lips, known as vulvitis. The problem may involve deeper tissues of the vagina, the vestibule (vestibulitis). Chronic burning and knife-like pain are common as is low abdominal pain. Symptoms can be intermittent,

Vulvodynia or vulvar pain syndrome—Severe pain, burning, and/or itching in the vulvar area (the vulva is the area of the female's external genitalia). This area is extremely sensitive to touch, and may or may not be red and visibly irritated. Vulvar vestibulitis syndrome (VVS) is less common, and applies to women who have pain only in the vestibule, a smaller area than the vulva.

localized, or diffuse. In the past eleven years, we've tabulated the incidence of vulvodynia and associated symptoms. Out of 5,468 consecutive new female patients, about 40 percent had pelvic complaints. In the early stages, pain may initiate only after intercourse, but later can occur without apparent provocation. Vulvodynia can appear at any age, including in young girls. It's not necessarily a sign of sexual activity. Intermittent bouts are the norm initially but in time become chronic and provoke overwhelming symptoms.

Like fibromyalgia, vulvodynia is somewhat a diagnosis of exclusion. Some conditions must be ruled out: infection, yeast overgrowth, genital warts, and herpes. The appearance is quite different from what is seen in those conditions. The skin retains its normal texture although it might be slightly red, suggesting a chemical burn. Diagnosis is usually slow coming. Patients get acquainted with a few gynecologists after several pelvic exams and failed therapies, often for yeast, before the condition is suspected. Vaginal smears, cultures, or more painful testing ultimately exclude infection, nerve damage, and dermatologic abnormalities. Using a simple cotton-tipped probe, the Q-tip will detect exquisite sensitivities of certain vaginal tissues. Physicians may also do a quite painless colposcopy to magnify and better visualize painful vulvar surfaces.

Though present at any age, the diagnosis seems obscure

until, on average, women are in their forties. It's commonly stated that between 150,000 and 200,000 women in the United States suffer from this facet of fibromyalgia. We think that's a huge underestimation. If there are 30 million women in the United States with fibromyalgia and we've documented that 40 percent of them have vulvodynia, significant misdiagnoses are rampant. If so, treatments are being aimed at the wrong culprit; masking pain does not exonerate the guilty entity. Some specialists who deal almost exclusively with vulvodynia suspect that one woman in six has suffered from this syndrome at some point in her life. That's close to our estimate that 15 percent of the women in the world have fibromyalgia. From the thousands of patients we've treated, we can unhesitatingly attest that of all the symptom clusters we encounter, the vulvar pain complex produces the most consistently painful and heartbreaking impositions on a woman's life.

As we've pointed out, fibromyalgia regularly affects the inguinal ligaments that connect hip and pubic bones. They, too, cause pain in the pelvic region. We've already mentioned that spasms may occur in the perineum and add to already overwhelming symptoms. In addition, the irritable bowel syndrome with all of its lower abdominal and rectal problems is present in 60 percent of fibromyalgic women. Twenty-five percent of those with vulvodynia report recurrent bladder infections and/or IC. Therefore, it's not always easy to separate bladder complaints from the vulvodynia complex because of the commonality of symptoms. The same nerves affect all of those regions to spread overlapping symptoms. Because these seemingly separate conditions kept appearing in the same patients, we finally linked them into a single entity. Though we're allocating each a chapter in this section, they're all part of the one big syndrome.

Informed professionals agree that fibromyalgia and vulvodynia are often connected but not always in the high percentages we

Oxalate—A chemical found in the human body as part of the energy production cycle. It is excreted in the urine, and is known as a topical irritant that can cause burning in the tissues. Foods of plant origin, such as fruits and vegetables, are high in oxalates.

contend. You've already read a statement from John Willems, M.D., head of ob-gyn at Scripps Clinic in La Jolla, California. He continues to do pioneering work and has considerable success in easing vulvodynia while acknowledging that those with fibromyalgia must treat that condition as well. As a result, we have many patients in common. Clive Solomons, Ph.D., a research chemist, worked for many years with The Vulvar Pain Foundation (www.thevpfoundation.org) to develop protocols for symptomatic relief for sufferers. Also spearheading education and awareness is the National Vulvodynia Association (www.nva.org). Support is offered through both these groups to help spouses of affected women cope.

For couples, perhaps the most horrible part of all of fibromyalgia is the dyspareunia or painful intercourse that is so common with the vulvar pain syndrome. Women with vulvodynia soon become conditioned to expect excruciating and long-lasting pain during and following intercourse. Soon many become afraid to initiate any contact, even cuddling, for fear that even this bit of intimacy might lead to pelvic disaster. Libido is so dulled and lubricant flow so minimal that just the thought of making love hurts. There's a high incidence of separation and divorce within this subset of fibromyalgia, often due to lack of communication that closes doors. Many women freely admit that they avoid forming new relationships knowing they must eventually perform sexually. A typical story appears below:

Prior to the guaifenesin treatments and my proper diagnosis, the most debilitating pain I would experience was the vulvar pain. The muscle pain could be significantly minimized with pain relievers but not the vulvar pain. In 1989, the vulvar pain became extreme and frequent. It was so severe at times that I would miss work. Because of this pain, I avoided intercourse with my husband and rejected the thought of having a baby.

My only relief from pain was warm baths, but I could not live in the bathtub all the time, so I sought help from my family physician. Even though [he] ... was aware of my other symptoms (acne, muscle pain, insomnia), he focused on each symptom as a separate medical condition and sent me to a variety of specialists. Since he did not focus on the body as a whole and was ignorant of the existence of fibromyalgia, he did not connect my cycles of muscle pain, and fatigue ... with my vulvar pain.

During the first few weeks of taking the guaifenesin I did experience vulvar pain an average of about two out of ten days, and the pain was severe. As I continued to take the guaifenesin, both the frequency and the severity of the pain decreased ... Since January 1995, I have not missed work due to fibromyalgia or vulvar pain. I am not fearful of sexual intercourse, and maybe one day I will even think about having a baby.

—*Angela, California*

Given these obstacles, it's safe to say that the relationships that endure despite vulvodynia are some of the strongest we've seen. Patient and spouse must both be committed to openness and new nonpainful ways of expressing their sexual emotions and drives. (See figure 11.2.)

The blatant and basic assault on these women's fundamental quality of life and the toll it takes on relationships have driven many to embrace drastic "cures." Those who simply purchased miracle creams and lotions were the least harmed by these measures, because for the most part they've suffered only from a wounded purse. Others who may have submitted to repeated injections of synthetic cortisone, alcohol, interferon, and local anesthetics directly into the painful areas may be left with painful scar tissue as a result. Most shocking and horrifying are the reports on file at The Vulvar Pain Foundation describing the unsuccessful and sometimes mutilating and multiple surgeries women have endured. Parts of the labia or vaginal lining were excised in an attempt to eliminate pain-producing tissue. Surgery is too often followed by recurrences and scarring that actually intensified symptoms. In some circles, surgery remains "the thing to do," but more prudent gynecologists hesitate and cut as a last resort. As long as there is the hope that another therapy can reverse symptoms and treat the root cause, it should be the preferred course. With guaifenesin, we are offering just that.

Unfortunately, vulvar pain symptoms are often subjected to treatments based on an incorrect diagnosis. It's common for women to be told (or think they have) a yeast infection that won't quite go away. It's important to remember that not everything that feels itchy is candida. If you don't see the distinctive cottage cheese discharge and your symptoms don't yield to a prescription yeast medication such as oral Diflucan or vaginally inserted boric acid capsules, further investigate the cause. As Dr. Willems says, "If the treatment doesn't work, reconsider the diagnosis." If you're prone to yeast infections, boric acid capsules can be used whenever you suspect a problem. Pharmacists will make them up for you, or you fill size 0 capsules yourself. Get them from a pharmacy or from a health food store. You can insert them nightly for a week or so when you have an infection and once a week if you are prone to them. Some women notice a flare-up of yeast activity the premenstrual week. If so, use boric acid prophylactically.

Dr. Willems has developed a treatment protocol that includes several therapies with refreshingly effective results. He

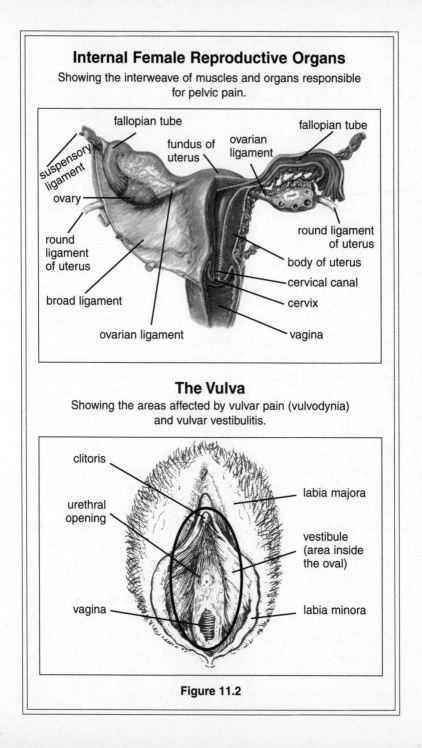

Internal Female Reproductive Organs

Showing the interweave of muscles and organs responsible for pelvic pain.

fallopian tube

fundus of uterus

ovarian ligament

fallopian tube

suspensory ligament

ovary

round ligament of uterus

broad ligament

ovarian ligament

round ligament of uterus

body of uterus

cervical canal

cervix

vagina

The Vulva

Showing the areas affected by vulvar pain (vulvodynia) and vulvar vestibulitis.

clitoris

urethral opening

vagina

labia majora

vestibule (area inside the oval)

labia minora

Figure 11.2

outspokenly condemns surgery done without clear indications or done before all else has failed. He has discovered that some compounds ease symptoms, and others even repair damage. Expert biofeedback and pelvic massage or pelvic floor therapy can make pain bearable and are highly recommended. His protocol is usually initiated using topical estrogen (estradiol) to rebuild vulvar tissue.[1] Fibromyalgic women should insist on hormones mixed with plant-free emollients to avoid undermining guaifenesin effects. There are safe commercial preparations, and compounding pharmacists can easily create them if necessary in a base of such substances as vitamin E—which has also been shown to help in a stand-alone treatment.

When it comes to topical estrogen, Dr. Willems uses Estrace cream as his compound of choice. He's said that Premarin or conjugated estrogen cream can achieve the same goal, but at a significantly slower pace. We stress that vaginal estrogen creams should be used in very small, pea-size amounts and don't significantly alter estrogen levels in the body. In this day of worry about the effects of hormone replacement therapies, topical compounds are not a concern. Once healing has occurred, the maintenance therapy requires lower doses still. (See figure 11.3.)

Emu oil is a natural anti-inflammatory that also has the ability to rebuild thinning, damaged tissue due to its content of fatty acids. For patients already on hormones, it can be used as an adjunct to that therapy. It should be noted that both the topical compounds that rebuild tissue take some time to work. They may increase pain and itching at first and simulate a mild yeast infection. That's fundamentally like the same itching you feel when an incision starts to heal. Some patience is required. Lidocaine in a 2.5 percent solution can be used to deaden pain. Combinations of local anesthetics called EMLA or ELA-Max may also be okay. For some, these are irritating and should be discontinued. Unlike estrogens, they provide only symptomatic relief of symptoms and do not restore tissue.

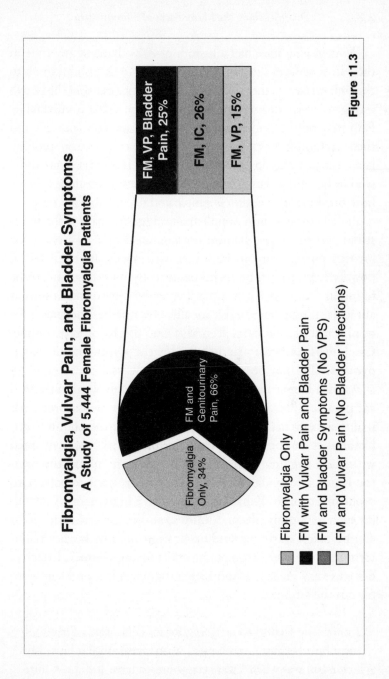

Fibromyalgia, Vulvar Pain, and Bladder Symptoms
A Study of 5,444 Female Fibromyalgia Patients

Fibromyalgia Only, 34%

FM and Genitourinary Pain, 66%

FM, VP, Bladder Pain, 25%

FM, IC, 26%

FM, VP, 15%

- Fibromyalgia Only
- FM with Vulvar Pain and Bladder Pain
- FM and Bladder Symptoms (No VPS)
- FM and Vulvar Pain (No Bladder Infections)

Figure 11.3

Women who have had a history of vulvodynia at any time in their lives or have extremely fair or sensitive skin should talk to their physicians as they approach menopause. Because the body's estrogen levels plummet, this supersensitive tissue is vulnerable. Pain may not be evident until tissue damage has occurred, and then rebuilding those tissues takes time. For this reason, prophylactic therapy should be considered. This is a disaster for those who've become asymptomatic on guaifenesin—recurrences are heartbreaking. Prevention is simple and dependably effective.

Prelief, the calcium supplement suggested earlier for interstitial cystitis, is also helpful for vaginal burning. When used for this purpose, it can be taken with meals. It's available in powder form so can be sprinkled directly onto food. It can be found in drugstores in sections displaying digestive aids such as antacids. If you can't find it locally, www.prelief.com has a list of pharmacies that carry it, and it can also be ordered online. Calcium is known to be helpful for the symptoms of vulvodynia, so this may be beneficial in other ways.

As with interstitial cystitis, mast cells are involved in the vulvar pain complex. To hinder their propensity to disgorge their irritating contents, both prescription and over-the-counter antihistamines can be used. Because it's often difficult for women with such nagging pain to sleep through the night, the over-the-counter formulas for insomnia can be used to solve two problems at once. Benadryl is the active ingredient in formulas such as Simply Sleep, Sominex, and in generic form. This can be taken during a flare-up or even nightly. It's not habit-forming and safe for pregnant and nursing women. Effective dosages vary greatly. If morning grogginess is a problem, simply cut the amount.

I know the feeling about going for a GYN exam. They told me it hurt because I was tense. I wasn't tense until it hurt. My first exam was when I was very young, a teen. It did not hurt at all. That is how it is supposed to be. Then came the FM and so came the pain there. Every person I have had do these exams has basically blamed me. One physician's assistant used a smaller device on me, which helped a little. Ask them to use the kids' one. I think this problem should improve on guai. I do believe it is the FM. You are still young so hopefully the guai will help before marriage. Most husbands are patient with us, or ask for divorce. It is a real sad thing either way.

—*Karen B., Massachusetts*

When simple measures don't adequately control pain, prescription medications may be used. We always view these as stopgap measures while we wait for the protocol to do its job. All but guaifenesin simply suppress symptoms and none are curative or change the course of vulvodynia. Antidepressants are often first selected as they are for other chronic pains of unknown etiology. The older tricyclics such as amitriptyline (Elavil) in dosages that vary from 10 to 50 mg daily are fairly effective because of their relaxing action on smooth muscle. Not all patients experience benefits: If so, quit it and try something else. That statement applies to most other drugs that are too often stacked up one on top of the other without thought of removing the previous, ineffective ones. The tricyclic antidepressant trazodone may help with sleep. Ativan (lorazepam) and Klonopin (clonazepam) should be used more cautiously since they may be habit-forming. Neurontin (gabapentin) is being supplanted by Lyrica (pregabalin); anticonvulsants are the newest class of drugs used despite the very common side effect of weight gain. Savella and Cymbalta, members of a newer class of antidepressants, may be tried although they are much more expensive and have not been shown to be more effective than older compounds. An important note: Older drugs are safer since they've had time to show their side effect fangs; the newer the drug, the less is known about its long-term dangers.

Another benefit of the older drugs, of course, is that they cost many times less.

Clive Solomons, Ph.D., whom we mentioned earlier in the chapter, found that a waste product in the urine, oxalate, was a potent local irritant. In conjunction with The Vulvar Pain Foundation, he developed a low-oxalate diet, which can be found on the website: www.thevpfoundation.org. The Foundation has borne the cost of analyzing foods and has published several cookbooks. If relief from the diet is incomplete, patients are asked to take calcium citrate and a supplement called Ox-Absorb if it is helpful.

There are other things you can do to ease symptoms. Women soon learn to avoid tight jeans, nylon underwear, and pantyhose. Seams press into the vagina and severely irritate or chafe vulnerable tissues. Obviously, wear only clothes that are loose in the crotch. Use unscented white toilet paper (aloe and dye-free) or avoid all toilet paper altogether and use distilled water spritzes (to avoid chlorine) and blot the area with a soft cloth. Urine is normally acid and therefore burns the already-irritated vulvae. Try pouring distilled water over the area as you urinate to wash the tissue and dilute the urine as you void. Do not use bubble bath or scented soaps, and make sure underwear is rinsed twice. Simply inserting a tampon can further damage the injured tissues. Instead, use white unscented cotton menstrual pads (such as GladRags). When you're well enough to attempt intercourse, stay with water-soluble lubricants such as Astroglide that are nonirritating. Bike riding and sitting for long periods without moving always make symptoms worse. Exercise and stretching may be painful at first, but with time they'll prove beneficial.

I have suffered from vulvar pain since 1990. I went everywhere for help. I even flew to Michigan for laser surgery from a now infamous doctor. I hooked up with The Vulvar Pain

Foundation and found out about the low-oxalate diet and citrate. I began this treatment and got a little better. I added Estrace cream per Dr. Willems at Scripps Clinic in La Jolla, California...I found out about Dr. St. Amand from the VP Foundation and read up on him. I firmly believed that I did not have FMS because I didn't have the body aches and pains. But as I read through the symptoms of FMS, I was astounded. I was reading my life's history. I began the guaifenesin, and the first thing that left me was the vulvar pain. Now I do indeed have the general aches and pains (but that's due to the cycling). I also realize that I have a high pain tolerance and just tolerated the aches. I cycled fairly quickly. Dr. St. Amand recently mapped me, and I'm almost cleared out!

—*Mary B., Alabama*

We've usually seen guaifenesin eradicate the above symptoms, given sufficient time. Patience and gentle management are required for healing the damaged tissue of vulvodynia. Some maintenance measures may be required for life, but none is particularly intrusive or demanding. Extremely sensitive women may wish to avoid Mucinex, the bilayered guaifenesin, because the blue dye can be a problem for them. A dye-free compounded guaifenesin is available from Marina del Rey Pharmacy (www.fibropharmacy.com).

Chapter Twelve

Dermatologic Symptoms

When I first started the protocol, my face and the back of my neck and upper back broke out *reallllly reallllly* bad. I was so embarrassed. I wore high collars at the back and tried lots of makeup to cover up my face. But around my mouth and chin were probably 50 bumps at one time and it lasted for a good six months. It was so awful. But it takes time for those phosphates to purge out and I think that's what was going on. As a teenager (and adult), I always had problems with my oily skin. I cycled there for a couple of months, but then after those first few months, I rarely had another breakout.

—*Jan, Kentucky*

WE'VE DEVOTED ENTIRE chapters describing the fibromyalgic assault on susceptible systems. Long before we wrote the first edition of this book, most experts in the field had realized that the musculoskeletal and central nervous systems were both victims of the same illness. Some are now becoming aware of the extent of gastrointestinal tract involvement. Newer studies are emerging connecting genitourinary tract problems with fibromyalgia. Almost none speak or write about the accompanying eye, ear, nose, and throat symptoms that most patients suffer. We'll describe that cluster in chapter 13. Meanwhile, we have clearly seen that FMS certainly affects the skin, nails, and hair—yet we know of no researchers or authors who are working on this connection. This chapter is dedicated to our observations on this subject.

SKIN

I have had this consistently since I got sick; my first symptoms being fatigue, itching rashes, and hives. I have been a notorious complainer about pins and needles, tingling, and painful burning of the skin. The itching intensified when I started the guai in November 1996. I used to use Benadryl almost every night for this. I also tried Caladryl, Benadryl cream, cortisone cream, etc. I have found several things that help: (1) dry brushing with a bath brush before a shower; (2) using a bath brush in a bath with 1 cup each of Epsom salts, sea salts, and baking soda (take a shower afterwards to wash off the salt); (3) Lac-Hydrin or Aquaphor lotion; and (4) Benadryl or prescription medications for itching or sleep at night. It has started to get better for me after a year and three months on guai.

—Heather, Texas

Skin is made up of layers, the dermis and the epidermis, and one of subcutaneous fat directly beneath. The epidermis is constantly active and creates new cells as they push older ones up toward the surface, where they flatten to become squamous cells. Those, too, finally move farther outward to become the scaly stratum corneum that's ultimately sloughed off. The average life expectancy of a skin cell is one month. The dermis has large amounts of collagen that serves as supportive tissue. Obviously, the skin contains blood, nerve, lymph, and muscle cells along with hair follicles and sebaceous glands. As you might imagine, it takes a lot of energy to keep this huge system running properly. Fibromyalgics are energy-challenged everywhere, even in the skin.

Table 12.1
Dermatologic System

	Male	Percentage Male	Female	Percentage Female
Number of patients	596		3,444	
Skin hypersensitivity	183	31	1,741	50
Itching	414	70	2,478	72
Rashes	284	48	2,042	59
Brittle nails	188	31	2,480	72
Easy bruising	122	20	2,617	76
Excessive sweating	349	58	2,256	66

All types of rashes smear the skin of fibromyalgics, such as eczema, nonpustular acne, seborrhea, hives, rosacea, large red patches, tiny red bumps, scaly-dry areas, and small blisters. Diagnoses such as dermatitis and psoriasis are appended, as are mysterious, unnamed eruptions that don't quite fit into existing nomenclature. Nails crack, chip, or peel and are often ridged. Cuticles shred, get thickened, and tear. Hair is usually of poor quality, dry, short lived, and so falls out prematurely. All of these defects are interrelated and well comply with our explanations.

In 1998, a scientific paper reported mast cell involvement in fibromyalgia. These are highly specialized white blood cells that produce more than thirty identified chemicals and proteins. There were twenty-two women in that study. They underwent skin biopsies that showed such cells disgorging themselves of their contents into the epidermis, the deepest layer of skin. Their stockpile includes histamine, a strong perpetrator of allergic reactions, including itching, hives, and other rashes. They're also involved in the immune response. People with hay fever can certainly attest to histamine's handiwork: swelling of affected areas; itchy eyes and nose; excessive tearing; cascades of sneezing; congested sinuses; wheezy lungs; and a faucet-like, runny nose. Other studies have also found higher-than-normal blood and tissue levels of histamine in fibromyalgic individuals. The compound also attacks the lining of bronchial tubes, lungs (asthma), bladder wall (interstitial cystitis), and vaginal tissues (vulvodynia). Mast cells are also implicated in facial flushing, cramps, and diarrhea. They gradually attract another type of white blood cell, the eosinophil, which intensifies these body-wide disruptions almost to perpetuity. Sound familiar? These findings have been documented system by system and merely lack the unifying theory that fibromyalgia provides. It's estimated that about 20 percent of the population has suffered from hives at one time or another.

Interesting but disconcerting is the tiny foot of immunoglobulin G that suddenly protrudes through the wall of a stimulated mast cell. It sticks on to a willing receptor in the epidermis. Immunoglobulin G is a known stimulator of auto-immune reactions. Do you wonder that, in combination with histamine, the skin can be supersensitive, on fire, itch, and explode over a person evoking strange sensations? Mast cells are also activated by a brain factor called CRF (corticotropin releasing factor) secreted into the bloodstream under stress conditions. Starting to make sense? The body triggers its cells, including the brain, to respond to anything irritating, injurious, or deemed foreign in its tissues.[1]

Only in recent years have we realized the variety and extent of skin symptoms in fibromyalgia. Nowadays, we expect patients to report tingling sensations in their fingers, toes, or scattered areas such as the face and lips. All kinds of other weird effects appear. Crawling feelings anywhere on the skin feel like errant hairs or insects that are never there. Burning can be felt anywhere on the surface of the body, commonly on the back of the neck, arms, or thighs; sometimes the opposite, a cold swatch of skin joins in. Fibromyalgics ritualistically cut irritating tags off their clothes before putting them on for the first time. Fiery hot, itchy soles and palms are relentless. So intense is this burning sensation that I would pull my feet out from under the covers even on a winter night. Symptoms in my hands were best relieved by holding bagged ice wrapped in a washcloth. I'm certainly not the only one who has made such improvisations.

> Sensitive skin is something many of us feel. Just a breeze on my skin feels like knife blades cutting me. Just a touch on my skin is painful like a blow. I'm always having traveling pains and shooting pains. Weather changes make it worse. I can't stand extra weight on my skin so I sleep with light covers. Heavy ones hurt. I can't tolerate synthetic fiber clothing at all. So I wear 100 percent cotton everything. I have to wear my underwear inside out so the seams don't hurt. I put all my clothes through about four extra rinse cycles because any detergent left over will irritate my skin. I cycle rashes.
>
> —*Ron C., California*

Nearly all fibromyalgics experience itching. It's generally worse and spreads at night because of the warmth generated under blankets. Humid weather is also a trigger. I soon learned not to scratch. Even gentle rubbing seemed to set in motion a seven-year itch that didn't stop even when my skin was bloody from scratching. When itching began in the evening, I knew I was in for a particularly sleepless night. It signaled another distressing round of fibromyalgia.

Generalized hives (urticaria) are among the worst rashes. A woman flight attendant was the first to show us how intensely those could affect a person. For many years, she suffered bouts of a strange type of giant hives that oddly involved only her face and neck. Each patch was accompanied by an underlying redness and an unusual amount of swelling. She described herself looking "like a gargoyle." We finally saw her during one of those cycles and I reluctantly complimented her on the accuracy of her description. On hive days, she had to call in sick to cancel flights. She'd undergone exhaustive testing for allergies and autoimmune diseases. We had never thought there was a connection between hives and fibromyalgia. Under treatment, the mystery unraveled.

She was the first to realize that hives always appeared during her pain cycles. In between attacks, her skin was clear. As you'd expect from the story, there's a happy ending. She's now almost totally free of fibromyalgia attacks, and in her rare and mild reversal cycles, she no longer has to deal with the unwelcome skin intrusions. Less fortunate as of this writing, we have another, more severely affected patient who is covered from head to toe with never totally remitting hives (chronic urticaria). She, too, is distinctly worse during her more intense cycles of fibromyalgia. To our knowledge, she has never totally overcome this perpetual torture.

Cortisone or topical steroid creams are often suggested for hives but generally are not very effective. The reason is that hives are caused by dilation of the capillaries, which allows fluid to leak into the surrounding tissue. Angioedema is the result of a similar but deeper process in which fluid seeps ever deeper, permeating the dermis, epidermis, and subcutaneous tissues. Since creams can't penetrate very deeply, they only improve the appearance of surface layers. Yet neither cortisone creams nor topical antihistamines (example: Benadryl cream) are blockers as long as no plant derivatives have been added.

Hives can be acute (episodic) or chronic as mentioned above. Chronic hives are those that have appeared at least twice a week for longer than six weeks, although that number is somewhat arbitrary. In 75 percent of patients, hives last longer than one year; 50 percent, longer than five years. In 70 percent of those cases, no cause is ever identified. Sometimes they're accompanied by an autoimmune thyroid condition that can be confirmed by blood tests. Allergy skin testing isn't much help because most people with hives react to most substances applied to their skin.

Chronic hives are less responsive to treatment and much harder to relieve. Once released, histamine effects are not easily blocked even by antihistamine taken on a regular basis. Antianxiety drugs have been used with some success in select patients, but they cause fatigue and are not used long term. Histamine-2 blockers such as Pepcid and Zantac, or Nexium and Prilosec, work by a different mechanism and may undependably benefit hives. One of the tricyclic drugs, doxepin, powerfully blocks histamine release, so is often used for patients with allergic skin eruptions. Brief courses of oral steroids may be given for particularly severe outbursts of hives. They're counterproductive in the long-term usage because of risky side effects such as causing osteoporosis, immune system depression, cataracts, ulcers, diabetes, and high blood pressure. Ephedrine is a powerful histamine blocker, but raises blood pressure and speeds the heart. Beta-blockers help a bit (propanolol, atenolol, metoprolol etc.), but they may too effectively slow the heart rate and drop blood pressure.

About 16 percent of patients with chronic hives can identify a physical stimulus for the rash. Exercise is one such trigger for histamine release as is anything that induces sweating. A few people are sensitive to cold, sun, heat, and or prolonged skin dampness. Topical doxepin is marketed as Zonalon, and will not interfere with guaifenesin.

I just got over the itching. It lasted for three weeks. All the Benadryl and prescriptions for itching didn't help it much at all. What helped me was just plain Tylenol or Advil. Heat seemed to make it worse but ice did help. I was also given a prescription for a lotion to use that would keep the skin from looking too bad from all of the scratching. It was Aquaphor ointment. After my itching was finally over, I did go into a pain cycle and am now coming out of it. In fact, today I feel pretty good. Yay Guai!

—*Katy, Arkansas*

Most of our fibromyalgia patients have visited dermatologists and learned that their scattered, dry, and scaly patches was eczema or neurodermatitis. The worst case we've ever seen was in a young attorney. His entire body was affected, but most distressing were his cracked, bleeding, and scabby hands. He was so embarrassed that he stopped offering clients a handshake. His appearance so overwhelmed him that he virtually ignored his muscular aches, fatigue, and minor cognitive difficulties. Upon mapping, we found the telltale lumps and bumps of fibromyalgia. While we could at least reassure him about the anticipated muscle recovery with treatment, we couldn't promise resolution of his skin issues. On guaifenesin, his rash became worse during each of the early reversing cycles. We took that as a good sign. Patchy improvement soon appeared and eventually cleared, never to return.

In my own case, patches of seborrheic dermatitis tormented me. Despite the superficial scaling, some tiny, broken skin areas constantly burned and felt raw. They were concentrated in my scalp, eyebrows, the sides of my nose, and adjacent cheeks. I would also get intensely itchy, tiny blisters on my fingers. I deliberately burst them since I much preferred the burning of the denuded base I'd left behind. Patients have described similar eruptions on other body surfaces. Psoriatic lesions often worsen during attacks of fibromyalgia. Psoriasis is characterized by small areas of red-pink, flaky, itchy, and scaly patches. They occur primarily on the scalp, backs of elbows, knees, and lower spine. They're ugly to look at, but at least aren't contagious. Like many other rashes, stress, alcohol, and climate changes make symptoms worse. However, short sun exposures help. The vitamin D derivative, Dovonex, coal tar preparations in cleansers, shampoos, and baths are safe to use with guaifenesin.

One night I was speaking to members of a support group and found it hard to avoid staring at one woman's face. She had been diagnosed with rosacea, which produces a distinctly red color, but hers was a deep magenta. It's another skin problem related to eosinophils, mast cells, and histamine cohorts that sting and burn, but don't itch. Eyelids and skin around the cheeks may be worst hit. Red bumps and pimples may emerge, and thread-like blood vessels become visible over time. During treatment, this woman soon observed that her most intense displays cycled in step with her fibromyalgia. She's now symptom-free, and the rosacea has cleared. Rosacea currently has no known cause, but things that cause flushing, such as extremes of heat or cold, rubbing or scrubbing, spicy foods, and alcohol, make it worse. Dermatologists sometimes prescribe metronidazole cream; that does not block guaifenesin. Some patients keep diaries to help identify triggers. Most of them find that the number one is the fibromyalgic flare.

A less dramatic, restricted or generalized flushing of the face or upper torso may appear only during adverse cycles. People with this problem can use a fingernail or blunt instrument to write on their skin and leave an inscription that remains legible for several minutes. This condition is called *dermatographia* and is caused by a linear swelling of capillaries that force edema into the skin.

Approximately eighteen to twenty-four months before I was diagnosed with FMS, I was diagnosed with rosacea. I was devastated. Now looking back on it, I see that a lot of things were going wrong back then, but it was the symptoms on my face that got me to the doctors originally. I took tetracycline daily for three years. I hated it, but if I stopped, I broke out so bad, and my skin would peel away, and I was red!!! Within a few weeks of starting the guai, I gave up the tetracycline as an experiment. I have not used it since. The symptoms have been manageable, although stress will trigger the rosacea again. Right now I am in a bit of a flare over a new job, but not enough to send me back to the tetracycline. My eyelashes grew back, and fell out, and grew back. I am very confident that the longer I am on the guai, the scare of rosacea will be behind me.

—*Dawn, California*

Many fibromyalgia patients suddenly experience outbreaks of acne. It's not uncommon to hear, "I must be in my second childhood," or "I never even had pimples in high school." Acne, whiteheads, and blackheads may be caused by blocked pores that are induced by the pubertal, hormonal surges of testosterone. Acne recurrences are frequent in fibromyalgia, but not pustules or blackheads. Patients connect acne to cyclic fibromyalgic assaults. Sufficiently bothersome, it may be effectively treated using a mild antibacterial cleanser. During troublesome outbreaks, spot treatment with benzoyl peroxide or triclosan might work. Acne products should be carefully screened for salicylic acid, which is regularly used in soaps, washes, cleansers, toners, scrubs, etc.

Common sense should be exercised by those with irritated, fibromyalgic skin. Expensive is rarely better than cheap when buying skin products. Itchy eyes, facial flushing, or flushing of the upper torso and rosacea are quick reminders that mast cells are active. Avoiding triggers is an all too obvious suggestion. Here are just a few: sun exposure, excessive heat, irritant botanicals, citrus extracts, alcohol, hot drinks or foods, biting spices, dyes, strong fragrances, and warm baths. Appropriately, many women who purge their products report improved skin tone and texture when they dump multiple ingredients. A good admonition: Keep it simple.

Treat dry, flaky skin by regular use of an alpha hydroxy acid cream or lotion. My coauthor, Claudia Marek, advocates AmLactin or Lac-Hydrin. They contain lactic acid, the skin's natural alpha hydroxy. Pamper such skin with gentle moisturizers and by avoiding bad items listed above. Some waxy compounds seal in moisture. Surgeon's Secret (www.jamarklabs .com) and Elta (www.buyelta.com) are companies that manufacture several helpful products. Prescription retinoids are also okay with guaifenesin: Both Retin-A and Renova soothe acne breakouts if your skin can tolerate them as will triclosan and benzoyl peroxide compounds if not.

FINGERNAILS

Nearly everyone in my support group can identify with having bad fingernails that break. Lots of us have dry fingertips that are always cracking. My nails finally got so weak that I could not even wear acrylic nails because my nails would bend and break underneath them. It took several years on guai, but now my nails are much stronger. I know they will never be glamorous, but at least they are normal and look presentable.

—*Janeen, Idaho*

During a new patient visit, we have a checklist of sequential questions and check off answers. That's how we get the statistics we quote in this book. Patients relate some of them spontaneously so we only have to further quiz them about the ones not mentioned. That's how we can state with considerable accuracy that "among the last 6,000 patients, 75% will have..." such and such a symptom. One slot on the list asks about the status of their fingernails. Some have them hidden under acrylics that hide the mangled, underlying nail.

Thinning, chipping, and breaking are extremely common in fibromyalgia. Sometimes defective nails don't break, but just peel off like sheets of mica. Early in the FM game, nails do fairly well, but they eventually lay down alternating good and bad layers, and suddenly four or five of them break all at once. In long-standing fibromyalgia, they're forever broken or don't even grow. You'll understand this phenomenon by comparing nails to concentric rings in trees. During untreated fibromyalgic cycles, there's an abnormal concentration of debris in the bloodstream. These minute excesses visit all parts of the body, as you've seen in earlier chapters. Tiny clusters of calcium phosphate hunker down in the nail root as fragile and unstructured sediments. Outward growth over the next eight to ten months brings the brittle, horizontal ring to the nail tip. Like so much dried mortar, all it takes is minuscule pressure to chip it off from the adjacent, healthier layer. Even during successful treatment, nails keep doing the same thing. It's from the same fundamental mechanism. When debris pulls out of muscles and other sinews, it sails into the bloodstream destined for renal excretion. Kidneys are a bit slow responding, as we've theorized. Delayed urinary extraction permits blood-borne calcium phosphate to linger just long enough to repeat past performances at the nail bed. Under treatment, nails stay solid for ever-longer periods of time until they become as strong as individual genetic makeup allows.

Hangnails are common because the softened fingernail easily tears at its edges. I also remember dry, thick, cracked skin around my nails and knuckles before I treated myself. It was hard to explain since the problem lingered throughout the seasons regardless of weather. Cuticles may get dry, irritated, or shred, and the whole area may crack and bleed. Rubbing vitamin E, lanolin, or emu oil into the affected sites is helpful. Immersing fingers into warm paraffin helps somewhat.

Some fibromyalgics have problems with nail fungus. It's not

really related to fibromyalgia except that the immune system might not be quite up to par. Drugstores sell topical compounds that should be checked for salicylates; the prescription drug Penlac is compatible with guaifenesin. Oral antifungal medications need to be taken for several months since nails are so slow to grow out. It may be unsafe for patients already on multiple oral medications to add another: It's safer to stick with topical products.

While waiting for the lengthy correction, soothe the areas by gently massaging nails, cuticles, and adjacent skin with the oily substances we mentioned above. Disguising the glaring defects with artificial nails is tempting, but lack of aeration further weakens the underlying bed. Best to let nails regain their normal strength and flexibility. It takes twelve to eighteen months for toenails to grow from the root to the free edge, and eight to ten months for fingernails. Certain paint-on nail strengtheners add synthetic fibers to hold the defective nail together. Use them as first-line treatments to protect vertical fractures from extending down into the nail bed. When you're applying expensive treatments to dead tissue, remember the visible part of nails lacks nutritive blood supplies. Ignore extravagant claims and just accept that you're coating for cosmetic effects.

HAIR

You will notice [after beginning guaifenesin] your hair is getting back to normal, actually better. Mine used to be dry, but got to where I could go a few days before I had to wash it (when I was sick, I didn't wash it for three days and it wasn't greasy). My hair is very healthy now. Just give it some time. I am taking 3,600 mg of guaifenesin a day, and have been totally pain free for about three months.

—*Mary B., Florida*

Fibromyalgic hair is often limp, poor textured, slow growing, and willing to make split ends. Defective energy production extends even to hair follicles. Hair normally falls out in cycles, but now, a whole bunch may come out at one time. Maybe you understand that when you're sick, but it may also get worse in the fourth or fifth month on guaifenesin treatment. Fibromyalgia reversal goes faster than did the slower accumulation of the compounds that cause it. Convalescence is also accelerated, but defective hairs come out sooner than normal ones take their place. It's a good general rule for the entire body: Mainly sick tissues participate in the cleansing process. Test results are usually normal and scalp pathology is rarely found, so we've given up referring to dermatologists unless someone needs a reassuring consultation. Luckily, expert hairdressers are our allies. They're used to instructing clients about periodic hair loss though perhaps not when it's as flagrant as in fibromyalgia. They easily spot healthy new growth to reassure patients and inspire them not to panic.

Many compounds are advertised to help hair growth, but when dealing with hair loss caused by fibromyalgia, patience is the best medicine. Gentle shampoos, conditioners, and a good stylist are the best weapons, along with time. Minoxidil (Rogaine) is the only product approved for female hair loss. It needs to be applied daily, which is a burdensome chore for someone too tired to make such efforts. Any favorable growth is abruptly lost if applications are stopped. Younger women with hair loss should avoid contraceptives that contain testosterone or DHEA—both have masculinizing effects on the body.

Two thirds of women and most men lose hair with aging. Don't expect the quasi-miraculous guaifenesin to produce a full head of lustrous hair you never had. Though quality may improve, there's a limit imposed by your age and genetic makeup. When you're reading promotional advertising, remember that, like nails, only roots are alive: Nails are dead. So nothing can improve beyond nicer touch and surface appearances. Lots of products accomplish exactly that, and they don't have to be pricey.

With the exception of chronic hives or psoriasis, most dermatological problems are not serious. They can be managed with gentleness, routines such as using lukewarm water instead of hot, and dabbing in place of scrubbing. A few gentle, unscented products are enough. Over time guaifenesin may render all this attention unnecessary.

> I have been losing a lot of hair. The part that I minded most is all of the little hairs that are coming in. I walked in the snow the other day, and when I got home, there was all of this fuzzy dandelion fuzz sticking out—my hair is very curly-frizzy. Then I went to the hairdresser and she was pleased that I had so much healthy new hair coming in. I didn't know that it was new hair growth and that I am on my way to healthier stuff.
>
> —*Jan, Kentucky*

Chapter Thirteen

Head, Eye, Ear, Nose, and Throat Syndrome

YEARS AGO IN medicine, there was a specialty in head, eye, ear, nose, and throat (HEENT). Then eyes became too complicated to remain part of the grouping, and it's now a stand-alone discipline. Perhaps as a reflection of my years in medicine, this chapter will deal with the all-inclusive cluster of symptoms, all of HEENT. Most fibromyalgics find at least a few problems in their heads: Not the psychological kind, just the outer structures! Some physicians in this limited field are beginning to connect them to the underlying disease. We've added this chapter so that you can!

> I could always tell when my younger son, Sean, was in a cycle, although he did not complain much of pain. When I would wake him up for school in the morning, his eyes would be almost glued shut with gooky stuff. I would have to put a wet washcloth over his eyes and let it sit for a while to soak this off. The clumps in his eyelashes were stiff and incredibly hard to get out. Those were the days when he would wake up irritable and tired, and have the most trouble in school.
>
> —*C.C., California*

Fibromyalgics have problems with the inner skin, the mucosa, the name given to all moist membranes of the body. These areas are subject to the irritating effects of fibromyalgia.

Table 13.1
Head, Eye, Ear, Nose, Throat

	Male	Percentage Male	Female	Percentage Female
Number of patients	596		3,444	
Frontal headaches	320	54	2,202	64
Occipital headaches	279	47	2,150	62
Generalized headaches	214	36	1,412	41
Dizziness	442	74	2,921	85
Vertigo	113	19	1,305	38
Imbalance	498	84	2,716	79
Faintness	113	19	992	29
Blurred vision	284	48	2,194	64
Eye irritation	365	61	2,486	72
Nasal congestion	410	69	2,610	76
Abnormal tastes	291	49	2,157	63
Bad taste	223	37	1,829	53
Metallic taste	190	32	1,639	48
Ringing ears	351	59	2,139	62
Unusual sensitivities	137	23	1,371	40
Light	154	26	1,071	31
Odors	86	14	1,236	36
Sounds	83	14	844	24

One reason is that the watery secretions that keep them wet become acidic and create surface burning. Eyes react with excessive tearing that dries during the night. As water evaporates, it leaves behind mucus and calcium phosphate crystals. By morning, only a sticky, sometimes gritty "sand" lies in the corners of the eyelids. It's a mistake trying to rub it away since lids get scratched and then remain irritated for a few days. It's better to rinse and gently dissolve them using a wet washcloth.

It's tough not to keep fingering itchy lids. Imperceptible, soapy residuals are forced into already damaged tissue. That further removes protective mucus, and if the eyeball shares the irritation, vision blurs. Even dim light from TV screens makes patients wince, and brighter sources are downright painful. Contact lenses are extremely irritating at these times, get cloudy, and need constant cleaning. Light sensitivity occurs, and patients instinctively shove sunglasses into place, anticipating the sunlight. Ophthalmic-safe creams help the lids, and artificial tears provide a protective corneal cover. Hold something cool over the eyes; use chilled cloths or well-wrapped ice inserted into plastic bags and keep water from further marinating the lids. Such tissues are very sensitive and may get "burned" by anything excessively cold.

Blurred vision can have other causes as well. There are four eye muscles attached to each eyeball. They're hooked into the orbits and coordinate eye movements. Any of the eight can be affected by fibromyalgia. In my early years with the disease, I could feel swelling, spasm, and tenderness in any one of them at different times. Blurred vision results when these fibromyalgic muscles tire from trying to synchronize focus.

The lens of the eye is a living gel-like structure. It participates in fluid shifts and admits nutritive substances through its membranes. Blood constituents move in and out under tight control. Just as glucose can enter to excess, so can calcium phosphate. Any ion intrusion has to be accompanied by water to guarantee safe dilutions. Extra water loads thicken the lens and alter the focal point to induce temporary nearsightedness. When they're eventually sucked out, the lens flattens to a more farsighted state. Ever-changing lens thickness causes blurring, and fibromyalgics periodically fight to maintain focus. This is not a good time to get a new eyeglass prescription—it will be wrong for you. Remember, reversing cycles reproduce symptoms, so blurring will occur whether the disease is getting better or worse.

At other times, both eyes get dry and red, what we call injected. Tears don't stream out adequately; even the mucous channels get dammed up. When inner eyelids desiccate, patients blink excessively. It doesn't help much since few coating lubricants are there to meet the challenge. Eyelid muscles share the upset, blink and twitch with rapid winking, suggesting a nervous tic. The only way to stop this performance is by holding light finger pressure on the offending lid. Since dryness may provoke this scenario, wet with artificial tears. There are many over-the-counter brands and prescription formulations such as Bion Tears, GenTeal, Lacri-Lube, etc. Watch out for those that contain castor oil.

I am forty-seven and have had dry eyes for what seems forever. I recently had to go to the doctor it got so bad. My left eye first turned so red I thought I had an infection. Then because the antibiotic dried it even more than normal, I scratched my eye with my own eyelid. That was corrected, but the dryness continued. My doctor gave me a prescription for an eye drop. This I use in the a.m. and p.m. In between for lubrication I use Bausch & Lomb artificial tears. My eyes still get "glued" in the a.m., but not as bad. So it has gotten somewhat better, just not cured. I do believe it is the fibro. I always had dry eyes, just not as bad. They will probably start to get better at times and worse at times.

—*Christine, California*

EARS

I, too, have noise sensitivity that comes and goes. Some days I cannot tolerate the sound of the TV or radio. I cannot tolerate noisy neighbors who play the radio with the bass blaring into my home. It drives me crazy and I have been known to tell some of them off for it. Sometimes I cannot tolerate the noise in restaurants of people talking, kitchen clattery, etc. Other days noise does not bother me. I can say now that after these years on guai, it is getting better. But I was raised on a farm, where there was no noise, and to this day, I miss it.

—*Char, California*

Women have more acute senses than men, and they're kicked up an octave during bad flares of fibromyalgia. Regardless of sex, heightened sensitivities to light, sounds, and odors often surface. Any of the three can trigger headaches and, oddly enough, nausea. For some reason, television noise is sometimes unbearable, especially when shows have built-in laugh or augmented sound tracks. Anyone with a fibromyalgic spouse is familiar with the anguished shout from the next room: "Turn the TV down!"

Ringing in the ears can start suddenly out of nowhere. It's almost always brief, but occasionally it persists for hours. If that sound is steady and unchanging, it's usually not due to fibromyalgia. Less frequently there's a buzzing or the sensation of flapping insect wings deep in the auditory canal.

Hearing is at times dulled, and momentary deafness may follow. Many years ago, I lost my hearing in one ear for two days. I was in my thirties, and the sudden onset was frightening. A colleague looked into the canal and found nothing. My premature deafness cleared as quickly as it appeared and never returned—except maybe a bit with old age!

Externally, the ears may turn a glowing red like a Christmas tree ornament that's been plugged into a light socket. They feel burned and, at times, sensitive to touch—forget about trying to wear earrings. The canals may itch and invite a Q-tip misadventure that temporarily satisfies, but usually resurrects the same discomfort within a few hours. If flakiness and dry skin are visible, a gentle oil may be applied. Emu oil, because of its anti-inflammatory properties, is a good choice.

Generally, the symptoms arising from the ears need little intervention because they come and go so rapidly. Tinnitus spells become most unwelcome intrusions that make it tough to get to sleep. At quiet times, noises in your ears are unnerving especially if unrelenting. There are counterbalancing, noise-producing gadgets that mitigate the steady drone; quiet music may also render offensive sounds less audible.

> Someone recommended the book to me *Too Loud, Too Bright, Too Fast, Too Tight: What to Do if You Are Sensory Defensive in an Overstimulating World*, by Sharon Heller, Ph.D. Whether my sensory defectiveness came along with the FMS, I am not sure, but this book sure helped me understand these things better. It also helped explain things to my nine-year-old son.
>
> —*Kathy, Florida*

NOSE

> My sinuses have cleared up considerably—I used to have a tissue in my hand twenty-four hours a day. Now I'm not even taking Allegra except during ragweed season. I used to get colds or sinus infections three to four times a year. I haven't been sick since I started guai.
>
> —*Karen, Texas*

Nasal membranes are not immune to fibromyalgia. Histamine release can cause sudden bursts of liquid mucus either from the nose or as postnasal drip. Waking hours may be spent sniffing, blowing noses, or clearing throats. Mucus drainage is usually clear, but the appearance of yellow or green phlegm can indicate a superimposed infection that requires treatment. Because of the excess mucus, affected individuals mistakenly blame their sinuses for the frontal headaches of fibromyalgia. Antihistamines may dry some of the offending discharge; during the day be sure to use nondrowsy varieties. It's not likely that an allergy medication will contain natural salicylates because plants are often the culprit that causes them. We've mentioned that the bodily secretions of fibromyalgia are acidic. Delicate nasal membranes are easily burned by surges of watery mucus. Inopportune bursts of sneezing are triggered by such irritation and represent nature's effort to blast out some particulate offender. Itching of the nasal tip emerges out of nowhere; even with rigorous rubbing, relief is scant.

Facial rosacea also attacks the nose, causing it to light up and swell a bit. It's slightly suggestive of Rudolph's dilemma and requires a lot of powdering to dim the glow. Patchy areas of pimples and irritation can occur anywhere on the body but are most annoying on the face. The dry mucosa of the nose may crack and easily bleed. Mineral oil, vitamin E, or plain Vaseline can soothe, coat, and protect the area from repeated assaults by Kleenex. If you have sensitive skin, you may prefer a soft cloth handkerchief.

Some odors are amazingly oppressive. Sensitive patients become ill from exposure to scented lotions, colognes, and perfumes. It often takes some effort to find personal and household cleaning products that don't irritate them or set off symptoms. Headaches may spring up after a brief exposure, sometimes accompanied by nausea. It's difficult to totally avoid exposure because of the prevalence of fragrances and heavy perfumes in public places. Some patients have to submit requests for participants at planned events to abstain from using scented products. Some patients are actually disabled because of their sensitivity.

THROAT

I've...found that sinus problems and IBS can both cause bad breath. For at least ten years, I've finished brushing my teeth by brushing my tongue and brush way to the back (I have no gag reflex). My daughter commented how I don't have bad breath anymore as I used to have from time to time. I don't have the chronic sinus drainage that I used to have before guai, nor the allergies and such, either. IBS is fading, too. Guai is changing my life one step at a time...or is that one pill a day.

—*Sandy, California*

The entire surface of the mouth and throat is lined with almost equally sensitive membranes. Salivary glands secrete digestively helpful and also unwanted compounds, which include phosphate (phosphoric acid) excesses. Such acidic secretions can scald like an excessively hot cup of coffee leaving a burned sensation. We can blame similar outputs for the sour or metallic sensations that invade our taste buds. Saliva leaks out during sleep and causes rashes around the corners of the mouth (more often visible in small children and fair-skinned people). More distant membranes aren't impervious to the acid wash, which can cause a sore throat or dry, hacking cough. Menthol-free cough drops, such as Fruit Breezers, xylitol "mints," Halls Fruit Flavored Drops, or old-fashioned Luden's are some products that won't block guaifenesin. The same caveat: Avoid mint, mentholated, and medical-strength herbal lozenges.

Let's not forget dental calculus. We discussed the nature of tartar crystals very early in this book. You may remember that they're largely made up of calcium phosphate, components pouring out from saliva. These small crystals wedge between the teeth and invade surrounding tissues to cause gingivitis. Salivary glands may swell slightly, ache, and become tender when irritated by their own acid contents. It's not uncommon for gums to bleed when brushed, especially in the early stages of reversal as tartar softens.

The tongue shares the bathwater. It sports the largest number of oral taste buds. Like any other muscle, it may become tender or feel as though it were cut. Sometimes only the borders are affected as if they'd been abraded by an emery board and unduly sensitive when rubbed against the teeth. Foods may seem altered, tasteless, or distressingly foul. During fibromyalgic flare-ups, mouth sores may revisit, suggesting a herpes resurgence; often they're of unknown, not viral origin (aphthous stomatitis). Smaller sores can be chemically cauterized using an old-fashioned, styptic pencil. Various compounds will shorten a true herpetic cold sore onslaught, e.g. Abreva, acyclovir, and zinc lip balms.

> As a dentist who treats patients with fibromyalgia, I often get complains of constant battles with bad breath. There are many reasons why this occurs, including medication, oral hygiene habits, the foods you're eating, the dental products you use, and old, defective fillings, crowns (caps) or dentures. Many medications have a side effect which leaves the mouth dry. This is a major contributor to bad breath. In general, bad breath is caused by sulfur gases that are given off by bacteria. If you clean your mouth thoroughly—flossing, brushing the gums and cleaning the tongue—bad breath will be history.
> —*Flora Stay, D.D.S.*

A common complaint in fibromyalgia is dry mouth, with or without dry eyes. It's sometimes part of the illness, but just as often it's a side effect of medication. Antidepressants, sleeping pills, and muscle relaxants are such offenders. Physicians should be consulted before altering the dosage of a causative medication. Treatments include toothpastes designed for dry mouth such as Cleure unflavored (www.cleure.com) and their nonmint xylitol breath fresheners which increase salivary flow. Strong flavors such as cinnamon may further irritate the oral tissue. *The Fibromyalgia Dental Handbook* written by Flora Stay, D.D.S., addresses fibromyalgia's effects on the mouth.

Sensitive teeth haunt many patients, especially after they've had chemical bleaching. Topical fluoride gels may be painted on surfaces as a restorative treatment. Again, get a nonmint brand such as marketed by Cleure or Colgate (Prevident).

The sore throat of fibromyalgia is usually unlike that of an impending infection. It's more superficial and not helped by swallowing, clearing, or coughing. Patients may raise only the usual, clear mucus. Spastic outside, mid-neck muscles may impinge on nerves and cause an intense sore throat indistinguishable from a strep infection. The absence of swollen glands upon examination can differentiate between the two. Swallowing is sometimes downright painful, as though a foreign body or tablet were locked in some deep recess. This sensation can last for weeks, but causes no tissue injury.

> My ENT says my larynx is swollen but other than that couldn't find anything wrong. I've been really hoarse all this time and the left side of my throat is also swollen. (He saw that it was swollen also when he did the scope on my throat.) He is sending me to a voice specialist in Salt Lake. I've had throat problems a lot in my past. I'm fifty-six years old. My tongue has had sores on the left side and on front that come and go. I have been diagnosed with fibromyalgia and my regular doctor says this is all part of it, maybe from a swollen tendon in my neck.
>
> —Elaine, Utah

Let's review the fate of these various symptoms. Recall how they came and went while you were developing the illness. On guaifenesin, they'll also resurge when you're clearing. Since they keep popping up, how will you tell whether you're improving or further regressing? Don't focus on just one problem, but survey all of the components of fibromyalgia at one time. If you can't get a decent mapping, the only method you have is to evaluate any systemic benefits of treatment to date. Alternating progressively more good days and less intense down ones are reliable, directional measures.

MISCELLANEOUS SYMPTOMS

Profuse sweating—I'm thirty-five now, [and] this started when I was around twenty-three. I thought it was peri-perimenopause. It wasn't. I always felt like I was burning up inside from the inside out. I would be dripping with sweat. It was very embarrassing.

—*Chantal, Michigan*

Every time we write a paper or book, we have leftovers, symptoms that don't fit into any category. They reflect the overall metabolic problems facing the body. Let's take a moment to look at them here.

WEIGHT GAIN

Most fibromyalgia patients gain some weight, and about 35 percent put on twenty or more pounds. We mentioned the loss of mitochondria that occurs in sedentary people. Muscle biopsies have shown up to 80 percent fewer mitochondria when compared with well-toned athletes. Lacking a full complement, we're left with fewer food-burning stations to eat up calories.

Table 13.2
Miscellaneous Symptoms

	Male	Percentage Male	Female	Percentage Female
Number of patients	596		3,444	
Weight gain	174	29	1,197	35
Allergies	146	24	1,007	29
Palpitations	270	45	2,058	60

Insulin to the misdirected rescue: If you don't burn it, store it. And fat cells are very accommodating. (See table 13.2.)

Just about the only success we've had with weight loss in fibromyalgia is by using the low-carbohydrate diet that we detailed in chapter 6. Low-calorie diets may further slow metabolism by recruiting resources against perceived starvation. By contrast, carbohydrate restriction doesn't have the same effect because of fat and protein substitutions. Wouldn't weight loss improve your self-image and mobility? Once you get moving, you'll re-create mitochondria and, thereby, replenish your stamina and energy storage capacity.

You have to push the envelope to see how far you can go. If you don't, you will not make progress. I have said for years [that] Dr. St. Amand's protocol is not about taking a guai pill and then hitting the couch to wait to get better. You have to do the work to build your body back up. The good news is that once the first hard months are over, it just keeps getting easier and better all the time.

—*Gretchen, South Carolina*

TEMPERATURE REGULATION PROBLEMS

Patients complain of low-grade fevers, and in rare cases the thermometer may register over 100 degrees. The majority of fibromyalgics sweat excessively at any time. Even minor fevers break at night, interrupt sleep, and drench bedclothes. Hot flashes are common in both sexes—I joke that I went through menopause at age thirty-two. The body's thermostat malfunctions in various ways, and you may feel comfortable only in a very narrow temperature range. You may rapidly switch from too hot to too cold. Layer clothes that easily go on or off for fast coping; keep a jacket or shawl handy.

WATER RETENTION

We've previously discussed water retention, so we won't review the physiology here. The body holds on to what only seems like excess water. It has to retain two or three pounds during attacks to facilitate the ionic shifts of calcium, sodium, phosphate, chloride, potassium, and magnesium as well as larger-sized compounds. Water accumulation will go into either direction: depositing or reversing attacks. It's the same chemistry going forward or backward. During cycles, fibromyalgics are accustomed to swollen eyelids and hands upon awakening; rings temporarily don't fit. During the daytime, gravity rules, and fluid dutifully slips out of the arms and torso to the legs. By late afternoon, shoes may not fit well. Without obvious swelling, skin is stretched from within. Internal edema tugs on millions of tiny nerve endings and indeed makes legs restless. Add foot and leg cramps for a miserable night. Vitamin E (800 mg) or magnesium at bedtime undependably ameliorate symptoms. The FDA no longer allows physicians to prescribe quinine tablets for cramping, but you may certainly drink a few ounces of sugar-free quinine water at dinner. A quarter cup of pickle juice has been shown in studies to stop foot and leg cramps. Medications should be reserved as second-line therapy because of their side effects. The two currently used medications for restless legs are Requip (ropinirole) and Mirapex (pramipexole). Both were developed to treat Parkinson's disease. Nausea, light-headedness, and fatigue are the main side effects.

Each reader could probably add to this symptom list. Remember the sudden leg kick or arm jerk just as you're falling asleep; intermittent nightmares; boil-like tenderness of your scalp; sudden toothaches though nothing's wrong; sharp stabs that run through your ears; unexplained shivers or total-body chilling; vibrations that come out of nowhere; electric currents that zigzag down your extremities? They're all real and not figments of your imagination. Always remember that our theory supports the notion that many cells in the body are struggling to fend off the sieges of fibromyalgia.

Chapter Fourteen

Pediatric Fibromyalgia

When I was growing up, my nickname was "Slow as molasses in January." As I grew older, the sense that I was not like other children deepened; I could not stand still and hold my arms out to have my clothes fitted; I needed more sleep but could not seem to get it; I had little energy and took refuge reading, lying down, on a window seat instead of playing outside. Burying myself in books, I felt the pain and difference of my childhood less acutely, but the guilt was always there; I felt that I was failing everyone around me by not being like them, by not being able to do what they did so effortlessly. My parents, after taking me to the doctor for thyroid tests, concluded that my tiredness was a character trait and not an illness, and I grew up believing them, never having heard anyone say otherwise.

—*Cynthia C., Michigan*

FACING THE PROBLEM: DID I GIVE MY CHILD FIBROMYALGIA?

As we learn more about fibromyalgia and reflect how it's affected our lives, we become aware of similar symptoms in those around us. Some will confide that they have the illness by name; others we can diagnose if we just listen to their complaints. And since fibromyalgia runs in families, it's inevitable that it lurks close to home.

During the process of guaifenesin reversal, it's inevitable that we stare face-to-face at the child we once were—a child with abdominal pain and side stitches; unexplained headaches; baffling irritable bowel syndrome; growing pains in the lower legs and knees that woke us crying at night; wrenching charley horses the day following gym class; endless days with fatigue and that horrible, drifting brain that just wouldn't concentrate in school. Such reminiscing is healing. Looking at that former kid lets us forgive the alleged hypochondriac. During the nostalgia process, we may sadly realize that one or more of our children are facing the same struggles. Nearly every day, a parent asks, "My daughter has bladder infections and growing pains—is it possible she has fibromyalgia?" "My son used to love sports, but now he won't even dress for PE. Something's always bothering him—does he have this fibromyalgia thing?" The list grows as each warms to the task of recall and we're asked about lethargy, headaches, former A students who suddenly don't achieve—all in the same anxious tones. Parental suspicions usually translate into accurate diagnoses: They know their kids!

Older children with fibromyalgia slowly realize they're not like other kids, but why? "Why" is recurrent: why was schoolwork easy yesterday; why still tired after sleeping twelve hours; why so little stamina when my friend can go and go like the Energizer Bunny? You can be sure they think about these yokes, but how can they shed them when grown-ups, including doctors, flounder about and can't free them? Lacking comprehension, youngsters soon become adept at making seemingly valid excuses. By the time they're teenagers, many have really good reasons why they hurt or why they no longer want to participate in activities they once enjoyed. But look closely: Those excuses don't really hold up.

Younger children have a different perspective. They've never felt any other way. They think it's normal to feel pain and fatigue and assume their peers feel the same. It ultimately becomes their persona to be weaker and lacking in determination, which they can incorrectly assume is a character deficit. Since they can't grasp the reality of their situation, they often become less assertive and let others take charge.

We know one little girl who began painful cycles at the age of two. She awakened during the night crying from leg pains. Her parents soon learned how to handle her complaints. They'd soak her in a tubful of warm water, dry her off, and then massage her. That was the only way to save them all from another painful and totally sleepless night. This family of six—mother, father, and four children—all have fibromyalgia. Having two parents with the illness has made it practically genetically inescapable for their offspring. The youngest three began having appreciable symptoms by the age of four. The only difference was the extent and severity of their complaints and physical findings.

Becky, the eldest, was severely affected by the time we first saw her at age eleven. Already suffering from unrelenting symptoms, she had seen chiropractors, physiotherapists, and physicians. No one could explain why, and few would believe that she sometimes crawled on the ground as the only way to get home from school. Leg pains and weakness were so bad that she couldn't keep walking or even stand. We also had trouble with that one. We had never encountered a crawling fibromyalgic or one so young with such intense symptoms. We began to suspect she was highly neurotic and using her illness for some emotional gain. Yet there were sobering balances to redress our thinking. Becky was a straight-A student and strikingly intelligent. She knew when she could study effectively and rested when she had no other choice. She took pain medications and antidepressants as prescribed by her family physician, but even in her sedated state, she continued to excel. Her mother was unwaveringly supportive and staunchly insisted that Becky was truly as ill as she described herself. Yet she gave Becky as normal an upbringing as possible. Becky attended public school and even in her back brace lived as normally as her symptoms allowed. She was never permitted to withdraw from life and, with full family support, fought through pain and fatigue with singular success.

Time, Mom, and Becky taught us about how severe symptoms could be in children. But it was a slow process. Her response to guaifenesin demanded precise adjustments. She simply couldn't tolerate much worsening of symptoms. She, therefore, improved very slowly. Tiny increments in dosage set off such intense reversals that she couldn't make it to school. Even had she struggled to get there, it wouldn't have been worth the painful effort: She couldn't possibly sit for even the first hour of class. Becky's personal war against fibromyalgia continued for more than three years; each tiny advance was a major battle won. Our first edition of this book reported that she was an A student completing her senior year in high school. She's now a college graduate enjoying life as a wife and full-time mother. Since she lives out of state, we haven't seen her for a few years, and I hope Becky will read this new edition and realize we ever remember her starring role.

Becky's story is heartwarming, but there are also very sad ones. Too many children have ended up invalids because of faltered parental determination or bungled physician treatments. Some parents accept defeat too easily and crumble beholding their suffering child. They're kept from school without much provocation. They condone the child's mounting inactivity and the loss of friends. Family life eventually revolves around the child's symptoms. The search narrows down to something for immediate relief—forget the future. The required effort and dedication to a protocol such as ours don't exist. They don't anticipate that the "usual" medications eventually won't help. Drug tolerance mounts with each new, powerful tablet. Waiting in the batter's box are the heavy hitters, narcotics and sleep prescriptions. Nothing much changes, and the child progressively withdraws. Morphine patches or pumps, followed by stimulants such as Ritalin or Provigil to overcome their superimposed lethargy dictate disaster.

When my younger son, Sean, was small, his father took him to a pediatric rheumatologist, who diagnosed him with a "pain syndrome." The doctor hesitated to make the diagnosis of fibromyalgia, he said, because Sean did not seem to have a sleep disorder. This doctor, who admitted he had never heard of guaifenesin, was willing to write a prescription on the spot for Elavil and Flexeril—for a seven-year-old child who was far from being in intractable pain. I could not believe this. He did not even know what was wrong with my son except that he was in pain, and admitted it, yet he was willing to change the chemistry of a seven-year-old child's brain.

—*C.C., California*

We don't have to belabor the fact that school absenteeism destroys a child's academic edge. The new information age grants little mercy in today's fierce competition for college. Slowly, the fibromyalgic youngster loses his or her perpetual catch-up race. Though determined parents may manage to wrench homeschooling tutors out of their budget-conscious school districts, it doesn't compensate for the well-rounding effects of extracurricular activities. Only social interactions with peers can provide certain skills during teenage years. The self-esteem and confidence we desire for our children is hard to come by when successes are isolated and they've been taught to believe they're too ill to compete.

Time is oddly suspended in the present for these families. There are few discussions about the future. What happens when Mom and Dad can't continue as caretakers? Adulthood doesn't end drug dependency or social isolationism. All too quickly parents share their home with an introverted adult who has few skills. At a certain age, nonstudent offspring can no longer be carried on the family medical insurance plan. It's impossible to qualify for substantial disability when you've never worked.

Recounting these stories brings to mind a little boy I remember vividly. When we met, Joe was sick, and he was afraid of both doctors and having more pain. Bravely he undertook our protocol and gradually reversed most of his complaints, although his mother was tentative and thought it might be too difficult for him. As time progressed, I learned to appreciate his good qualities. We became friends. One day he brought a poem of gratitude he had composed especially for me. I hung it on my office wall and saw him glow as he looked up at his masterpiece.

Joe and his family moved away. When he came back a few years later for a checkup, he wasn't Joe anymore. He was sadly changed. He wasn't following the protocol and had been off his guaifenesin for some time. Because of severe headaches, his mother and his new doctors had put him on narcotic pain medications. These were the very drugs I had steadfastly refused to prescribe because I didn't want to sap his already low energy. I wasn't even sure they were safe for growing children. But now, narcotics were Joe's new friends that made him feel better about his life. They certainly gave partial relief for the headaches and much faster than the gradual improvement I could offer if he chose to resume guaifenesin. I argued in vain with his mother. I don't know what happened to him after his last visit. I'm guessing Joe never fulfilled his boyhood dreams of playing college basketball. Narcotics had become his companions. Hardly my choice of friends.

These two are contrasting stories at very opposite ends of a spectrum. Becky's story always makes us smile, but it only partially offsets Joe's failure. She owes a great deal to her mother, a strong supportive parent who didn't shy away from a rather long road to health. She never gave Becky the option to quit, deny her illness, or stop her medication. She wasn't afraid to parent. Joe's mother was motivated by the same love and determination for her child, but she made an unfortunate choice. It seemed wrong to her to make her child work back through his problems as others have successfully done.

More recently we were presented with a talented young man named Jason, whose life was becoming increasingly circumscribed by the very potent prescription medications given to him to control his considerable pain. As a result, he was also suffering from depression. Both he and his parents were quite aware that his future wasn't very bright, and that he was descending into a cycle of stronger and stronger drugs that were working less and less well. They all came to see us and spent the afternoon listening to what we do and how we do it. Even before guaifenesin lessened Jason's symptoms, it gave him hope. And when he started to respond as we predicted he would, for the first time in a long time, Jason dared to dream.

Luckily Jason proved to be a low-dose responder. Because he was a dancer, despite his heavy narcotics he was aware of his body and able to feel it changing. And we are overjoyed to announce that he graduated from a top university and has a dream job in the computer social network industry. As he improved, he cut back on his potent pain medications, including morphine, which is not easy to do. With courage, determination, and hope, he was able to win the battle. Odds are against kids like Jason, but they do exist, and hope under any circumstances is a powerful ally. Another is strong, compassionate parents who keep the faith even when frightened themselves.

It's imperative for physicians and parents to make an early diagnosis of fibromyalgia, and attack the cause, not cover up the symptoms. It will take persistence to accomplish this but the stakes are high. Our children don't really have many formative years, and it's never too early to show them how to accomplish things by determination and hard work. In general, children haven't lived long enough to see impact on many tissues so there's less disease to reverse. Recovery is much faster than in adults.

Perhaps the only reward for fibromyalgic parents is the bonus of recognizing themselves when they were in the early stages of their own illness.

I do not remember a time when I did not have headaches. Since my mother had always suffered from migraines, my headaches seemed to be part of my destiny. The pain in my head was, at least, taken to be real by my family. Not so by the outside world, in which, during my adolescence, I would often hear: Just relax, lie down in a dark room for a few minutes, and take an aspirin. Fasting glucose tests, an electroencephalogram, an electrocardiogram, and other tests at the university clinic showed nothing. I had migraines, and not much could be done beyond living with them. Expensive shiatsu and acupuncture gave me sporadic relief but no more than that. I lived my life around my pain, as frustrated as my doctors. I hid my pain as best I could, but I could not hide it from those closest to me. By the time my daughter was three, every week I was taking a bottle of naproxen sodium and Tylenol, and as much sumatriptan as I could get my doctors and medical plan to provide, and yet I was still helplessly spending my afternoons on the couch. I had severe headaches every day, and most of them were migraines. I felt isolated by my pain, unable to even begin to communicate to anyone what my life was like, and increasingly devastated and guilty from the effect my pain was having on my family.

—*Cynthia C., Michigan*

THE FIBROMYALGIC CHILD

I remember clearly the moment I knew my son had fibromyalgia. And it was not his complaints of pains or nervousness that tipped me off. I didn't know that children do not normally complain of headaches, because I had them all my life. I didn't know there was no such thing as growing pains. His aches and pains did not disrupt his life, and I did not think much about them, either. But one day I was standing in the doorway watching his trumpet lesson, and I heard his trumpet teacher say: "At this point I shouldn't have to tell you how to play a B note." And I looked at my son's face, and I knew that at that moment he had no more idea how to play a B on a trumpet than I did, although he did know. All the times in my childhood when I was yelled at, told I knew things I could not bring out of my mind because my mind just wouldn't always work to produce them on demand, came flooding back. I knew then and there Malcolm had fibromyalgia, too, and I would have to get him help.

—*Claudia Craig Marek*

If you or anyone in your family has fibromyalgia and you're suspicious, look as objectively as possible at your child. No doctor on earth will ever know that little person as well as you. What should you look for? We've mentioned that kids don't very often fake pain; if they do, it's usually to get out of doing something obvious. They're not seasoned actors, so the put-on is fairly transparent. Not well coached in the role they're playing, they can be easily distracted. Part of your challenge is that they may be fairly inarticulate and nondescriptive. They won't say much more than "it hurts" or "I've got a headache." Younger children, or anyone who's had the disease a long time, can't recall being without this or that symptom. As we said before, they don't identify themselves as unusual or abnormal.

Always tired? Just constitutionally weaker than their peers. Having no wellness point of reference, what's unusual about growing pains and daily headaches?

You're the parent trying to peek in. Focus on your observations. Are your children exhausted some mornings even though they've just had a substantial amount of sleep? Have you seen them leave off playing with friends or siblings and lie down for a spontaneous rest or nap? Have you witnessed intermittent difficulties with memory or concentration? You might notice that they easily complete tasks one day but badly fumble on the next try. Do they have abdominal pain, constipation, and diarrhea? Does your daughter have bladder infections, painful urination, or vaginal irritation? Do they complain of leg and knee pains by day and seemingly more vicious ones by night? We've even wondered about a colic connection in babies who draw up their knees while bellowing, possibly reacting to abdominal pain. There are no follow-up studies on such ailing children as they age, or on the prevalence of fibromyalgia in their parents.

Children with fibromyalgia may begin adverse cycling from an early age, a few even before preschool years. We've had the opportunity to diagnose and treat four two-year-olds and fifteen four-year-olds. In almost all of these cases, a parent with the disease, not the physician, first suspected the illness and brought the child to us for confirmation. The youngest kids can't articulate where they hurt, but cyclic whining, crying, and irritability are all too eloquent. Slightly older children can at least alert their parents about pains in their knees and adjacent structures. These are often dismissed as "growing pains," especially if grandparents are consulted. Since they're often the earliest recognizable symptoms of fibromyalgia, we record them to pinpoint the onset of the disease. In children with higher pain thresholds, fatigue, irritable bowel, or bladder symptoms may be the first clues. Some little girls may begin with vulvar irritation, itching, or pain.

Affected children may begin hurting between the ages of seven and ten, but sometimes as early as four years old. Pains come and go without rhyme or reason and are recurrent for a few months or even years. As in adults, early attacks are sporadic and unrelated to growth periods. About 40 percent of the fibromyalgic adults we question recall having pains in their legs when they were young. Remember, there are no such things as growing pains! The term is actually a misnomer because the hurting begins well before the enormous growth spurt of puberty. Growth is not painful. A baby triples his or her size in the first year of life and doesn't seem to experience any discomfort in the process.

A significant fact is that boys and girls are equally affected before puberty. When we wrote the first edition of this book, we were just beginning to assemble statistics on our pediatric cases. Of course, since that date, many more families have come in to be examined. While working on our book *What Your Doctor May* Not *Tell You About Pediatric Fibromyalgia*, a chance observation by my coauthor that we were seeing as many boys as girls struck me as odd. But when we pulled the records from our charts, we documented that indeed the sexes were evenly divided. We've since found that other physicians have made this same discovery. Statistics from pediatric pain and rheumatology clinics have made their way into print. Most adult patients are female, but since that's not so before puberty, what changes at that time to skew the incidence to 85 percent women? We finally realized that adolescent muscles and bones soak up great quantities of phosphate. Though both sexes get more massive at that time, boys get much bigger and will have to sustain that size for most of their lives. They may be taking in more phosphate than they can excrete, but suddenly their bodies can use every bit of it.

Later in life, pain and fatigue may resurface to become the 15 percent male incidence. So the disease will probably regenerate later in life, sooner in women, maybe in the teenage years, or well beyond that time. We don't have space to outline them here, but many factors determine how soon symptoms resume. At first, only a bit of nagging during the premenstrual week: Cramps, PMS, and headaches, often of migraine intensity, uptick and strike more regularly. Soon enough, it becomes impossible to keep step with peers in gym activities or on playing fields. Formerly promising athletes tire far too soon and lag behind less capable prospects. The thought of expending energy terrorizes these children, who know that muscular pains will surely follow within twenty-four hours. They barely comply with compulsory physical education requirements, but that's as far as it goes.

Pain waxes; stamina ebbs. Brain haze sneaks in and textbooks might as well be written in hieroglyphics. Without reason or warning, they're upset with dizziness and exhaustion. What good are fourteen hours of sleep? Backpacks weigh a ton. Eyes go in and out of focus; that glassy look is interpreted by teachers as deliberate inattention. We used to call them lazy teenagers, but now everyone is "with it" and makes the diagnosis of attention deficit disorder (ADD). What a rotten conclusion! Everyone's suddenly baffled when all of the symptoms disappear—for a while.

Now that we've treated several hundred children under the age of sixteen, we earlier suspect the diagnosis of pediatric fibromyalgia. My three daughters suffered their first cycles at ages eleven, thirteen, and sixteen. In the next generation, I found lesions in my grandson, Nick, at age twelve. Coauthor Claudia's sons required treatment by age seven. Sean, the younger, has a high pain threshold and complained of only minor aches. His illness jumped out at us as irritable bowel syndrome, but there were unmistakable, telltale body lumps and bumps that clinched the diagnosis. The elder, Malcolm, my guaifenesin guinea pig, was fully articulate (seemingly from birth) and able to express himself very forcefully. He had the full mess of symptoms, including those affecting his brain, musculoskeletal system, and gastrointestinal tract. He posed no diagnostic dilemma! If you think grandchildren, nieces, or nephews are prospects, you can certainly hand information to the parents and hope they're receptive.

Physicians must depend on parents for crucial information and observations. Even then, they may not recognize the early intrusions of pediatric fibromyalgia, much less grasp that there's effective treatment. Parents are on the firing line. They must trust some instincts and long-term observations. Since we can't just sit back and watch our children suffer, discovery and the solution are up to us.

TREATING CHILDREN

She was not like my other two children, who ran and played all day long. She would always sit on the sidelines watching or "holding" other people's things for them. She started to complain of constant neck and shoulder pain. We tried everything but nothing consistently worked. We watched a very profound change in her from when she was eleven through thirteen. She became very foggy in her mind and could not remember the math she had done the day before. She also got discouraged, and every day became a "burden" to her that she felt was becoming too great to bear. We started her on guaifenesin and soon she was sleeping and kept telling me how different she felt. She was able to do her schoolwork and remember what she had learned.

—*Wendy M., California*

Someone sent us a paper written in 1928 by a family practitioner. He described children with growing pains, "great mental and body fatigue," "cold extremities," and "feeble digestion."

He listed so many other symptoms that the diagnosis of fibromyalgia is obvious in retrospect. He successfully treated his small patients using a tree bark extract called guaiacum. For some reason, not many pediatricians paid much attention. Sixty years ago, one ingredient was purified to guaiacolate and included in some cough preparations. Five years later, it was synthesized as guaifenesin for another brand. Thirty-five years ago, several companies pressed the compound into tablet form and marketed it in long-acting formulations. Sadly, those preparations went off the market when the FDA demanded that "long acting" when applied to guaifenesin meant twelve-hour duration of action. None of the companies had research facilities and stopped making them.[1] We addressed that problem in chapter 3.

There's no need to go into great detail about the treatment of children, since it's not much different from adults. As we've stated, guaifenesin is an over-the-counter medication and is available in various strengths. Younger children may need a liquid form. That's formulated in two strengths: 100 mg and 200 mg per teaspoon. Slightly older kids may be able to swallow small tablets or capsules, which are more slippery when wet. Those can be found in 200, 300, 400, and 600 mg concentrations. Tablets may be broken to create smaller doses. Crushing is not advisable—without a capsule, guaifenesin lands directly in the stomach in sudden release, and nausea may follow.

All guaifenesin is bitter, so it takes a bit of ingenuity to hide the taste. Liquids can be disguised in juice. Capsules may be opened and the contents hidden in applesauce or pudding. You may have to delay treatment until children can swallow tablets or mask the distasteful liquid preparations. It's very difficult to force a choking child to keep trying especially if larger quantities are necessary. We start children at 300 mg every twelve hours and gradually raise their dosage until subsequent mapping shows reversal. If that technique is not locally available, parents have to wing it and make conclusions based on complaints and behavior. Simple notations about fatigue and pain levels on a desk calendar are really sufficient to monitor progress in most cases.

Unless the situation is desperate, it's sometimes wiser to initiate treatment at the beginning of summer vacation or the long winter break. This allows more time for rest and avoids simultaneously struggling with reversal cycles, school, and homework. Within a few weeks, most children demonstrate noticeable improvement before classes resume. Parents should not hesitate to begin guaifenesin for a student who, because of impaired memory and concentration, is getting failing grades. Initially, it may be helpful to cancel music or dance lessons for a month or two, depending on the severity of the illness and individual stamina. It's also counterproductive to remove just-for-fun activities so that a child feels left out and weird. If a temporary break is necessary, assure your child that he or she is getting well and will soon resume normal routines. It's also wise to consider resuming activities one by one without waiting for a complete response. Most children can cope just fine even when they've only partially purged. Getting back with friends prompts confidence, takes the focus off the illness, and convinces them that they're not really different from their peers.

It's tough to watch an ailing child, especially if you're the one who transmitted the defective gene(s). The first few reversal cycles are disturbing, but you should use all of your parental skills to make them tolerable. Preschoolers can rest and take warm baths; most can swallow liquid Tylenol (acetaminophen), Advil (ibuprofen), or the likes for pain relief. Insomnia and frequent waking can be countered with Benadryl (diphenhydramine, as in Simply Sleep or Sominex), which is available in various pediatric strengths. The many over-the-counter medications for symptoms such as diarrhea, gas, and painful urination need only be checked for salicylates. In general, children's compounds don't contain aspirin because of the danger of Reye's syndrome. (Pepto-Bismol is a rare exception, but is clearly marked.)

Because children use fewer products than adults, older ones might actually enjoy helping you find salicylate-free items as you simultaneously teach them. Tom's of Maine makes two children's toothpastes—Silly Strawberry and Orange Mango. Kids may also enjoy the citrus, pineapple, or cranberry flavors produced by Cleure (www.cleure.com). Oral B's children's line, Zooth, does not contain mint, and Colgate Watermelon is also okay. Janelle Holden, D.D.S., created a children's line called Tanner's Tasty Paste (www.tannerstastypaste.com), which, like Cleure, contain no mint and no sodium lauryl sulfate.

Children should be encouraged to interact with friends and stay as active as their illness allows. No matter how often you have to repeat, it's encouraging to hear that nothing's so seriously wrong that time won't fix. Parents walk a bit of a tightrope at this point. They must display compassion while remaining resolute that some symptoms will be revisited and must be endured. They might need the wisdom of Solomon and the patience of Job to steadfastly hold a sick child to certain standards of achievement and behavior. But in truth, applying common sense and an attentive ear to the child's needs serve as admirable substitutes. Older children quickly learn how to pace themselves and work hard during better periods and rest when they feel worse. Smaller children can't be expected to understand—but then their lives are less stressful, and missed opportunities have fewer negative consequences.

Most children test the system once they're feeling well. At some time or another, expect them to stop their medication. Each of our children has done exactly that; even Malcolm, the original guinea kid, has done it more than once despite his pride at being the first person treated with guaifenesin for fibromyalgia. We have to expect that, as they grow older, they feel that great surge of invincibility required to propel them into lives of their own. Rest assured, they'll grope their way back to the medicine shelf and that bottle of guaifenesin when they feel bad enough. Luckily, since they're young and haven't fallen far behind, they respond as before and quickly make up lost ground.

In summary, guaifenesin is safe at any age. The return road from fibromyalgia enjoys a higher speed limit. The journey is even shorter if begun early. For the sake of our children we, their parents, must trust ourselves to diagnose the illness perhaps sooner than can physicians. We're fortunate to have a reliable medication that so swiftly restores our youngsters to normal. Looking at our affected family, those of us with fibromyalgia will inevitably reflect on our own past. We'll always wonder how different our lives might have been had we been provided an early diagnosis and effective treatment. For most of us, life would certainly have included considerably less suffering and fewer broken relationships. Instinctively, as parents, we can surely appreciate that our sad experiences gave us insight to help our children, and were thus not entirely wasted.

I suggest you get and read Dr. St. Amand and Claudia's book *What Your Doctor May* Not *Tell You About Pediatric Fibromyalgia*. Because they clear so quickly on guai if started early, I would rather my child had FMS than many other chronic illnesses. We were thrilled when Dr. St. Amand diagnosed my fourteen-year-old granddaughter with both FMS and HG. Otherwise she would have been labeled bipolar and on meds the rest of her life. Instead she is phasing off her antidepressant and doing so well in many ways. No more hating PE or being unable to go to school after walking home six blocks the day before. She also has the energy to do her homework and the memory to turn things in on time.

—*Sandy, Idaho*

Part III

❦

Strategies for the Road Back

Unlike the chapters included in part II, the following chapters are not specifically about treating fibromyalgia. Rather, they are about practical, everyday matters that affect your life, such as coping with your job, family, home, and other medications that are commonly used.

We hope that the information and suggestions in the following chapters will help you contend with your illness on a daily basis. Undoubtedly, you will learn some things that your doctor has not told you, or that you have not learned through other sources. We hope this part will help you while you're waiting to begin (or are in the early stages of) guaifenesin treatment.

Chapter Fifteen

Medical Band-Aids

*Currently Promoted Treatments for
Fibromyalgia—What You Don't
Know Can Hurt You*

Ms. W. presents today in follow-up for depression. States she is significantly better. Feels like a different person and thinks she may have fibromyalgia and has been taking guaifenesin twice a day from a book she red [sic] and states that she is doing much better also. Patient is eager to discuss this novel or book by someone in California about the treatments of fibromyalgia which she states "has saved her life." A/P 1) Depression: Patient is significantly better and I am happy for her.

2) Myalgias: Also better. Encouraged the patient to continue to take the guaifenesin if it is effective for her.

—*Actual medical records of patient, Durham Medical Center*

THERE IS NO mystery to the standard approach to treating fibromyalgia. The party line is echoed throughout medical literature over and over, and little or no dissent is heard. Therapeutic options arise in scholarly journals such as the *Journal of Rheumatology* and work their way down into publications for general practitioners, chiropractors, nurses, and physical therapists. All footnote the same studies, and the same advice is given, tailored slightly for each target audience.

It's virtually impossible to get published in medical journals when your ideas differ from the accepted norm or if you are an outsider—not a researcher at a university. The peer review process is part of this obstacle. Before being approved for publication, manuscripts are peer-reviewed by experts in the field for comments and recommendations. These "peers" are generally editors of other publications or professors in their respective fields. Their main function is to scrutinize papers for fraudulent conclusions or plagiarism. By nature, then, they are leery of new and contrary ideas that spring up from any source other than full-time academia or other well-known researchers. What peer reviewers and editors say goes; there is no place to appeal their decision except to seek publication in another journal. While, for the most part, this is an admirable system, procedurally sound, and designed for patient safety, it also stifles innovations that might arise from practitioner rank and file, or those in the trenches who treat patients full time and don't have access to laboratories.

I've commiserated with more than a few colleagues who've unexpectedly stumbled onto something not offered in textbooks. Physicians are trained to be alert and respect their own serendipity and the experiences they've acquired dealing with real live patients, but most avenues are closed for propagating their observations. This is unfortunate. I believe it's rare to find a physician who, after a lifetime of practice, couldn't relate at least one better way of doing medicine. As we'll discuss later in this chapter, the FDA trusts physicians to use medications in any way they feel is appropriate once they are on the market. However, if they stumble upon something that works, there's no way to share this information with others. Lacking laboratories and funding, it's not an option for them to explore the chemistry or reasons that would explain what they've learned.

Medical journals have a gold standard when it comes to introducing new therapies—called a *double-blind study.* In this setup, half the patients are treated with a certain modality and the other half are given a sham treatment, or placebo. *Double-blind* refers to the fact that neither the physician nor the subject knows who is actually being treated. At the end of a predetermined time, results are tabulated; if those who were treated have improved more than those who were not, the study is considered a success, and suitable for publication. It's been documented time and time again that placebos help patients about 30 percent of the time, so that's the actual number a new discovery has to better. If that's accomplished, a paper can be written and submitted to journals for publication.

For practicing physicians, this is an all but impossible obstacle to surmount. No matter how interesting their observations, they have no way to instigate a clinical trial. Writing the proposal, getting permissions, and doing other paperwork require specialized knowledge as well as a huge investment of time and money. And without a drug company or a research grant, financing a large study with lots of patients, positive outcomes are hard to come by. Seeing ten or fifteen patients improving is just not going to cut it, and then there's the problem of having to give half the patients who come for treatment a placebo.

Top researchers or big names in the field routinely get hefty sums of money to be consultants to test new medications. Since they're well known, it's easier for them to get published when the study is done. A private physician can't possibly compete. There's no hope at all when the therapy in question isn't a potential moneymaker for drug companies or institutions. A new use for a drug still under patent or exclusively produced would probably titillate interest, but barring that, the establishment just isn't interested. It's these limitations that keep many physicians from investigating previously unexplored problems—no matter what their potential benefit.

It's no secret that medical research in the United States is driven by a huge respect for the financial bottom line of drug manufacturers rather than for patients' welfare. As a result, very few of the "new" medications brought to market are actually innovative, or different. Instead, research money is invested in producing chemical cousins of existing drugs: variations on antidepressants, statins for cholesterol, stomach acid blockers, or blood pressure drugs. As we've seen, new medications are tested against sugar pills, not against existing drugs. To be approved by the FDA, they simply have to be better than nothing, not better or safer than something already on the market. Negative studies are usually not published and often suppressed, while a new research trial is designed to rearrange the results so the new compound can pass muster. With a huge percentage of drug testing done around the world far away from the FDA's eye, this is easy enough to do.

As Dr. Sharon Levine, an associate director of the Kaiser Permanente Medical Group, put it: "If I'm a manufacturer and I can change one molecule and get another twenty years of patent rights, and convince physicians to prescribe and consumers to demand the next form of Prilosec or weekly Prozac instead of daily Prozac just as my patent expires, then why would I be spending money on a lot less certain endeavor which is looking for brand new drugs?"

We've encountered these obstacles for many years. Facing this reality in 1999, we wrote the first edition of this book because we knew of no other way to get our observations and results in the hands of patients and their physicians. We didn't want our protocol to die with this physician. Enough patients now have the message and energy to teach physicians and to help each other when necessary. And as we'd hoped, this reverse approach is working from the bottom up, from patients to professionals. While this certainly rubs some professionals the wrong way, others are delighted to find something that actually offers patients a chance for improvement. When they see the results for themselves, they, too, become believers. Each year, physicians from all over the world fly to California to work with us in our office and to learn firsthand what it is we do. There's no doubt that there's hope.

THE ACCEPTED TREATMENT

> It may well be better not to treat patients with our well-known but hardly effective armamentarium of drugs...Treatments with antidepressants, tricyclics, formal exercise programs— particularly because they do not seem to work—prolong medi- calization and dependency, the opposite of what we should wish to accomplish.
> —*Frederick Wolfe, M.D.,* Journal of Rheumatology[1]

So what's the accepted treatment for fibromyalgia? We already know that at best it's only partially effective, because disability claims, alternative treatments, and self-help groups abound. To make matters worse, the deplorable choices patients are being offered by many doctors are not great improvements over simply suffering in silence. We might say that at least these practitioners admit there's an illness and they're trying to help, but that doesn't much change the outcome of their approach.

The current party line for treating fibromyalgia is to:

- Maintain a positive attitude about the chances for recovery.
- Assure patients that fibromyalgia is not going to kill or maim them.
- Advocate exercise for resurrecting energy.
- Endeavor to restore normal sleep patterns.
- Relieve as much pain as possible using medications the physician feels comfortable prescribing. (This varies greatly from doctor to doctor.)

- When those fail to restore health, help patients file for disability.

On the surface, we can't imagine anyone quarreling with these noble goals. They sound simple enough, and if achievable, they'd be a solution. Or would they? Look closely and you'll notice that despite their appeal to common sense, not even one aims at correcting the basic metabolic malfunction of fibromyalgia. Except for exercise, none of them will keep patients from getting worse. But it's unlikely that sick people can push through the pain of even a minor workout. If they can't, what's left is a life of prescription medications that over time will need to be stronger, and with side effects that add more complaints to their already long list. On top of that, the very last item—"Help a patient to file for disability"—implies that despite the optimism recommended in item 1, it's accepted that many will have to face getting more and more incapacitated until they are disabled. Patient and doctor end up mired in a legal battle to document just how ill he or she has become and testify that there is no possibility of improvement. We must ask ourselves, finally, should disability be a desired goal of those who come to a doctor looking for help and guidance?

PAIN

The official position of the American Medical Association is to use the lowest possible dose necessary of a medication for as short a duration as possible.

By the time patients visit doctors, they have more pain than they can manage by themselves. The brain gives pain priority over other sensations because it is such an important warning signal. Tissue destruction is what triggers the alert, and the body demands an immediate and dramatic response with the goal of preventing further injury. Reflex withdrawal of fingers from flame illustrates that principle. Yet as we've seen, there is no damage in fibromyalgia: The pain is chronic, or something that goes on day after day. The result is a brain that has exhausted its resources. Evidence is ample that the body responds in a different way to pain that is consistently present. We just don't get the benefit of the potent hormones and neurotransmitters released by a body in an acute scenario.

Even before their initial consultation, patients will have tried over-the-counter analgesics such as aspirin, acetaminophen (Tylenol), and nonsteroidal, anti-inflammatory drugs such as ibuprofen (Motrin, Advil). A physician may have already prescribed mild muscle relaxants such as carisoprodol (Soma) or cyclobenzaprine (Flexeril), Many have been offered an antidepressant. Confused as to why when they don't feel sad patients often initially refuse this choice.

The relief most patients feel with these medications quickly wears off. Before tossing up his hands, the doctor may have raised the doses a bit—accepting collective medical wisdom which concludes that, in this case, a little more can be better. But still the patient is in pain and complaining. Now the frustrated physician has no choice but to refer the patient to a specialist who is more comfortable writing stronger prescriptions after, of course, conducting further testing that will point to nothing except fibromyalgia.

Hopes are raised: a new doctor! Simply taking the complicated history will fill the twenty to thirty minutes. Then, in a testimonial to the age of computers, the hopeful patient produces a file stuffed with documents listing every doctor who's been seen, each medication that did nothing much, and even the sequential dates when symptoms first appeared. There's always a sheaf of blood test results, often with saliva, hair, and stool analyses thrown in. Perhaps included are surgery and radiology reports or gruesome details of accidents. Added to the stack are results of X-rays, MRIs, ultrasounds, scans, and copious notes inscribed by a variety of medical examiners. Nearly all these tests are normal, but here and there slight deviations have been dutifully circled. Everything is there.

Last night before going to bed I took some sleeping pills (trazodone) and an anti-inflammatory (Voltaren). By the side of the bed I put some Bonine because I was feeling a little dizzy, Ambien because I come wide awake every night between 2:30 and 5:30, and if it's earlier rather than later, I knock myself out so I can get a little rest, Tylenol because my spine aches terribly after lying in bed, Pamprin because menstrual cramps can be awful in the middle of the night, and a heating pad (because a few nights before I woke up with a severe calf cramp that crippled me for three days afterward). I ask you, is that normal? I've always hated taking pain pills; even after I ruptured a disc, I refused to take painkillers and sleeping pills. I got through it with difficulty but I survived. Now I am so worn down that I'll take anything if it will help me get some sleep. Every morning I wake up expecting to be normal again. It's a bad dream.

—*Susannah, Maryland*

The physician must think quickly. He knows people in the waiting room are rechecking their watches and have finished last year's magazines. Just about now one of them must be plaintively asking the receptionist, "How much longer do you think?" There's probably a bored patient in an adjoining exam room staring at the ceiling while freezing to death in a crumpled paper "gown."

"She needs pain relief; she's already tried a bunch of over-the-counter drugs. I've got to do something." Out comes the prescription pad; now it's time to try something more powerful, something different from what the patient has had before. It could be tramadol (Ultram) or perhaps the new expensive form of naproxen (Naprelan)—something that isn't on the patient's intimidating, already-done-that-doesn't-work list. The patient leaves clutching the new prescription hopefully.

Unfortunately, if the medication works, it won't work for long. Pretty soon, the physician must pull out the prescription pad again. It's time to get serious and turn to bigger guns—narcotics. They're all close cousins with different names, some natural and some synthetic, and are marketed alone or in combination with aspirin, acetaminophen, or ibuprofen. Readers may already be closely acquainted with some of them: Vicodin, Lorcet, Lortab, hydrocodone, OxyContin, Percocet, Norco, or Fentanyl, for example. At first, the pain is certainly dulled, and patients learn to deal with side effects: a little fatigue, nausea, dizziness, and constipation. With the exception of constipation, these lessen over time as the body becomes accustomed to the compound.

The first problem with narcotics is that the body gradually builds a tolerance to them. There's only a certain amount of time nature allows for the efficacy of any particular pain reliever. So they aren't really designed for long-term use. But faced with unyielding pain, physician and patient succumb. What choice is there but to raise the dose when the drug no longer gives relief? And here comes the catch. The path toward stronger, longer-acting narcotics is one well trodden. When searching for relief from pain, danger lurks at every step, and patients are given contradictory information. They take what are marketed as "safer" pain pills, achieve temporary relief, develop tolerance, and move on looking for more powerful help. Unless fibromyalgia is treated at its root cause, the hourglass runs down. Even doctors quick to prescribe narcotic drugs admit "nearly all patients on opioids become physically dependent."[2] Some physicians neglect to tell patients their new prescription is an opiate that will surely make them physically drug dependent. Often they are prescribed by brand or chemical names that unsuspecting patients, in their desperation for pain suppression, don't recognize.

After just a few weeks of using narcotics regularly, many

patients may not be able to muster the willpower to stop. Even if pain levels improve, the brain doesn't see it that way. It has adapted to its marriage with the narcotic, which occupies receptors in the emotional part of the brain, where it produces pleasurable feelings. The body doesn't have to work to produce its own feel-good chemicals, endorphins, anymore. A pill is doing it the easy way. When the plug is pulled, the brain becomes petulant: You ration me and I'll give you pain like you've never felt before! Withdrawal means greater fatigue, insomnia, cognitive wipeout, severe anxiety, and even salivation or itching as parts of the ploy. That's true drug dependence, a physical reaction beyond the control of the conscious mind. The plot is this: When it's time for another dose of narcotic endorphins, the brain reproduces every mental and physical symptom the individual has ever experienced. Fibromyalgics can't discern the difference, since their brains have been expressing identical complaints for years. The reasoning goes: I feel all the same things, so my fibromyalgia isn't a bit better. It's nevertheless brain-speak and duplicity. No longer are muscles, sinews, gut, and bladder sending distress signals; the brain now initiates them. Even after guaifenesin has sufficiently reversed the illness, the brain keeps trying to get the narcotic endorphins. And once these have been discontinued, it takes some months for the body to begin producing its own natural endorphins again, which makes this period very difficult. Other hormones related to the hypothalamus (such as estrogen) are also reduced and may be one of the reasons for fatigue and weight gain. A growing number of new studies are showing a link between opiate derivatives and the growth of cancer cells.

In medicine, we sometimes play with words. *Habituation* and *dependence* versus *addiction* are examples of this. Like everybody else, doctors like clear separations—black and white suits us much better than gray. We have a preference for findings and solutions that can be accurately filed into distinct categories. When fibromyalgia presents its spectrum and hops disconcertingly from one system to another, we're far less comfortable. We're very insecure if we have to handle a conglomeration of symptoms all at once. We know we should relieve pain. That's part of our oath, but *primum no nocere*—"above all, do no harm"—should supersede our need to be heroes trying to curb every discomfort no matter what the cost.

Since escalating drug use often ends up badly, we direct you to an old medical maxim: For chronic diseases, avoid giving addictive drugs if at all possible. In fibromyalgia, this can be accomplished only by early diagnosis and treatment. Some of you probably want to slam this book down thinking that we don't understand, but we do. Hear us out. We judiciously prescribe pain medications if we must, but only nonnarcotic varieties. We stress to our patients: Bear with us and let's treat the disease instead of masking worsening symptoms that will eventually break through.

On this emotionally charged topic, it's hard to get both sides to listen to scientific fact and reason. Narcotic side effects are certainly easier to tolerate than never-ending pain. Dependency is not the same as addiction, which by definition means that drug use is causing a problem in certain social ways. Dependency simply means that the body has come to depend on an outside chemical to fulfill a normal function. The body converts narcotic pain medications to morphine, which occupies pain receptors in the brain, ones that were designed for natural endorphins. When this happens on a daily basis, the brain is duped and cuts production levels drastically, and especially in fibromyalgics, this can be down to next to nothing. There's no problem as long as the body continues to get the artificial supply, but when a dose is skipped or delayed, there is no longer any natural chemical to replace it. Since endorphin receptors are largely in the emotional part of the brain, depression and apathy also occur. This is the reason that patients are put on even more potent and long-acting narcotics such as OxyContin or morphine. The rationale is simply that since these compounds don't wear off as quickly as, say, Vicodin, the patients are spared the discomfort of rebound pain every four to six hours.

There are no medications in the *Physicians' Desk Reference* (*PDR*) designated for long-term relief of chronic pain, defined as lasting longer than six months. That's because these medications aren't safe or devoid of serious side effects. In general, chronic pain is more difficult to treat than the acute kind. In normal responses to trauma, the brain masterminds the release of endorphins and other specific hormones to deal with hurting. Nature's idea is to blunt pain enough for the injured body to get to safety. Also, pain is a necessary warning signal that persuades the injured to rest and heal by respecting necessary limitations. The brain isn't programmed for dealing with prolonged hurting because it expects its pain to be a self-limiting messenger.

Long-term releases of endorphins promotes desensitization to their effects. As we've seen before in other systems of the body, unrelenting messages are eventually ignored, construed as crying wolf. In this case, they wear down endorphin-producing cells, which finally refuse to respond. The brain gradually produces less, and unneeded receptors recede into the depth of cells, where many are destroyed. Steady narcotic use meets that same kind of ultimate stonewalling: Brain cells tire, reject the opiate signals, and keep right on hurting. Mounting complaints make doctors think patients must be overly sensitive to pain and obviously need heavier dosages. Eventually, most physicians balk at the quantity they now must prescribe for even modest relief and send the poor patient packing.

Tramadol (Ultram, Ultram ER) is a narcotic-like pain medication that has been studied and shown to be of some benefit in fibromyalgia. It is also manufactured with acetaminophen under the name Ultracet. It binds weakly to opiate receptors and is related to antidepressants The most common side effects are drowsiness, slow heartbeat, weakness, and light-headedness. Convulsions have occurred at higher doses or in patients who have combined the drug with other medications that raise serotonin levels. Originally touted as not being habit-forming, it is now conceded that it can be, and therefore, it should not be stopped abruptly.

In May 2009, the FDA issued a warning letter alleging that its manufacturer had "overstated the efficacy" of the drug, and "minimized the serious risks." This year a warning was added to tramadol's label stating it may cause an increased risk of suicide in patients who are also taking antidepressants, muscle relaxants, or tranquilizers. There's a long list of medications to be avoided with tramadol because it is loosely related to many other classes of drugs.

A very small preliminary study recently showed that low doses of an old generic drug, naltrexone, might help with fibromyalgia pain. At high dosages, it's used to treat opiate and alcohol addiction. It simply blocks opioid receptors and voids their narcotic effects. As a result, opiates and alcohol should not be taken while on naltrexone, or nausea, vomiting, cold sweats, chills, and numbness in the limbs may occur. Naltrexone may also interfere with or counteract over-the-counter NSAIDs.

Use of naltrexone initially increases pain. Narcotics cannot be taken for two weeks at the beginning of this treatment. Side effects include vivid, bizarre dreams, fatigue, spasm, and pain, which usually recede after a few weeks. It is unlikely that large studies will be mounted to test this generic drug since little financial gain would accrue to any drug manufacturer.

Complete relief from fibromyalgia pain is not always possible. If your pain is moderate but you're living a normal life, going back to work, we've made progress.

—*Doris Cope, director of pain management*
at the Pittsburgh School of Medicine

So what do you do if you don't want to take narcotics? Cumulative studies are showing that acetaminophen (Tylenol) can lead to kidney or liver damage if taken regularly over several years. That same study found no such problems with some non-steroidal anti-inflammatory drugs (NSAIDs) such as ibuprofen or naproxen. However, this entire group may induce bleeding ulcers, liver damage, and symptoms that mimic fibromyalgia or even disrupt deep-sleep patterns. The newer anti-inflammatories (Cox-1 inhibitors) that are kinder on the stomach appear to be harder on the heart. One of them, Vioxx, was recently pulled by its manufacturer. Celecoxib (Celebrex) alone of the Cox-1 inhibitors remains on the market but with a warning label suggesting it, too, may have cardiac risks.

Recent references suggest that all NSAIDs, along with acetaminophen, can interfere with energy production in mitochondria. If taken before exercise, they can actually interfere with some of its strengthening benefits. However, when compared with prescription compounds, over-the-counter medications certainly have less potential for side effects. The most important thing to remember is that the warnings for excess intake should be heeded.

AN OVERVIEW OF MEDICATIONS COMMONLY USED FOR FIBROMYALGIA

The doctor who diagnosed my FMS asked if I was depressed. I was not happy about being in constant pain that seriously disrupted my life so I said yes. He said that pain and depression are like the chicken and the egg—which came first? He explained it was a cycle, one feeding off the other. He prescribed amitriptyline because it has been known to ease pain. Simply put, I felt drugged: sluggish, detached, hollow, empty, and very unlike myself. I felt no benefit on my pain. I couldn't wait to get off it but I followed directions and tapered off. My senses gradually reawakened and I felt present in the current moment again, better able to appreciate the colors and simple sensations like the wind on my skin and the warmth of sunshine.

—*Jody D., North Carolina*

Since the mid-1980s, low-dose antidepressants have been used for fibromyalgia. Side effects include weight gain, dry mouth, constipation, and fatigue. Studies suggest that the oldest type, the tricyclics, gave relief in only 30 to 40 percent of patients (see the quote by Dr. Goldenberg below)—clearly not much better than the placebo response. Newer, specific serotonin-reuptake and norepinephrine-reuptake inhibitors are being prescribed as though they were no more dangerous than after-dinner mints. A very recent paper suggested they had no advantage over placebo. That's suspect because at least clinically, significant numbers of patients have surely been helped. In those for whom such drugs are effective, sleep patterns are somewhat restored, depression eased, and pain perception may be diminished up to 50 percent. Notwithstanding, some people get adversely wired up and suffer serious disruption of stage 4 sleep. Because they don't seem to be as dangerous as narcotics, physicians continue prescribing them despite the unpromising statistics; making combinations of the various types of antidepressants is increasingly popular. Side effects for these newer classes vary greatly, but most common are drowsiness, nausea, headache, and dry mouth. For fibromyalgics, particularly disturbing can be hair loss, significant weight gain, and lowered libido in both males and females. SSRI antidepressants have been linked to the increased risk of cataract formation.

The above paragraph is discouraging—and it gets worse! Antidepressants have no lasting benefits for fibromyalgia, even though pain and depression are temporarily masked. Their effectiveness lessens after about nine weeks, and unfortunately, the disease marches on. Nothing has been done to alleviate the cause, and symptoms simply burst through the drug suppression at some point. Dosages should not be titrated upward. Studies show that if low potencies don't work, then higher amounts won't prove much more effective.

The new "selective" SNRIs (serotonin and norepinephrine reuptake inhibitors) are increasingly prescribed as first-line drugs for fibromyalgia pain. Since these are the newest class on the market, there are fewer of them available. Cymbalta (duloxetine) and Savella (milnacipran) are the only antidepressants approved by the FDA specifically for fibromyalgia. Other drugs in this class include Effexor (venlafaxine), which is an older drug and available as a generic. Studies have shown these to be ever so slightly more effective for depression than the older SSRIs, but the two classes haven't been studied head to head for fibromyalgia. Both types have about the same side effects because of their similar action. These range from insomnia, anxiety, sweating especially at night, muscle pain or cramps, weight gain, fatigue, drowsiness, headache, raised blood pressure, nausea, and problems with judgment, thinking, or coordination. Another common side effect is sexual dysfunction. The latter side effect might be slightly less common with newer drugs, but it remains a major reason for discontinuation. Some male patients have reported swollen testicles when taking milnacipran.

This brings us to the so-called discontinuation syndrome (or withdrawal), which occurs when one of these drugs is discontinued abruptly. Effexor (venlafaxine) is considered to be the most difficult one in this class to stop because of its relatively short half-life. All these drugs should be stopped only under the supervision of a physician.

According to the FDA, all antidepressants have a very serious increased risk of suicidal thinking and behavior, especially in young adults. All antidepressants now carry a black box warning on their packaging. This is the strongest tool the FDA has to issue consumer safety warnings. They are almost always issued for an entire class of drugs because side effects broadly apply to all those related compounds. Unfortunately black boxes are becoming so common that patients don't always understand their gravity. Investigators recently looked at the twenty different drug classes that made up two-thirds of the 200 top-selling drugs in America. Half of them carried these serious warnings, but the packaging wasn't always clear. (Not every drug that's been withdrawn from the market first had such a label.) It's important for consumers to check this information because these warnings are considered enough of a safety precaution to protect manufacturers from liability in the case of adverse events.

I have tried Savella. The side effects are pretty horrible. Although it did help my pain, it was just not worth it. The nausea, sweating, hot flashes (to the point of feeling like I was cooking in my oven), fevers, and dehydration were not worth it to me. I was on it for about twenty days until I couldn't take it anymore. Everyone I know has had the same nasty side effects. I have yet to meet someone who has had good luck with this medication. Your doctor might prescribe either Lyrica or Cymbalta or maybe both. I will forewarn you that Cymbalta will give you horrible headaches for about a week. Most doctors don't offer Lyrica because with most patients it causes serious weight gain or bloating.

—*Melissa, South Dakota*

Drug interactions are another concern with all antidepressants, especially the newer classes. Quite often they are contraindicated with other therapies. The triptan migraine medications (Imitrex, Maxalt, Axert, and Frova) should not be used within five weeks of some antidepressants. Used with sleeping medications, both prescription and over-the-counter versions may cause over-sedation. Other therapies that have an effect on serotonin levels such as 5-HTP are considered dangerous in conjunction with any antidepressant. Tramadol (Ultram) is also considered risky in combinations. Narcotics, central nervous system depressants such as muscle relaxants (for example, cyclobenzaprine), and benzodiazepines (used for anxiety) should be used with great caution if you are taking an antidepressant.

> Although tricyclic medications, notably low doses of amitrip-tyline and cyclobenzaprine, have been beneficial in controlled therapeutic trials in fibromyalgia, overall effectiveness in patients has not been impressive. Patient self-rating of medici-nal therapy has been no better than such nonmedicinal treat-ments as physical and chiropractic therapy. Only 30 to 40 percent of our patients described medications as very effective. In the only long-term longitudinal study reported in FMS, we surveyed 39 patients for three consecutive years. Although 83 percent of them continued to take some medications, usually multiple, during the three years, only 20 percent felt well.
>
> —*Don L. Goldenberg, M.D.,* Journal of Rheumatology[3]

Muscle relaxants, sedatives, and anti-anxiety drugs are all commonly prescribed for some of the many symptoms of fibromyalgia. Patients tolerate them only in limited quantities because of the hangover fatigue they generally induce. That and mental fogginess are two reasons patients give for discon-tinuing them. Confirming their value by double-blind studies is difficult, because sedative effects are too obvious compared with placebo. They don't interfere with our protocol and are helpful for those who handle them well.

Antiseizure drugs have worked their way into the fibromy-algia arsenal. Beginning with Neurontin (gabapentin), a drug designed for epileptic seizures that do not respond to other medications, these began to be used off-label for nerve pain. Lyrica (pregabalin)—a more recent tweak of the molecule— was the first medication indicated for fibromyalgia. It was originally approved for nerve pain from such conditions as shingles. Lyrica carries a special warning for men, who should not take this medication. Animal studies showed lowered fertility in males and could cause sperm abnormalities. Birth defects were reported in some of their offspring. It is unknown if pregabalin would do the same in humans, but until further studies, it would seem prudent for men to avoid it. Ativan (lorazepam), a benzodiazepine often used for seizures, is currently being studied to see if it can best placebo for pain.

Topiramate (Topamax) is a medication that was originally designed for epilepsy and is now approved for the treatment of migraine headaches in adults and teenagers. It is often used off-label for nerve pain and fibromyalgia. Doses are titrated up especially when used for controlling migraines, but the side effects of fatigue and dizziness, burning and tingling often preclude patients reaching an effective dose. A recent study linked topiramate to a fourteen-fold increase in birth defects.

ENERGY

An alarming trend has begun largely in response to the fatigue, mental slowness, and lethargy caused by narcotic pain medications, especially the more potent ones. It's becoming all too common to see patients of all ages on potent combinations of painkillers offset by a stimulant. Most commonly used are the newer class called by the cheerful name *wakefulness promoting agents*. These are: modafinil (Provigil, Alertec, Modavigil), armodafinil (Nuvigil), and adrafinil (Olmifon). Common side effects are dizziness, insomnia, and diarrhea.

Even stronger stimulants, amphetamines such as methylphenidate (Ritalin, Concerta, and Metadate), amphetamine salts

(Adderal), and dexamphetamine (Dexedrine) are still used in many patients with severe fatigue. In other cases, patients may be taking them for attention deficit disorder, which might be caused by fibromyalgia (problems with memory and concentration) or the side effects of other medications. In fibromyalgia, where energy formation is faulty, these drugs are particularly problematic, especially when used for long periods. Although they'll work initially, the cells eventually become exhausted and fail to respond to even higher doses of stimulants, rather like beating a dead horse. The body's energy stores are dragged farther back into deficit spending, and it takes time to recover when the drugs are finally stopped because of lack of efficacy. Side effects of stimulants are pretty obvious: jitteriness, anxiety, and insomnia. They may also raise heart rate and blood pressure. Patients with fibromyalgia, because of the nature of the disease itself, may be more susceptible to rebound fatigue, depression, and anxiety. Other less potent compounds that are sometimes used to promote daytime alertness are the antidepressants fluoxetine (Prozac) and buproprion (Wellbutrin).

Prescription drugs aren't the only thing commonly used for fibromyalgia. In response to the lobbying efforts of the multibillion-dollar "dietary supplement" industry, Congress in 1994 exempted their products from FDA regulation. Since then, products of all description—animal, vegetable, and mineral— have flooded the market, subject only to the scruples of their manufacturers, who promise all sorts of miracles in carefully worded infomercials. The so-called scientific facts on labels are often indistinguishable from advertising jargon because they are! Dietary supplements may contain the substances listed on the label in the amounts claimed, but they need not, and there is no one to police them and prevent their sale if they don't. The well-advertised coral calcium products, for example, which claimed to treat everything from cancer to fibromyalgia and arthritis, were found to contain dangerously high levels of lead when finally subjected to independent laboratory testing.

> In an analysis of ginseng products, for example, the amount of active ingredient in each pill varied by as much as a factor of 10 among brands that were labeled as containing the same amount. Some brands contained none at all… The only legal requirement in the sale of such products is that they not be promoted as preventing or treating disease. To comply with that stipulation, their labeling has risen to an art-form of doublespeak.
> —*Marcia Angell, M.D., and Jerome P. Kassirer, M.D.,*
> New England Journal of Medicine[4]

According to a recent survey, about 40 percent of Americans use some sort of medical alternative treatment, and most of these are chronic pain patients looking for relief. A new development is that more insurance companies are advertising these services. Only a few actually cover herbs and other dietary supplements because they are of unproven safety and worth. Yet they let sellers advertise their products to members, which can imply benefit. Some HMOs allow doctors to prescribe them although the patient must pay for them out of pocket.

What does this mean? It means that patients who pick these alternatives pay more for health care because they aren't using their drug cards. Every person who uses St. John's wort instead of Prozac or red rice yeast instead of a statin pays for it out of pocket and saves the insurance company money. So is it a coincidence that several large insurers are contracted with dietary supplement companies to "deliver discounts" to their members? And the criteria for promoting a product? "If a healthy person can safely take it, we will sell it."

It's not within the scope of this book to agonize over herbal medications, their safety, and their efficacy. Since plant concentrates totally block guaifenesin, it's a moot point for us. We've previously questioned the wisdom of taking tablet concentrates from crushed leaves, roots, or other plant parts that contain at least one hundred thousand various compounds. The dangers of individual idiosyncrasies mount with that volume of chemical contents. While herb users are seeking help from just a couple of these chemicals, they are consuming many more by ingesting the entire extract. The sheer number of components exponentially raises the likelihood of hypersensitivity reactions as well as liver or renal damage. The potential for harm is increased with frequent dosing and questionable purity and potency.

While some herbal formulas with a doctor or health practitioner's guidance can certainly be beneficial, the vast majority of users self-medicate, which can be a recipe for disaster. As these supplements are used more widely, interactions with prescription drugs have been documented as well as side effects—the same as with any medicinal compound, no matter what the origin. Despite what advertising would have you believe, *natural* is not a synonym for *safe*. Medications, quite simply, are poisons judiciously administered. We suggest that any compound that has a medicinal effect on the body should be treated with respect.

Hormones such as DHEA, thyroid, progesterone, testosterone, growth hormone, and estrogen will not block guaifenesin. These must be prescribed by doctors. Too often they're given because one of them turned up low on a single test, and sometimes not even the appropriate one. Just as often, they're handed out for reasons such as "boosting the metabolism" or for hot flashes not caused by a hormone imbalance but by fibromyalgia. As an endocrinologist, I strongly suggest that patients do extensive research before considering hormone therapy of any kind. These are powerful and too often mishandled without respect for their full effects. Always be sure your levels are abnormal on repeated testing, done at the proper time of day, before considering hormone adjustments. Also bear in mind that many hormone levels are meant to decline with age, and boosting them to youthful levels in older patients may cause severe problems. "Bioidentical" sex hormones are a case in point. Although these have not been shown to have the same risks as synthetic or animal compounds, they also have not been studied to the same extent. *Bio* means nothing and *identical* signifies that these must attach to at least most of the same receptors in the body that other hormones do. Attaching to an estrogen receptor, for example, means that it has the same effect on the cells as any other estrogen, including your own. It also carries the same risk. Lifetime exposure to estrogen, even the most natural form of all—the one women's bodies make themselves—increases the risk of cancer.

Some hormones such as growth hormone cannot be taken orally but must be injected because it is destroyed by the gut. Thus any oral preparation touted as growth hormone isn't that but a concoction said to stimulate it. Abnormalities of other hormone levels (such as cortisol) must be diagnosed by tests administered at appropriate times of the day, as normal levels vary widely depending on the hour. Again, caution should be the rule.

There are numerous new warnings about ingesting excess vitamins and supplements. These won't block guaifenesin, but they can interfere with prescription drugs, especially the absorption of thyroid hormone. Very little is known about the effects of consuming large quantities of any substance and unbalanced components may interfere with the others. Yet vitamins are consistently marketed as life extenders and necessary for good health. Americans take some 23 billion dollars' worth of them a year and yet not a single one has been actually proven to reduce deaths or illness. Fat-soluble ones such as K and E pose minor risks because overabundance can't be excreted. Vitamin A (beta-carotene) seems downright dangerous in the quantities customarily marketed. Calcium is known to partially block the action of some antibiotics, and magnesium the effects of Neurontin. Very recent studies have cast doubt on the safety of calcium supplementation, showing an increased risk of heart attacks and strokes. Magnesium is often taken for muscle relaxation but can cause diarrhea. Larger amounts of others such as zinc have been questioned for safety by some Alzheimer's disease researchers. Vitamin C in large doses can increase the risk of weight gain when taken with tricyclic antidepressants.

Vitamin D deserves its own paragraph. It's now the darling of the vitamin world. Some well-quoted papers claim that 65 percent of American adults are D deficient and nearly every new patient we see is taking or has been told to take large doses of it to help with pain and other complaints.

But is this true? Can it be true? Of course not—how could it be? This conclusion is based on plasma measurements of 25-hydroxy D3 (25-OH D3), which is made in the liver after the sun has radiated certain fatty substances in the skin. 25-OH D3 undergoes further transition when a kidney enzyme piggybacks another hydroxyl (OH) onto the liver version. This produces 1-25dihyroxy D3 (1-25 OH_2) D3, a vitamin turned hormone that is four times more potent than the original compound the liver produced. A recent paper in the *Journal of Nutrition* clearly demonstrated that the liver's vitamin D had only a 3 percent benefit to promote intestinal calcium absorption whereas the more potent form had a 97 percent rate. This clearly shows that the free form of each vitamin (that is not bound to a blood protein) is what matters. It turns out that many tissues including the bones seem able to make the more powerful vitamin D form and can meet the body's needs easily.

Parathyroid hormones, estrogens, and certain bone-kidney

liaisons do the delicate balancing of the body's vitamin D. The amount you can create from exposure to the sun depends on your skin tone. For lighter skins, fifteen minutes in the sun during the middle of the day provides 4,000 units of D. Think of 1,000 units as a safe number. If you're not sure whether you need supplemental D, make sure your doctor tests for the 1-25 variety. If it's normal, you don't need additional D.

I should tell you that not only have I improved due to guaifenesin, I have also thrown out all the other stuff I was on. Now, I use no sleeping pills, no antidepressants, no steroids, and I used to think I needed all three of them for the rest of my life. I only take a little Tylenol now and then for headaches, and of course, guaifenesin.

—*Jeri Lynn, California*

SLEEP

Difficulty falling asleep and staying asleep long enough to reach the stage 4 phase of restorative sleep is the first major hurdle that we face in dealing with the other symptoms of FMS. I absolutely cannot nap no matter how hard I try, and going to sleep at night requires a ritual of sleep aids, a calming atmosphere, total darkness in the room, numerous pillows piled around my body, a lightweight cover. I would like to trade a day with a normal person who goes out like a light, sleeps deeply, and wakes refreshed. Oh, I wish...

—*Elizabeth R., Georgia*

The desire for restful sleep eventually leads exhausted fibromyalgics to demand sleeping pills. By that time, an expensive mattress, contoured pillows, blackout curtains, and white noise tapes haven't made much difference. Pre-bedtime rituals that initially helped, such as warm baths, dimmed lights, soothing music, or meditation, no longer work. My own experience was that nighttime inactivity further stiffened my already contracted muscles, tendons, and ligaments. Every time I'd lie in one position for a few minutes, my pain mounted progressively. At first it was subliminal—just enough to make me restless. As the night progressed, I hurt enough to awaken from whatever stage of sleep I'd managed to reach. My nights were a bit like the Indianapolis 500, moving to and fro, constantly steering for position. I could make a rare victory lap only if I got a good night's rest. As I recall, I rarely won.

The earliest study of modern fibromyalgia by Drs. Moldofsky and Smythe explored the complaint of sleep disturbances, documented in 70 percent of patients. Because articles about sleep disturbance were the first to make it into medical journals, nearly all physicians are willing to prescribe sleeping compounds and are aware that fibromyalgics have problems getting enough rest. It's so prevalent that those who don't complain of poor sleep are often told they don't have the disease!

We urge patients to begin with the over-the-counter sleeping aids—diphenhydramine and doxylamine. These old antihistamines made people so drowsy that, when better compounds came along, they were abandoned as allergy treatments. Once available over the counter, they were rediscovered as sleeping aids. They are non-habit-forming and safe in small amounts, even for children. Diphenhydramine is often allowed by obstetricians during pregnancy. It's marketed in 25 mg capsules and tablets, but the dosage can be titrated up to 100 mg a night. Diphenhydramine is the sleep-inducing ingredient in products such as Tylenol PM, Simply Sleep, Benadryl, Sominex, and Unisom. It helps reach delta, deep-sleep levels. About 10 percent of people get adverse effects such as jitters and excitability, and for those, these two antihistamines should be avoided. Others find that these compounds make them excessively tired the next morning. If this is the case, you should purchase them in liquid or tablet forms so that very small doses can be used and titrated on a nightly basis if needed.

Melatonin is a hormone released by the pineal gland. It has many effects in the body, where it's eventually converted to serotonin. It's safe and helps reset the sleep clock in the brain. Travelers have used it for years to offset jet lag. Levels of the hormone decline with age, which may explain some of the insomnia of the elderly. Its safety has not been established for children or teenagers because they already produce large amounts. We concur that it works best for older individuals, who may require a higher dosage than younger patients because their own levels are considerably lower to start with. Various papers recommend trying the hormone for at least two months before abandoning it for lack of success. A new study found best effects if taken six to eight hours before bedtime since the hormone doesn't often cause daytime drowsiness. Its function is to reset the clock restoring natural sleep, the so-called circadian rhythm. High dosages of melatonin may cause vivid or unpleasant dreaming; if that is the case, a lower dosage should be tried. Depression has also been listed in various places as a possible side effect when higher amounts are taken.

If taken at bedtime, the sublingual form of melatonin provides quicker action and makes for smaller dosages. This introduces it directly into the bloodstream and avoids the digestive tract. The pill dissolves and absorbs within ten minutes under the tongue. Fibromyalgics should be aware that the minted variety will block guaifenesin, but orange flavoring is also available. (The tablets, which are swallowed, contain no flavor at all.) We've had some success combining melatonin with diphenhydramine when neither worked as a stand-alone therapy, and there's also evidence that it enhances the action of amitriptyline (Elavil).

Another nonprescription compound is 5-HTP, short for 5-hydroxy-tryptophan, one of the chemicals in the process leading to the formation of melatonin and serotonin. Doses generally begin at 20 mg before bed, but lower doses are sometimes taken by day to help control pain. Doses as high as 100 mg three times a day have been studied; doses should be started very low and moved up slowly. Side effects include dry mouth, daytime fatigue, dizziness, and constipation. Most pharmacies and health food stores carry 5-HTP, which has been used since L-tryptophan was taken off the market when contaminated batches caused some fatalities. This product should not be used within five weeks of treatment with an SSRI antidepressant because of its effects on serotonin.

If patients still can't sleep or don't tolerate the above compounds, they must turn to prescription medications. These all have the potential to create dependence although they vary greatly in this capacity. If our patients must take them, we suggest taking the tiniest effective amount and diligently avoiding nightly use. Sleeping medications are more effective when used sparingly for short-term situations. In as little as three weeks, benzodiazapines can completely lose their effectiveness if used nightly. Using them on alternate nights lowers the probability of habituation and loss of efficacy. Before turning to stronger compounds, first the exact type of sleeping problem should be identified. Do you have a problem falling asleep or remaining asleep? Is early-morning awakening the problem? Different medications may work better on these various problems so that solutions can even be addressed on a night-by-night basis if necessary.

Sedatives work by depressing the central nervous system, which in turn leads to a morning hangover. This compounds the problem for fibromyalgics, who already have difficulty functioning at that time of day. Sleeping pills may also cause rebound effects the next afternoon when the fatigue can actually be intensified. If patients are forced to nap as a result, they may get into a vicious cycle that further intensifies nighttime insomnia. Other side effects are mental confusion, slowed thinking, dry mouth, dizziness, and malaise. The overall quality of sleep can be reduced when using medications that produce less restorative deep sleep and dream sleep. There are some other recently publicized serious side effects of the sedative-hypnotic drugs. These include sleepwalking, sleep driving, and sleep eating. Patients may have no memory of these events, and especially for those who live alone, these are dangerous scenarios. If your body is accustomed to sleep medications, insomnia will be worse when you don't take them.

Many medications, such as muscle relaxants, tranquilizers, antianxiety drugs, antidepressants, and narcotics can add to an already overwhelming fatigue. Fibromyalgics are given these compounds in diverse combinations. Some of these are used to promote sleep because the side effect of drowsiness helps patients fall asleep and remain so for hours. It's a toss-up whether or not the enhanced sleep they provide is worth the energy-sapping side effects. We urge patients with unrelenting fatigue to review their medications with their physicians or pharmacists. Ever-present exhaustion should not always be blamed on the illness—symptoms of fibromyalgia are usually variable from day to day. Even over-the-counter anti-inflammatories and analgesics must also be viewed in context, since they can contribute to the problem by cutting energy production.

COMMONLY PRESCRIBED MEDICATIONS FOR SLEEP DISTURBANCES IN FIBROMYALGIA

The most common group of sleeping pills are known as sedative hypnotics. In general, these medications act by working on receptors in the brain that slow down the central nervous system. Some are used more for inducing sleep, others for staying asleep. Some last longer than others in your system, and some have a higher risk of becoming habit-forming. This is why you should work with your doctor to carefully decide which choice(s) would be best in your particular case.

Benzodiazepines are the oldest class of sleeping pills still in use. As a group, they are thought to be the most highly addictive. Although primarily used to treat anxiety disorder, they are also approved to treat insomnia. Because they are older drugs, generics are available so they are preferred by insurance companies over the newer compounds. They have longer duration of action than some of the newer medications, which may result in more morning fatigue. In addition, they can quite quickly lose their effectiveness if used longer than several weeks. The most common of these are estazolam (ProSom), flurazepam (Dalmane), temazepam (Restoril), and triazolam (Halcion).

The newer drugs designed for insomnia don't have the same chemical structure as benzodiazepines but act on the same area in the brain. For some reason, they have fewer side effects and a lower risk of dependency, although they are also considered controlled substances. Ambien (zolpidem) has been on the market the longest of this group. It is available as a generic although the controlled-release formula is not. Zaleplon (Sonata) has the shortest half-life of all and is used to help patients get to sleep. It's especially effective for those who wake in the early morning and need only a few more hours of sleep. Owing to its shorter half-life, it has less rebound fatigue but is not designed to help patients sleep for a full eight hours. Getting a good night's sleep may pose dangers for people with mild heartburn and the more than 40 percent of Americans with gastroesophageal reflux disease (GERD). A 2009 study found that people taking Ambien were less than half as likely to wake up during bouts of acid reflux, increasing their exposure to nighttime stomach acid. This backwash can cause damage to the esophagus that may not have occurred had the person awoken and swallowed, thereby neutralizing the acid with saliva. This type of damage to the cells lining the throat may increase the risk for esophageal cancer.

In 2004, Lunesta (eszopiclone) was approved by the FDA for difficulty falling asleep as well as staying asleep. It is nonnarcotic and not limited to short-term use like other compounds for insomnia. It is available in two strengths but not as a generic so insurance companies don't always cover it. Lunesta has an additional side effect of a bitter or bad taste in the mouth the following day.

The most recent addition in this category is Rozerem (ramelteon). It is the first novel drug in thirty-five years of sleep research and is indicated for insomnia. It targets specific receptors in the brain, MT1 and 2, which are critical in regulating the body's sleep-wake cycle. In other words, it mimics the action of melatonin. Rozerem is considered safe even for those with a history of drug abuse—it is the only prescription sleep aid that is not classified as a controlled substance. Because it does not work by slowing down the central nervous system, it isn't as likely to cause daytime grogginess. It is not available as a generic, which brings up a question of cost effectiveness. In a government-sponsored study, patients who took Rozerem fell asleep sixteen minutes faster and slept eleven to nineteen minutes longer than those taking a placebo. Another concern is that Rozerem works by increasing the level of melatonin by about sixteen times in the brain. Melatonin is a hormone that could potentially alter testosterone levels. It's possible to experience changes in your sex drive as well as your menstrual cycle.

In fact, Rozerem isn't much different than its chemical cousin, plain nonprescription melatonin. The primary difference is that prescription drugs are held to higher standards when it comes to ingredients and potency than are dietary supplements, which are not, as we have seen, regulated by the FDA.

If you suffer from severe restless legs syndrome which keeps you from sleeping, the newest treatment is to use a dopamine agonist such as ropinirole or pramipexole. These two medications were developed for use in treating Parkinson's disease. The most common side effects are nausea and dizziness, but these medications have also been linked to compulsive gambling, eating, and altered sexual habits. This is because dopamine agonists target receptors in the brain associated with motivation and reward; researchers suggest that anyone taking these drugs be screened for compulsive behaviors and then monitored carefully. Another problem with taking these compounds for restless legs is that over time they may lose effectiveness. The problem is intensified because symptoms can return more severely and begin earlier in the night than before. Patients should be aware that the medications may lose efficacy; patients may need to switch to a different class of drug or take a few weeks off.

Another medication we see more frequently used for sleep disorders is Xyrem (sodium oxybate), which is currently only indicated for narcolepsy and is tightly controlled. It's not available in regular pharmacies but is distributed from one central pharmacy. The reason for this is that sodium oxybate is another name for GHB, the so-called date-rape drug. Small studies of fibromyalgics demonstrated some benefit in pain reduction, but the FDA refused to approve it, saying benefits did not outweigh the great potential for abuse. Sodium oxybate can cause serious side effects even when taken as directed. It cannot be taken with antidepressants, alcohol, or benzodiazepines, and withdrawal generally occurs when it is discontinued.

Sodium oxybate must be taken twice a night because it has a short half-life and won't last long enough. The first dose is taken once in bed as it begins to work very quickly. The second dose must be placed near the bed and an alarm clock is used to awaken the patient for the second dose. Users are cautioned about getting out of bed at all during the night, which makes it inappropriate for most fibromyaglics, especially those who are parents and may be called on by their children during the night.

Tricyclic and polycyclic antidepressants (the most studied drugs in fibromyalgia) are often prescribed to help patients sleep. Possible weight gain is a side effect, as well as early-morning grogginess, constipation, and dry mouth. Benefits are seen two to four weeks after initiation. If efficacy starts to fade, a month-long break may be taken every four months. The most common are amitriptyline, doxepin, cyclobenzaprine, nortripyline, and desipramine. Side effects include drowsiness, nausea, headache, and constipation. Trazodone—both a sedative and an antidepressant—is the most commonly used. Small doses should be used in the beginning, and often that's all that is necessary. Other classes of antidepressants such as the SSRIs generally do not help as well with sleep problems.

Some patients can use muscle relaxants to allow for better sleep. This is because their effect is to depress the central nervous system and thereby they have an overall sedating effect on the body. The majority of these drugs do not act on the muscles, but on the brain. This same fatigue can make them problematic for daytime use.

Most common are the older cyclobenzaprine (Flexeril) and carisoprodol (Soma), which have been well studied. Most of the research done on muscle relaxants was done on Flexeril, which has been shown to increase stage 4 sleep. Increasing this sleep stage does help patients feel more refreshed in the mornings. Studies have also demonstrated that this action helps reduce pain in some fibromyalgics. Other medications in this class are methocarbamol (Robaxin) and metaxalone (Skelaxin), which is newer so it's available only in brand form. Carisoprodol is not recommended for older adults or for those with a history of drug addiction. Metaxalone can cause nausea, irritability, nervousness, and upset stomach. Comparisons have not shown either of them to be superior to the other.

A newer addition is the much more potent Zanaflex (tizanidine hydrochloride)—actually marketed to decrease spasticity of muscles in serious spastic conditions. Side effects include mental confusion and hallucinations; this one especially should be used with care. It can also lower blood pressure, causing light-headedness and dizziness. Other side effects include dry mouth, blurred vision, constipation, frequent urination, runny nose, speech disorders, and vomiting.

Although we've learned that it is better to take only guaifenesin, for many it is difficult to do so. Many of us started on a number of different medications. I was diagnosed with FMS in 1988 and have been on plenty of medications since then. My symptoms began in 1977. I was taking Elavil for three years and Ambien for two. I tried to stop taking both of these a number of times before guaifenesin but I was in such sad shape I would have to start up again. I very slowly weaned myself off the Elavil. That was not very hard to do. I had no real reaction from stopping. I was concerned with the Ambien because I needed to sleep, so I cut way back, usually only taking 1/4 of a tablet at night except when I was feeling well. Then I stopped taking it. The first few nights I used Benadryl, it made me very groggy. Then I tried melatonin and got the same results. I also tried a combination that made me groggy, too. So after a week of messing around, I went to bed without anything and I fell asleep just fine...

—*Linda P., Ohio*

EXERCISE

Exercise is one of the most effective treatments for fibromyalgia. It benefits all of the symptoms of fibromyalgia, including pain, fatigue, and sleep problems.

Exercise can help maintain bone mass, improve balance, reduce stress, and increase strength. Getting regular exercise can also help control your weight, which is important to reducing the pain of fibromyalgia.

—*Daniel Clauw, M.D., professor of anesthesiology and medicine, University of Michigan*

The recommendation for exercise is one of the few truly useful ones made by nearly every physician. It's near and dear to the hearts of researchers and medical practitioners alike, and is the most commonly prescribed treatment for fibromyalgia. Endless studies have proven its benefits as well as the difficulty in persuading patients to begin a program and stick with it. Guaifenesin can reverse your fibromyalgia, but it takes exercise to rebuild your body and maintain your health. You need both and you can start to experience benefits from even a small amount of activity fairly quickly.

Advice is soundest when gentle stretching, simple walking, and pool workouts are suggested to begin the process. We heartily endorse these types of gentle movements, which don't overstress an already weakened body. The problem is that well-meaning physicians try to push patients into an immediate athletic program that very few can handle even though it may be labeled "low impact." A huge number of fibromyalgics can't even tolerate walking a few blocks without bracing for the physical price they'll pay the next day. There are good reasons for this. The aches and pains of fibromyalgia are caused by intracellular metabolic debris as a result of steadily working cells. As long as those residues remain in the affected cells, they remain in a perpetually contracted state. Any significant workout creates more of this debris, which must then recruit other tissues to act as dump sites. This intensifies the condition because the body doesn't have the capacity to make enough energy to clear the problem. Further malfunction follows: more pain, fatigue, and finally, systemic collapse.

The rationale behind prescribing heavy exercise is understandable. Stress releases our natural brain opioids—endorphins—in response to muscular aching. As they latch on to receptor cells, pain perception is dulled, allowing patients to push on with the activity. But the positive effects are nullified when the pain caused by exercise lasts too long. This is even more predictable when the patient has taken narcotic pain medication before exercise. As we've seen, narcotics depress the brain's ability to produce natural endorphins and grow new mitochondria to produce energy (ATP). It should also be remembered that upon discontinuing narcotics, it takes the body some three or four months to begin producing natural endorphins. During this period, if you begin an exercise program, be aware that your tolerance for pain will be abnormally low. Muscle aches, which under normal circumstances would be minor, will seem more intense until endorphin levels return to normal. Many other pain relievers—especially nonsteroidal anti-inflammatories—slow or block the body's ability to form new mitochondria so it's best to use them sparingly if at all prior to exercise. Endorphins also reduce tension and anxiety.

Physical activity has been proven to raise serotonin levels, a neurotransmitter which helps regulate mood, appetite, and the sleep-wake cycle. High levels are associated with an elevated mood while low levels are associated with depression. Thirty minutes of exercise raises blood levels considerably. Approximately 75 percent of the body's supply of serotonin is located in cells of the gut, where it regulates intestinal movements.

Another benefit of exercise is that it naturally raises growth hormone levels. Some well-known researchers have focused entirely on the effects of this hormone, which may be low in some fibromyalgics. It stimulates growth of muscles, tendons, and ligaments. Aerobic exercise induces its release by the pituitary, to promote important effects on protein, lipid, and carbohydrate metabolism.

A 2010 study published in *Arthritis Research & Therapy* found that regular daily activities, such as taking the stairs, gardening, or doing chores, can help reduce pain and improve daily functioning for those with fibromyalgia. This study shows us that every bit of activity is beneficial for fibromyalgia pain; it doesn't need to be a formal exercise program.

Moving your body at all may be difficult at first, but as you continue, you should notice that the activity gets easier. We can't emphasize enough that muscles, tendons, and ligaments must be treated gently until guaifenesin has cleared them. Until that time, care is needed. Exercise cannot heal tendons and ligaments, and as long as they are affected, they may not provide adequate support for joints. Until ligaments are strengthened and tight muscles are relaxed, endurance exercises should not be undertaken. In the beginning, a warm shower or bath may be helpful before stretching. Gentle walking is another way to begin an exercise session. The goal is not to yank hard on contracted structures which can cause injury and derail the program. The simplest prescription for healthy exercise came from the U.S. surgeon general: Accumulate 30 minutes of moderate activity on most days of the week. A 30- to 45-minute walk every day will help boost your immune system significantly, lower your risk of chronic disease, and make a dramatic difference in how you look and feel.

Disciplines that benefit healthy patients don't always work as intended when it comes to fibromyalgics. Exercise should gradually make you feel better, and that goal should be kept in mind. The rules are simple: Keep muscular workouts light and within tolerable discomfort zones. Treat the underlying disease, wait for improvement, and only then expand muscular efforts based on tolerance. When you feel better, you can go for the gold and finally begin to feel the full benefits of more energy and less pain.

Earlier we stressed that totally sedentary people wipe out up to 80 percent of the mitochondria in their muscle cells. As we've seen, without abundant power stations, the energy-generating capacity of the body is compromised and cannot be remedied. The problem is that you can't heal without energy and you can't make energy when you have fibromyalgia. Reversing fibromyalgia with guaifenesin restores the efficiency of the remaining mitochondria, but only endurance exercise can promote new growth, and resurrect dormant ones. Added mitochondria result in more abundant energy and growing stamina. While it doesn't happen overnight, exercise will begin the process of making both body and brain more functional. The key is to start with realistic goals and expand them as reversal makes more activity possible.

> If exercise could be packed into a pill, it would be the single most widely prescribed and beneficial medicine in the nation. Many health experts now feel that the single most important behavior you can adopt for good health (other than to quit smoking) is to get regular physical activity.
>
> —*Robert Butler, M.D., director, National Institute on Aging*

DISABILITY STATUS: A RAGING CONTROVERSY

> When it comes to disability determination, anyone who has to prove he or she is ill will be rendered more ill in the proving. When a physician participates in the process, it becomes worse than counterproductive, it becomes iatrogenic. At issue is the growing numbers...for whom self-respect in the workplace is so elusive that the gauntlet of disability determination seems an easier path.
>
> —*Nortin Hadler, M.D.*[5]

At the end of April 1999, the Social Security Administration issued regulation SSR 99-2p, which boldly announced that fibromyalgia and chronic fatigue syndromes *are medically determinable conditions*" capable of causing disability—defined as the inability to work at a job with regular demands. Despite this straightforward statement, qualifying for benefits remains a major challenge for patients and, by extension, for us, their physicians. Unique problems exist in fibromyalgia because of the subjective nature of complaints and total lack of diagnostic tests. It's impossible to prove someone is actually sick with the disease, let alone that he or she will not improve or recover. Obviously, and for good reasons, the judges are a little leery of "the patient says he [or she] hurts too much to work." There remains no way to measure pain—to prove it exists (or doesn't), or where it's located—and the same goes for fatigue. Equally elusive are the symptoms of irritable bowel, bladder discomfort, muscle stiffness, and problems with memory and concentration!

> It boils down to a judge's opinion about whether you could hold down a simple sit-down type of job that requires no training that also allows you to sit, stand, and adjust your position that is not production oriented.
>
> —*Jonathan Ginsberg, attorney at law, Georgia*

As physicians, we have an obligation to care for patients. That much is clear. If patients say they are too sick to work, how could it be our mission to prove otherwise? The conundrum is the absence of an unequivocally accepted yardstick to measure this illness. We are relegated to vague answers such as: "The patient states she is too tired to work, and describes daily headaches." "The patient says sitting at her computer makes her back hurt too much to concentrate." "Fibromyalgia is known to cause cognitive problems such as impaired memory and concentration."

Under pressure to control costs, insurance companies balk and demand proof of a disability that meets their criteria. The fact is, patients, doctors, lawyers, third-party insurers, and government agencies are locked in a complicated struggle with no easy solutions. Insurance companies and governmental agencies are justifiably terrified of the sheer number of potential claimants especially as the baby boomers age. Currently 11.8 million workers between the ages of sixteen and sixty-four report the presence of a medical condition that makes it difficult for them to find a job or remain employed. They comprise 6 percent of the population. (This does not include people with severe disabilities who have never been able to hold a job—another 12 percent.)

> Right now, I can work a full-time desk job, but if my brain fog gets worse, or my pain gets worse, I don't think I want to be at work. I have a highly stressful job. I work as a marketing/advertising manager for eighteen automotive dealerships, and I am under constant deadlines and pressure to get it done. Mistakes aren't tolerated, and I'm afraid of being fired if I start making too many. This automotive field of work is full of workaholics. I used to be the same way, but I just can't do it anymore.
>
> —*Debbie, Arizona*

Disability law is structured so that if you can perform a simple job, even though it hurts you or makes you tired, you're not eligible for benefits. The younger you are, the harder it will be for you to convince a judge that you can't do any kind of work. While it's easy for fibromyalgics to take this situation personally, it should be mentioned that only a terminal illness allows for immediate granting of benefits. Missing an eye or a limb or a hand doesn't guarantee you'll win your case—despite their obvious limitations. Everyone else is in for a struggle, especially one with an illness as invisible as fibromyalgia.

> Disability insurance companies certainly have the right to demand proof that a person is unable to work. Malingering and exaggeration are real problems with which insurers must contend. What's more difficult to understand is why some insurers also dismiss the judgment of those who know best, the physicians, friends, and neighbors of the patient, those who are best qualified to confirm how fibromyalgia impacts the patient's life. Instead, insurers seek "objective" proof by actually watching patients exert themselves. Fair enough, in principle, but not fair or reasonable as often applied in practice, especially for patients with fibromyalgia or chronic fatigue syndrome.
>
> —*Richard Podell, M.D., M.P.H.*

Physicians' letters are no longer all that's required to collect insurance benefits or Social Security disability. They're only the first steps in a long and costly process. Initial denials are routine, even with a lawyer's expertise. Second appeals are often summarily dismissed as well. At this point, persistent fibromyalgics who haven't already done so end up hiring attorneys for their third appeal or the trip to federal court that follows if that, too, fails. There is no question that this is a dismal and demeaning situation for a severely incapacitated individual who must face a long, expensive fight.

On the other side, extensive paperwork and phone interviews steal time from busy physicians, who are more comfortable treating patients. Records are copied multiple times, report upon report is demanded, for which charges must be made because of the time involved in writing them. These piles of papers are a real burden to a medical office when multiplied by many patients. Resentment can grow on both sides easily;

physicians do not always find it possible to answer questions the way a patient wishes. Doctors can expect to be grilled over the phone by "claim experts" who work for the insurance companies. Applicants can expect the ordeal of being examined by physicians working for insurance companies and the state. Physicians can expect their reports to be scrutinized and questioned by examiners who have never seen the patient face-to-face.

> FMS cases have reached near epidemic proportions in the courts, in U.S. Social Security disability claims, workers' compensation, and accident litigation. As many as 25 percent of U.S. patients with FMS have received some sort of disability or injury compensation.
>
> —*Frederick Wolfe, M.D.*[6]

One long-term disability insurance carrier notoriously maintains that fibromyalgia is a mental impairment, since nothing ever shows up on accepted tests. Records are combed for words such as *depressed*, *anxious*, and even *sad*. This permits enforcement of the fine-print clause limiting coverage for psychiatric illnesses. Dirty? You bet! There's a not-too-funny cartoon circulating of a physician reading the Miranda Rights to a patient sitting on an examination table: "Anything you say may be used against you in a court of law."

We badly need to replace the Functional Capacity Evaluation that's currently used to measure the level of disability in patients. While this form works for most ailments, it's commonly accepted by specialists that it's totally useless when it comes to fibromyalgia. Basically it relies on measurements of motion and strength over the period of a few hours. Among other things, patients are asked to touch their toes, walk, and crawl, sit in a chair for half an hour, and lift a ten-pound weight. It does not address the fact that it is the repetition of tasks that causes exhaustion and pain and results in the flare-up of other symptoms in fibromyalgia. Lawyers have managed to challenge the legality of these findings, but a better scale needs to be devised.

Michael's attorney, who herself had FMS, felt that this FCE testing protocol would give misleading results, drastically underestimating his disability. She pointed out that the test lasted just two hours, and it made no provision at all for seeing how Michael fared later that night or through the next day. She asked for my opinion. I agreed with Michael's attorney, and here's the reason why: Michael would have done the FCE on what he would view as a relatively good day. On a bad day he would stay in bed, and the FCE would be canceled. So almost by definition, the FCE results would not account at all for Michael's bad days, even though they occurred at least weekly.

More importantly, how Michael would do over two hours of touching toes and crawling had little bearing on how he would feel and function the next day, and whether he could repeat this kind of exertion day after day and week after week. The FCE claims to predict that, but there's no scientific basis for that claim. For those who live with this postexertion delayed flare-up pattern of CFS/FMS, to suggest that just two hours of observation could detect or predict this could be generously described as "silly."

—*Richard Podell, M.D., M.P.H.*

Bear in mind that no company is in business to go broke. As a result, disability insurers take the not unreasonable position that everybody with a job is tired, has aches and pains, and yet continues to function. Taxpayers and their legal representatives in the legislature are frightened, too. Some states have gone so far as to introduce legislation banning fibromyalgia as a compensable condition, at least under workers' compensation programs. As governments become more and more strapped for cash, this situation is going to become worse, not better. Even those already granted benefits can expect further scrutiny that will only get more intense.

We doctors also pay taxes and are aghast about the impact of fibromyalgia on the economy. Yet our concern is tempered by our oath to care for our patients, and what we should be asking ourselves: What is best for each individual? Is long-term disability really in a patient's best interest? We instinctively know that remaining active and functional in some capacity is an integral part of self-esteem. Pride in accomplishment is essential, and so is the sense of usefulness. A job well done, no matter how small, feels good. Long-term disability, like some of the other current solutions for fibromyalgia, begins or is party to a downward spiral. Too often, patients have no choice but to accelerate this slide by expending energy and resources trying to prove disability. Even after the long battle is won, victors must find ways to restore meaning and challenge to everyday life. They can't undertake restorative physical activity in public for fear of being videotaped by an insurance private eye. Out of legal necessity, they must behave sickly enough to merit regular medical attention. The cards are stacked against them: Even if improvement is managed, rehabilitation is out of the question. It's practically impossible to find a way back into the workforce if a patient is lucky enough to improve. Having been disabled, they are a poor risk for a potential employer to hire and train. Companies are not often willing to accept the expense of adding members to their medical insurance policy who have been diagnosed with fibromyalgia or chronic fatigue.

Most of all, as healers, our responsibility is to keep each person as productive as possible. The best way to accomplish this is by early diagnosis, education, and effective treatment. It's hard for us to side with a middle-aged person who just wants to stay home and uses fibromyalgia as an excuse to escape from the workforce.

Somebody's got to pay for the contemplated lifetime of relative leisure. Yet it is also an inescapable conclusion that we, the public, will have to rework the disability system if it's to survive. There are people who are truly ill who have fought long and hard to remain working at jobs they enjoy and cherish until the day that it just can no longer be done. Their reward for this perseverance is to have to fight even harder for help. The answer may lie in more flexible workplace policies mandated by law. More jobs should be tailored for employees with limitations that successfully bolster productivity and maintain self-esteem. We must do this for the financial survival of the government, and for patients and their doctors, it would be a real win-win situation.

Despite compassion, we physicians should feel that every patient requesting permanent disability represents a major defeat for medicine. If at all possible, we should fix them before they ever pick up an application form. Fibromyalgia reversal is swift in younger people and can be completed long before such thoughts are considered. Victories will come only with early diagnosis and treatments directed at the cause and not the symptom patchwork that's now so common. Too often disability is necessary because of the side effects of multiple medications that cannot be discontinued easily or effectively replaced.

Filing for disability is a long process with no guarantee of final victory. What's more, reports of depression beginning when benefits are granted are also common. With the fight behind you, the ramifications of what being legally disabled means can be very difficult to accept. Finding a meaningful life in the aftermath is a challenge in our society that on some level regards those who do not work as failures.

We know some of the preceding paragraphs will hurt readers who are on disability or in the process of trying to get it. But our bottom line is simple. Look back and remember what it was like to feel good. If you had known that it was possible to reverse your fibromyalgia, would you not have jumped at the chance?

We hope this chapter has answered some questions but, more important, that it has underscored our basic tenet. First and foremost, we've got to diagnose patients before they are incapacitated, and then fight for treatments that get patients well. Each and every patient should be offered the chance to have the most productive, successful, and complete life possible. Nothing less should be acceptable to us both as medical professionals and as human beings.

> Having a reversal protocol has changed everything. I now see it as a wake-up call and one I have used to empower myself and to heal myself. I feel strong and confident. Without [this], it would be a dreary time of self-blame if not outright depression.
>
> —*M.K., Hawaii*

IN CONCLUSION

To recap, we steadfastly advocate a single, simple medication for the treatment of fibromyalgia—guaifenesin. It's been around for a very long time and devoid of side effects, so we unhesitatingly prescribe it for persons of all ages. We're especially pleased when new patients come to us with the desire to stick to just one protocol. This way, there is no confusing what gets them well. In time, they'll know that guaifenesin is what got them there and not some complicated combination of things. Although it's tempting to reach for every new golden promise or astounding miracle, it's wise to stick with one modality at a time. Wiser still is to research the proposed treatments thoroughly for safety. When it comes to that issue, guaifenesin wins hands-down.

If there were any drugs that always worked for pain and fatigue, we'd all know about them. The vast amounts of drugs and supplements patients take are ample proof that none is very effective. People who come to us are frequently taking amazing combinations; it's common to see patients on ten or more medications. The saddest part is that even with all those compounds, they are still searching for relief. These days, five brain-altering drug mixtures are almost the norm. Even mathematicians couldn't calculate the possibilities of drug interactions in that interplay. For us, it's mind-boggling!

New patients arrive with their drug stockpiles, and in the beginning we don't try to interfere with their products. Once they're doing better, it's time to discuss the notion of purging their list one drug at a time. We're happiest with newcomers who are taking no such products. Luckily, we also see patients who have tried everything and concluded that strong medications are of no real benefit and only result in more symptoms from their side effects. Common sense dictates that you should avoid chemical Band-Aids when at all possible, especially because there is reversal treatment at hand.

Polypharmacy, or multiple medications, is a very real problem when suffering has gone on without relief for a number of years. Eventually, medications alone are reason enough for a patient to be considered disabled. For example, people taking heavy narcotics such as methadone, fentanyl, or OxyContin should not drive cars. Many states consider this "driving under the influence," and it is a crime. At work, narcotics certainly make people accident-prone and a possible danger to themselves or others. Some patients may not be able to pass drug screenings because of their medication list.

Are new drugs rushed to market without adequate testing? Do current methods of studying safety and efficacy of new compounds leave something to be desired? These questions remain to be answered, although books such as this one raise serious questions.

Recent withdrawals of Rezulin (diabetes), Lotronex (irritable bowel), Baycol (cholesterol), Zelnorm (IBS), and Vioxx (osteoarthritis) certainly underscore concern. There's really a dual issue: Is a new medication more effective than existing ones, and is it safer? In general, our feeling is that the longer the track record of a drug, the safer it is. Not even one study showed Vioxx more effective than ibuprofen for pain, and yet heavy advertising sold it and consumers assumed it was better because it was newer! The FDA, which was once considered too slow and too careful, now approves new compounds faster than corresponding bodies in other countries. Another problem is that while quick to approve, it moves slowly when it comes to withdrawing drugs that are unsafe from the market. Rezulin, for example, was withdrawn in England two and a half years earlier than it was in the United States. Avandia (diabetes) has already been pulled from the market around the world yet it remains on the market (although with restrictions) in the United States, despite some very serious concerns.

> More serious is the fact that many of us are taking a lot of drugs at once—often five, maybe ten, or even more. This practice is called *polypharmacy*, and it carries real risks. The problem is that very few drugs have just one effect. In addition to the desired effect, there are others. Some are side effects doctors know about, but there may also be ones we are not aware of. When several drugs are taken at once, those other effects may add up. There may also be drug interactions in which one drug blocks the action of another or delays its metabolism so that its actions and side effects are increased. When the function of an organ, for instance the liver or kidneys, is even slightly impaired, the problem of complications from one or other medication increases. And the more medications taken, the more likely it is that one of them will interfere with the normal function of some organ.
>
> —*Marcia Angell, M.D., former editor in chief,*
> New England Journal of Medicine

Chapter Sixteen

Coping with Fibromyalgia

What Will Help While Guaifenesin Helps Your Body Heal?

> I have been on guai [for fourteen months]—I probably have
> another two to three years to clear. These past months have not
> been hell at all. They have been the best fourteen months in a
> long time for me. I know I am healing. I have more energy. I
> have more stamina. I can do more things, socially, physically,
> and mentally. So for me, if this is hell—bring it on!
>
> —*Linda P., Ohio*

IN A VERY real sense, the first day you take guaifenesin is the
birthday of your new life. You've read testimonials throughout
this book. They're all good and true. Yet you must wonder:
Authors would hardly include bad ones, would they? It would
be more helpful if you knew someone who's run through the
protocol and is responding well to guaifenesin. If you aren't
that lucky, you'll just have to trust us and the online support
group. Wonderful possibilities lie ahead, and for the first time
in what seems forever, we hope we've given you hope. If so
many others get well, why can't you? But you may be one of
those who worry, "But what if it doesn't work for me?"

By now you're also aware there's more to this treatment than just swallowing a pill. We haven't hidden the fact that fibromyalgia reversal is demanding, takes time, and requires both perseverance and dedication. You may encounter people who think this protocol is too restrictive or too complicated. Guaifenesin is, after all, not for the faint of heart. If it's any consolation, we'll tell you straight out: Since you've bought this book and read this far, you've got the guts to persevere!

What's left now is to think about what you can do for yourself while waiting for guaifenesin to do its job. We think it important enough to repeat: If you're taking the correct dosage and you aren't blocking, guaifenesin will work. You don't need to take any other medications. Everything else, as far as we're concerned, is optional or only temporarily useful. But there are certainly things you can do mentally and physically to pave the way toward your new life.

> Nothing could stop me from trying guaifenesin. I was diagnosed in 1988—have tried everything—they all helped to some degree, but not like this. I've had symptoms since at least 1976. I leapt at the chance for this. I have been through so much with this disease over the years—I wanted a chance to get well. The fear of a little more pain was not going to stop me. Besides, what guarantee do you have now? My FMS seemed to be getting only worse over the years and here is a chance to change that.
>
> —*Jerri, South Dakota*

REDUCE STRESS

Poor stress! It's blamed for everything unpleasant that happens to us. For years, it was even thought responsible for inducing fibromyalgia. There's no doubt that chronic pain makes it a battle even to get up and dress in the morning. That's real stress! Add to this the other things you can't get done; things you regularly forget to do and the neglect you impose on your family and relationships. These are all enough to keep you on edge and at fever pitch. Undoubtedly, mental strain intensifies the symptoms of FMS or, for that matter, any chronic illness. That's no surprise, is it? Being sick is stressful. You may have already considered many of the coping strategies we'll suggest, but we think it still helps to see them collected in writing.

At the beginning, prioritize getting other health worries out of the way. Make sure your doctor has checked carefully for coexisting conditions. Treat anything that overlaps and confounds fibromyalgia. Thyroid function should be checked and treated only if it's abnormal. Anemia can make you feel tired and weak, and can greatly block the muscular clearing of fibromyalgia. If you're hypoglycemic, don't duck the issue. Start the corrective diet without hesitation. In just a few weeks, you'll have more energy, feel better, think better, and find your irritable bowel gradually placated. Within two months, all of the carbohydrate-related problems will be gone. That's your easier problem to reverse. Your worries about more serious conditions being the root cause of your many symptoms can be set aside by your doctor—so discuss these underlying fears with him or her. Remember that the Internet contains both accurate and not-so-accurate information and must not take the place of a qualified medical practitioner.

Review your medications and remember that some of them are certainly compromising your recovery, because of side effects. Some depression is normal in chronic illness. Do you really need to take an antidepressant? Such medications are often handed out with very little reasoning the minute a doctor suspects fibromyalgia. Maybe you can cut the dosage. Study the effects of the mood-altering drugs and tranquilizers that have stripped your personality of its highs and lows. We acknowledge you must make adjustments just to continue functioning, but it's also logical to question how much a drug is actually helping. For that review, you'll need the wisdom only your doctor can offer. Ask how you should go about sequentially reassessing your medications for both value and side effects. You might wonder what this has to do with stress, but it's pertinent for several reasons. Deep down you're probably worrying about the effects and long-term risks of multiple compounds. Most people really don't like taking drugs. Budgets are strained when paying high pharmacy bills each month, and this doesn't make life any easier. Finally, until you reduce drugs to minimal needs, you can't estimate how this polypharmacy is affecting your mental outlook.

Besides your prescription drugs, look at the over-the-counter stuff and the supplements you've added over the years. These may be more expensive if insurance doesn't cover them. Wonder more than a bit about side effects and safety, since they aren't often tested for interactions with prescription drugs. This is a new beginning: a good time to repack the baggage you'll carry into the future. If something hasn't been very helpful, ask your doctor's opinion about tossing it out. We understand the fear of omitting anything on the chance it might make you feel worse. Dwell on this thought a bit. If you stop something and you realize it was actually necessary, you can always add it back. Your target is to make your regimen as simple as possible. Removing the worry about what medications are doing to your system should certainly lessen stress.

Please don't worry about what may or what will be, and take each day/moment one by one. The anxiety you cause yourself will not serve you in a positive way, as you may be surprised how your cycling goes. Taking guaifenesin could quite possibly lift the symptom you are most worried about, and how you reexperience it may not be on the same level you already experience it. It was that way for me as I could much easier handle cycling depression versus depression caused by my past problem.

—*Kim, Pennsylvania*

STRESS AT HOME

One day I asked my husband what was the hardest part about being married to someone as sick as I was. I expected him to say working all day, then coming home to do the cooking, cleaning, and wait on me. But he didn't, he said it was the loneliness!! I had no idea. At that time I wasn't able to give anything to him, I was a blob. He took care of me and loved me unconditionally. Maybe not perfectly, [but] to the best of his ability. See, I am the luckiest girl in the world!

—*Susie, California*

Next, carefully examine where life is the sweetest—hopefully your home. Ask those who share that comfortable retreat to understand what you're about to undertake. If they're interested in reading about your illness and the protocol, you can share parts of this book or materials from our website: www .fibromyalgiatreatment.com. The site also contains a "Letter to Normals." Read and adapt it for your own use if you're interested in putting your feelings on paper and sharing them that way.

Everyone in the household should be given a chance to understand what's happening with your health. Keep explanations simple with children. Remind them you're going to get better. It may seem a bit scary at first for juvenile minds. The fear of losing a parent is always present. Let them know there'll be things you just can't do right now; it isn't your fault or theirs. If you express yourself simply, even youngsters can understand and face the circumstances by making up activities you can mutually share. Keep in mind that time spent with kids not only is instructive but will also go into their nostalgia files for review in adulthood. Our time is truly the most precious thing that we have to give. Long after cherished toys are broken and forgotten, children remember the day "Mom, hand on my shoulder, taught me how to bake cookies." Board games can substitute for outdoor playing. If your children are old enough, let them read to you out loud. Watch movies with them, or work on simple projects. On better days, as energy permits, short walks together can be marvelously bonding and refreshing.

Let family members know what help you need. Be specific and explain why you need it. If they understand that you are seriously beginning a demanding protocol for getting well, it will be hard for them to refuse you. There are three secrets for getting help. First, learn how to ask and be specific about what you want. Don't expect clairvoyance from your significant other when it's time to mop a dirty floor. Children won't automatically volunteer to haul trash all the way to the curb just because you wish they would. Second, if someone is trying to do something helpful, don't supervise the task. Not only does this expend energy you don't have, it's annoying to those over whom you hover. If it's not exactly the way you would've done it… oh well! There are more ways than one to accomplish things, and perfection in household tasks is not essential. And third, of course, say thank you. Express your appreciation even to a child who made you a cup of tea or drew you a picture. Be grateful to a spouse or friend who cooked dinner and even cleaned up afterward. Let each know you view their efforts as wonderful. "Do you know what that means to me?" goes a long way as a reward and installs them as participants in your recovery.

"Lower your standards" would make a good motto when you face house and garden chores. This last phrase might contain words of wisdom for the new millennium—even healthy people have too much to do these days. Everyone, not just fibromyalgics, feels stressed out and pressured from all sides. Changes you cultivate during guaifenesin treatment may turn into much healthier habits useful for the rest of your life.

Consider simple meals and eating them off paper plates. Save some energy by cooking bigger batches of familiar recipes when you feel up to it. Freeze the extra portions for the energy-deprived days that are sure to come. Find easy recipes—women's magazines and cookbooks have plenty of them; some are printed on package labels. Especially in the winter, Crock-Pots can be used for one-dish dinners without supervision, and require less cleaning up. Low-carbohydrate recipes are available on the Net and also in cookbooks if you're hypoglycemic, especially on the strict, weight-loss diet. But no matter which diet you are on there are lots of resources at your fingertips.

Stop worrying about what's accumulating behind the refrigerator or under the stove. Remind yourself over and over that there's a time for everything, and this is yours for healing. A spotless house should be low on the list of priorities in life, with health at the very top. You've already lost your well-being, so we don't need to remind you what you're looking for. When you regain that, you'll have plenty of energy to play catch-up with all of those dusty corners.

Perhaps you can afford to pay someone to help with housework. We're not insensitive to the fact that some budgets won't allow it. However, just having someone come in every two weeks or once a month to do the heavy stuff is lifesaving. Another possibility is to let your kids earn extra money by doing housework. You know it won't be to your satisfaction, but it'll be a learning experience for them. They'll undoubtedly do it in fits and starts, but so what? It's at least a little break when you're about to collapse.

Even my spouse could see the incredible difference. He now felt guilt-free to serve me with divorce papers. How kind of him. He was going to anyway, he says, but he had been feeling painfully guilty about it. Look how guai even helped his pain!

—*Iris, California*

If your relationship doesn't survive the symptoms of fibromyalgia, remember that it might have faltered anyway. Some couples get lucky and mend the rifts, but for right now, concentrate on getting well. As you reclaim your life, you'll have chances to find what it is you are looking for. Don't waste your precious energy being angry or confrontational. Instead, concentrate on yourself and making peace with yourself.

My energy levels are up and the fog lifted almost immediately and some of my hair is growing back! I am doing things now that I couldn't do a year ago. I wake up in the morning and my legs don't ache. I sleep. FM has taught me to appreciate the little things in life and that in and of itself is a blessing. I also make it a point to live life more fully and to take the time to do things for me. This protocol has worked and I hope that anyone out there who might be contemplating whether they should do it or not will "Just Do It!" This past week we hosted friends of ours in our home for a week. We were on the go all week long and I managed to get by on just two Aleves, which I took as a precaution since it was that time of the month and I was trying to avoid getting a headache. Yes, I am feeling tired today, but then again, we all are!

—*Susan, California*

STRESS IN THE WORKPLACE

Emotionally I'm still very depressed by having so little education, work experience, and future financial security at my age.

And I am simply lonely from so many years of isolation. I don't know how to make or keep friends. Dr. St. Amand assured me that my mind would heal along with my body and that I simply couldn't imagine the positive changes I would experience in my emotions. I hope this is true. I will simply have to rely on the same hope that caused me to start the guai in the first place.

—*Iris, California*

Job stress from overwork and anxiety about it are sure to magnify your symptoms and make fibromyalgia worse. It's important not to let work situations weigh you down. We don't recommend quitting, but perhaps a sympathetic boss will let you cut your hours temporarily. Or possibly you could do some paperwork from home. Computers have made it much easier for employees to telecommute or simply bring chores home, where they can be completed in a comfortable chair and preselected surroundings. Working at home, you can move around, stretch, and take breaks as you need them.

The problem with this simple advice is that by the time many fibromyalgics are diagnosed or begin treatment, they may already be having problems at work. Some have taken too many sick days; others have fallen behind and performed badly on days when fibrofog and other symptoms were at full fury. If it's feasible, schedule a meeting with your supervisor to discuss fibromyalgia and the treatment you're about to start. Keep it simple and honest but stress that you're going to improve. You can finally promise that in good faith; all you ask is for some tolerance in the weeks that lie ahead.

If you've been told that your job is in jeopardy were you to call in sick just one more time, you might need to take some specific actions when you start guaifenesin. Your possibilities will be different depending on the size of your company and your benefits package. It's not a bad idea to consider the option of taking time off at the beginning of treatment if you feel you won't be given any help. The Family and Medical Leave Act (FMLA) became law in 1993 and may apply to you if you work for a company that employs more than fifty people. It was enacted to permit up to twelve weeks of unpaid leave for you to reverse a serious health condition. It does require continuing treatment by a licensed health care provider. You'll need to provide documentation from your doctor. The law also mandates you be restored to the same or an equivalent position with the same pay and benefits. You can get better information from your state's Board of Equalization (by whatever name) or your employer's Human Resources Department, where you can learn about your personal options in detail.

On the other hand, it's still important not to be too frightened or overreact in advance, especially if your options are limited when it comes to time off. Despite what you may have heard or read, the vast majority of patients continue working during the initial days on our protocol. Only a few require a period of absence, and typically that means just a month or two off. We're not all endowed with the same strength, but certainly most of our patients cope with jobs successfully throughout reversal. That's one of the reasons why we've advised you to start on a small amount of guaifenesin and titrate up slowly to find your proper dosage. Taking more medication than you actually need will make you cycle harder. It's far better for you to take the correct amount and sooner attain good days. When these start appearing, it will make it possible for you to catch up with some of your work.

In the United States, employers are becoming much more sensitive to those with disabilities. There are now many resources available, and often a simple note from your physician will help you make changes. More comfortable chairs, wrist supports for computer work, footstools, and cushions are all things your employer might provide. New laws require them to make reasonable accommodations, and a little research on your part can promote cooperation. The best approach is to do some research on your own and present options that you believe will help you be more productive. Try to be realistic about what your employer can afford and keep demands at a minimum.

Relationships with coworkers might benefit if you simply tell them that you're beginning a difficult new treatment for your fibromyalgia. Share your hopes and fears and explain that you intend to do your best and continue working as hard as you can. Most people will respond to such a direct approach and will be more inclined to help. Try getting them to understand that a medical problem is the basis of your struggles and that you're doing your best to get it under control. Reassure them that you won't be ill forever.

Normal are the hours when I forget I am a sick person. Normal is when I keep up with a fit person my age and don't pay for it big time. Normal is when I cry for a normal reason. Normal is when I laugh without being macabre or cynical. Normal is when I don't burn when I think about doctors. Normal is when I want to do something besides watch TV. Normal is not being in pain all the time. I have these normals now and you will, too.
—*Janet, Canada*

THINGS YOU CAN DO FOR YOURSELF

I was told by my primary physician and rheumatologist that there was really nothing to do but exercise, eat well, keep my weight down, [and] take antidepressants, pain, and sleep meds as needed. I was advised to get a hot tub and have frequent massages. I was told that I wouldn't die from fibro or be cured. Gradually I got worse to where I had very few good times, and though I continued to work, life became almost intolerable most of the time.

One day at work one of the teachers asked how I was and I said, "Do you really want to know?" She said yes and I told her that I didn't want to continue to live if this was all there was going to be in my future. The pain, brain fog, fatigue, and depression were more than I wanted to deal with. She looked at me and asked if I had seen a doctor. I told her I had fibro, but other than that, everything always tested normal.

She told me the most amazing story about her friend with fibro who went to a physician named Dr. St. Amand, who had changed her life completely with his treatment and understanding of the disease. I am one of the lucky ones who is able to go see Dr. St. Amand, and I have lived an entirely different life since finding there is hope!

—*Cathy, California*

GET ENOUGH SLEEP

During our sleep we all clean out the metabolic debris created by simply existing. That's the time when cells do their housekeeping. Fibromyalgic muscles compile overabundant metabolic leftovers because they're kept constantly contracted and this prevents the restorative rest needed for a good nighttime cleansing. To a lesser extent, it's the same for the rest of the body, particularly the brain. It follows that a prominent complaint in fibromyalgia is insomnia and the dominant exhaustion that this imposes. No matter how tough you are, fitful sleeping makes it impossible for next-day function. Rest is crucial, so get as much as you can—but realize that it won't entirely solve the problem of fatigue.

When you've had a bad night, occupy the next day with less demanding tasks. Although this is not always possible, choose the simplest ones from your must-do list. On those bad days, send your kids on the errands they can do. Now is the time for simple meals such as grilled cheese sandwiches, soup, or takeout. If you've frozen a casserole or portions of a larger meal, this is the time to thaw it out. Conserve what strength you have for the most basic and urgent tasks. Remember that mental and emotional workouts are also tiring.

A good general rule is to grab what rest the disease allows whenever you can. Snatch naps when you have to if at all possible. Keep them brief and find a way to awaken yourself before you lapse into a prolonged coma. You've got to remain tired enough to sleep that night. When you start yawning in the evening, forget the next TV show and go to bed earlier than usual. Sometimes it requires a Herculean effort to propel yourself from your chair into the bedroom, but do it. Dozing in your chair or on the couch is not as restorative as sleeping in a quiet room. Your spouse isn't enjoying your company, especially if you're snoring. He won't mind if you beat a calculated retreat. Your workplace may have a back room or a private area where you can rest at lunchtime or during breaks. A small, inexpensive futon can be stashed on a shelf along with a small pillow. Even half an hour can make a difference if it's spent stretched out with your eyes closed.

Schedule sufficient bed hours; it's counterproductive to aim for seven hours when you know you need nine. Set your alarm half an hour earlier than usual if you really must finish some task from the night before. You'll complete it much more rapidly when you're rested. It may also help to set the alarm earlier, take your morning dose of pain medication, and then press the snooze button while waiting for it to take effect. In this way, you'll feel better when you finally have to get up and start moving.

If you're a light sleeper, relaxation tapes, quiet fans, and white noise machines can make it easier to stay asleep. Make sure your bedroom is dark and your mattress comfortable. When purchasing a new mattress, ask for a trial period and a money-back guarantee—there's no one kind that helps everyone with FM. On painful nights, little adhesive heat pads for muscle pain may be used or apply a simple old-fashioned hot water bottle. You don't want to use electric heating pads all night because of the danger of burning yourself. Don't overlook simple aids such as earplugs or sleep masks if your room has features that keep you from fully relaxing. Exercise in the afternoon will also help, as will gentle stretching after a shower or a bath before bed.

Without medical reversal of fibromyalgia, everything gets even worse, including insomnia, and nocturnal tissue cleansing remains incomplete. During guaifenesin reversal, you'll still have to temporarily make do with whatever downtime you can muster. Making rest a priority and finding workable solutions to avoid unwanted wake cycles are essential for restoring your ability to cope on a daily basis. (See chapter 15 for guidance on getting better sleep.)

> I am sleeping through the night right now without the aid of medication and I am dreaming again, oh what a wonderful thing! It's amazing what a good night's sleep does for a person! Speaking of sleep, last year I couldn't sleep on my sides because my hips hurt so bad. Now I only sleep on my sides. I can make it through a day without needing a nap or needing to lie down. Last year if I didn't lie down at least once in the afternoon, I couldn't make it to dinner. Restless legs plagued me for years. It was one of the first things to go so now my husband sleeps better, too.
>
> —*Gina, New York*

TAKE WARM BATHS

I recently spent a week at my mother-in-law's apartment in New York City. Because the shower had variable temperatures in the space of a few minutes, I couldn't deal with it, so I took a bath. I was immediately sold on the idea because it made me stop and relax and also made my muscles feel much better. I vowed to make the time for at least one bath a week, and I do. Bubbles in the bath help me relax more because I can't see my body and it's like being in a cloud.

—*Valerie, Nevada*

Hot or warm baths will soothe sore muscles or joints and ease the aching pains of the FMS day. They're quite relaxing and may help you fall asleep—not in the tub, please! Epsom salts, powdered milk, cornstarch, or mineral or emu oil can be added to the water. Do not use the oils if your skin doesn't need them, but buttermilk and powdered goat's or cow's milk contain a gentle exfoliator called lactic acid. It can also help to soothe irritation, and is a mild nongreasy moisturizer. Turn off or dim as many lights as possible to set a pleasant atmosphere in the bathroom or bedroom. If you have dry, itchy, or irritated skin, remember to use warm water rather than hot.

Heavy fragrances should be avoided in bath products. Even if you can tolerate the smell, the added chemicals can irritate the skin and even make it difficult to relax. Some patients report that a mildly scented candle is a wonderful addition to this quiet time. If you have noisy children or a spouse who likes a loud TV, play a relaxation tape or quiet classical music to make your bath more soothing.

Warm showers work best in the morning. That's when you must loosen muscles that stiffened during the night, yet not get so relaxed that you want to go back to bed. Baths do their best work at night, showers in the morning. Body lotions designed for use in the shower can soften and moisturize your skin for the entire day. They also help calm the itchy skin so common in fibromyalgia. If you have long hair, wear a shower cap: It will keep you from having to wash and style it each day. This alone can save a lot of energy. Some of you find taking a shower simply too exhausting; try gentle stretching for about ten minutes instead.

UNDERSTAND YOUR DEPRESSION

The fact is that FMS is a potentially debilitating inherited illness that not only affects our entire bodies but is progressive. It is nothing to take lightly and nothing that can be fixed with an antidepressant. I just had one of the best years of my life, am very active, very happy even with this illness, and yet my physician wanted to put me on an antidepressant to ward off hot flashes. Ridiculous. No way will I subject my brain to a mind-altering substance when I am very happy with my brain. I have had to take charge of my own health when it comes to fibromyalgia

It's my body and my decision.

—*Jody D., North Carolina*

A certain amount of depression and frustration is normal with chronic illness. Most patients instinctively understand and don't want to take medication for milder forms. Antidepressants certainly have a place in serious depression, but as we've seen, they have effects on the body that are less than desirable if there are other choices.

Try a few tricks to coax your brain out of a funk while you're waiting for guaifenesin's benefits. Easier said than done, but you can trick the brain to fend off some of the facets of your depressing thoughts. It's perfectly normal to chafe against your limitations, mourn losses, and feel sad at being deprived of stamina to do what you previously enjoyed. You can find new activities to replace some lost ones and, in less demanding ways, spend time with those you love. Overcoming such obstacles will make you feel better.

Depression in fibromyalgia may stem from feeling defeated in trying to meet some unrealistic standards, self-imposed at home or work. Recognizing limitations is a good place to start and might also lessen stress by letting you erase self-inflicted rules. Concentrating energy on doing what you do best helps immensely. Find relief from the tasks you dislike such as housework and save your efforts for what fulfills you. You're not alone: Many women say that looking around their unkempt homes puts them into an immediate tantrum. If the deplorable state of your house is a major cause of your anguish, put changing this at the top of your priority list. Lower your standards, however, and remember that most people with children and busy lives don't themselves live in magazine-picture-perfect rooms. We've addressed this, but get outside help if you can afford it. If being in an imperfect home is that depressing to you, paying for a little help should take precedence over less important things.

Worth thinking about is using your talents to supplement your income while doing something you enjoy. For example, if you're adept at sewing, you might earn extra money to help pay for a cleaning helper. Embroidering school and club uniforms or costumes might be right up your alley. Holiday tablecloths or place mats might be sold at craft fairs or accepted for sale by small boutique stores. You could even make presents of your wares. Besides just earning compliments for your skills, some recipients and their friends might well offer to pay you for similar productions.

Exercise is a fantastic way of fighting depression and feeling blah. Simply getting out for a walk can really make a difference. Walking to or sitting outside in a park, weather permitting, is a great change of pace. If you live in an area where outdoor exercise isn't a good option, check with local indoor shopping centers to see if they have a mall-walking program. Joining an exercise class at the YMCA or a local recreation department (many have programs tailored for arthritis) can get you out of the house and you may even make some new friends. Curves is a franchise popular with women who have fibromyalgia because the workout can be adapted to the day's stamina. It's also inexpensive, and if you have Medicare and a supplementary insurance, it may well be free. Water exercise classes are helpful, especially for patients who are overweight and may have joint issues. Here, too, you will find many classes for seniors or patients with chronic pain. Remember that any kind of exercise will trigger your feel-good endorphins, and don't forget to check with your insurance to see if they will cover costs. Many offer programs for patients with pain, stiffness, or arthritis.

JOIN A SUPPORT GROUP OR START YOUR OWN

Be careful. There are some groups claiming to be support groups that are actually venting grounds. That is, the people in the group do little more than moan and groan about what a lousy hand life has dealt them. A little venting is good for the soul and the health of everyone. But if the entire discussion is centered on moaning and groaning, it will drag you down into the depths of negativity. Avoid negative groups.

—*Devin J. Starlanyl,* The Fibromyalgia Advocate[1]

Communicating with other fibromyalgics is very comforting. Connecting with others is inspirational for you and them; it's encouragement you can all use. It hauls you out of isolation, and quite likely, you may help others in the process. Local newspapers publish calendars with weekly schedules of other groups dedicated to helping various medical conditions. If you have trouble locating one in your area, you may be able to find one through the National Fibromyalgia and Chronic Pain Assocation (www.fmcpaware.org) or the Arthritis Foundation (www.arthritis.org). Health care providers who deal with fibromyalgia may know of a group. Local hospitals are another resource; they often have meeting rooms used by local support groups. If you live in a sparsely populated area, remember that any chronic pain or arthritis group might serve just as well. Increasingly, face-to-face support groups are giving way to Internet chat rooms and online message boards. These work well for patients with fibromyalgia because they often don't feel well enough to get dressed or drive across town. There's an online group available for the guaifenesin protocol which you can access from www.fibromyalgiatreatment.com.

If you live in a large city, you may find more than one fibromyalgia support group. Visit each and select the one that gives you positive feelings. Ideally, a group serves two functions. First, it should afford members a venue for expressing feelings and releasing frustrations. Unfortunately, this is where too many of them stop. Meetings are full of sad stories strongly accentuated with moans and groans, week after week. Tales of pains, failed therapies, and poor spousal and family support are part of each person's litany. It sounds like a competition for who's the worst off! These are negative organizations. Forget them! You're already low enough emotionally. The second thing you want from a support group is dedication to improving the quality of its members' lives. It should be a forum for suggestions that help you cope with daily functions. Members can share resources and information about fibromyalgia, good care providers, and ways to make day-to-day life easier. Some even organize car pools, shared child care, or potluck meals. They do just what the name implies—offer support for members. When one individual isn't feeling well, others will come to the rescue. Helping with household chores, doing a little shopping for you while doing their own—just a few practical things that an understanding friend can provide. Loneliness is terrible, but your life brightens when you call a buddy and speak to an empathetic ear.

I call people by the wrong name. I called my new daughter-in-law by her sister's name and then a few weeks later I called her by my own sister-in-law's name. It's embarrassing. I must come across as a total idiot to a lot of people in those situations when I can't recall the simplest things; fumble, drop, and spill things; and ricochet off walls and doorways.

But I've learned that when I'm in a group of people who share my experiences, that all falls away. It is so wonderful to know that everyone there understands exactly what I'm talking about and why I can't remember my own name or what day it is and there is so much warmth and acceptance that I can soak it up and coast on it for a long time afterwards.

—*Anne Louise, Minnesota*

If no acceptable support group exists in your area, consider starting one of your own. We must stress *acceptable.* Many of our patients have gone to more than a few and left disenchanted. Discussions too often center on a new pain pill, sleeping potion, antidepressant, "my doctor said," and the hot new herbal concoction of the day. You're far better off with a guaifenesin support group devoted to a single protocol designed to heal you, not simply applying patches to your symptoms. Starting an organization is not an enormous task, so don't be frightened at this thought. As with everything else, simplicity is the notion of the day. You can start by getting together regularly with a fibromyalgic friend or two. You'll be amazed how quickly that sprouts into a sizable group—Jane will know Suzie, who knows her mother and a neighbor with fibromyalgia. Once under way, work on constructive things: Discuss the protocol and where to find good salicylate-free products; collect simple recipes and helpful tips for improving the quality of your lives. Groups from all over the world are now linking up, and soon there'll be an international organization. You and your friends can help yourselves and millions of others. It will take many missionary leaders to spearhead and support the awesome task ahead. As soon as you start your group, a simple post to the online support group or a member of the administration team will get you a listing so that others may find you and pitch in.

We've included it a number of times in these pages, but once more, here's the website: fibromyalgiatreatment.com. Claudia and the administrative team are dyed-in-the-wool guaifenesin protocol supporters and totally knowledgeable about the disease and our treatment. They answer e-mail inquiries regularly throughout the day. The same website will keep you up to date on any new research and information that will help you.

> I had to quit telling my mom things that I knew she wouldn't be supportive about. But it took me forty years! We always think that "surely" our families will support us and say the right things. Instinctively we know the truth. It's hard to accept. I rarely talk to anyone about my FMS but my support group.
>
> —*Kathy, Oregon*

GET SOME EXERCISE

I understand how hard it can be to exercise when you hurt badly but you must understand that even the slightest exercises such as gentle stretching will help you to be not so stiff. The more you can do without overdoing it, the better for your body. Everyone needs to learn what they can handle and celebrate the small victories, as the small victories lead to big ones in time. You may gain weight having this chronic illness, and some factors such as medications can cause you to gain. That may be out of your control, but you can still choose to eat right and exercise to the best of your ability. If you can control small things, you will not feel so depressed but feel instead you are

making steps in the right direction. Celebrate all your victories
no matter how small or insignificant they might seem.

—*Kim, Pennsylvania*

In this high-tech age, we often forget how simple things can
be. We've already beat this into the ground, but perhaps we
can embellish our suggestions. Exercise doesn't require fancy-
colored tight-fitting designer togs, shiny equipment, hundred-
dollar shoes, or a racing bike. You don't need to join a gym
or even buy weights that match your leotards and sweatbands.
The sight of well-toned athletes working out with huge resistance equipment is intimidating and looks too hard to try. The
reality is that very few people look that good. Most of us don't
have those perfect bodies or the money to buy fashionable out-
fits just for exercise. Many more people stay healthy by taking
long, peaceful walks, especially with a calming partner. There's
no doubt even modest exercising will make you feel better. We
discussed this fairly extensively in the previous chapter. Besides
improving pain thresholds, releasing endorphins, and rebuilding mitochondria, exercise has a positive effect in relieving
depression.

You can begin early in the treatment, but go easy and start
out moderately. Ambitious jump starts are predictors of certain
defeat. You can begin by walking around the block or gently
stretching on your living room floor with a computer program,
DVD, or book to guide you. Some are designed particularly
for fibromyalgics, and you can find these easily on the Internet.
You'll appreciate hints that help you recognize and abide by
your own limits of tolerance.

Exercise should never be done when your muscles are cold or
tired. Do some mild stretching, or take a warm-up walk, even
a warm shower before you begin. In her book *The Fibromyalgia Advocate*, Devin Starlanyl offers an excellent rule of thumb
for evaluating an exercise program: "If mild soreness disappears

after the first day, you can repeat it on the second day. If it persists to the second day, postpone any exercise until the third day. If soreness persists on the third day, your exercise routine must be changed. This rule of thumb is true for any treatment, such as massage or electrical stimulation."[2]

> I started slow, walking around the block. One day I walked five blocks to buy a lottery ticket (hope blooms eternal) and five blocks back. It almost did me in, but I survived. Now I can walk to the grocery store, and if I am too fatigued, I take the bus partway to save a few blocks. It's like Claudia once said—you will be in pain whether you are home or not. You will be worn out at home or you can get out and be just as tired. Sometimes it is like I am moving in a fog but at least I am moving. A few times I've called my friend in San Diego on my cell phone and the walk doesn't seem as long because we are talking the whole time.
>
> —*Janice, Minnesota*

For those who prefer structured programs, the Arthritis Foundation will direct you to those that meet your needs. Ask for descriptive brochures. The recommended aquatic program is often the easiest and most sustainable. It's designed for those with limited mobility and empowered by enlisting the soothing buoyancy of warm water. There are beginner group workouts that offer exercise in class-like settings. They're not hard to find. One secret is to join a class designed for senior citizens; the pace is usually slower. Yoga, tai chi, and other disciplines all have advocates. The value of any exercise is determined by the number of people who stick with that particular modality. We encourage patients to keep searching until they find a regimen they can all enjoy and tolerate. The consensus is: Carefully graduated workouts that avoid overdoing things progressively promote energy and a wonderful sense of well-being.

After about three months on the guai, I decided to try exercising on my stationary bike again...I have found that when I am really hurting, if I ride the bike for at least fifteen minutes, the pain begins to ease up. It is really hard to convince myself to get started when it hurts to even walk, let alone really exercise. But the benefits are worth it. Evenings are my worst times, and I find that if I ride my bike for about thirty minutes just before bedtime, I get rid of a lot of my pain and become very relaxed. This promotes a good sleep that often leads to a better day afterward.

—*Marilyn J., North Carolina*

TRY MASSAGE AND BODYWORK

I have had pain all my life but was told it was growing pains. I have chronic back pain at times so severe I can't function. The muscle spasms are so bad it feels like I have ropes in my back. This was much worse during pregnancy. I discovered then that if I roll on a tennis ball in the areas where it felt just like knots, it would make the pain radiate somewhere else or it hurt right where it was, but either way it always felt better. What I have read tells me I am actually rubbing on trigger points.

—*Liz, Kentucky*

Bodywork is done by licensed practitioners who use teaching, touch, and repetitive strokes for healing. Practically no one discounts the soothing power of human hands. Only a few hypersensitive people cannot tolerate being touched. If you're one of these, you know it and can skip this section until you feel it becomes applicable to you. For most people, trained therapists who understand fibromyalgia and use gentle massage can magically ease muscular pains and pacify jangled nerves. As long as you both bear in mind that the benefits are transient, you'll do fine.

Carefully avoid deep-tissue work and stay away from Rolfing—these techniques will increase pain. The wrong kind of massage can bring immediate pain that may last for days. Other times, you won't realize until much later how badly you've been hurt. Bear in mind that the lumps and bumps of fibromyalgia can't be jackhammered out by using bare-knuckled attacks. That can cause tissue damage and greatly disturb already distressed structures. Make sure that any practitioner you visit understands fibromyalgia. Read printed material about the proposed treatment before you submit to it and be sure it's appropriate for your condition. Some patients get relief from acupuncture, and many medical researchers support its benefits. As it is with chiropractic approaches, other investigators have found little lasting benefit. Ask your doctor and support group for recommendations if you don't know where to start. When using chiropractic services or acupuncture, make it absolutely clear that you cannot use herbal products offered as medications or on the skin. Even though you think you've explained this thoroughly, be vigilant to make sure that you were understood and your practitioners comply.

Highly endorsed by fibromyalgics is the Feldenkrais Method. In a series of lessons, patients are taught how to integrate their body movements so they can function with less effort and pain. Instructions are individually structured as a series of altogether smooth and gentle activities. Similar disciplines such as the Alexander Technique and Bowen Therapy also have staunch supporters, but our experience with these is minimal. After any kind of treatment, except massage, plan on resting. Your body has just had a significant workout. If your muscles are already getting tight, take a warm shower to relax them.

Unfortunately, the above therapeutic approaches are expensive. Not every patient has insurance coverage, and even sound, hands-on treatment is often rejected as unnecessary. Prepaid medical carriers usually regard massage as a luxury except following an accident, and not for extended periods. However frustrating this is, it will help to accept that these modalities will, at best, provide only brief comfort, and that none of these disciplines is required for healing.

> There are colleges of massage therapy that charge much smaller fees than do the professionals. I had my second visit at my local school and I am still sold on the idea. I even took my sisters-in-law and the four of us got in on a two-for-one special: $10 a person! They are now sold on the idea, too. One important note: Although there may be one main address for the school, there are often additional locations of that school in different cities in your state. Take Utah, for example—there is one school but it has three different locations throughout the state. Contact the schools in your state for more information on additional locations.
>
> —*Sharon H., Utah*

DO SOMETHING YOU LOVE EVERY DAY

> I used to put "baking cookies with my son" on my list almost every week because we would talk while we were cooking, and he loved that. I would tell him about when I was a little girl and how I used to watch my mother bake, and it made me happy to remember good things. If I did nothing else at all that day, at least I did that. I made a vow not to flog myself for what I could not do—not to sit and watch other mothers running after their kids and beat myself up anymore. Instead I focused on the tasks I had made for myself... and counted myself lucky when I could do them.
>
> —*Cathy, California*

Most detrimental of all to your emotional health is to stop doing things that are important to you. You must somehow keep in touch with yourself and the person you were before fibromyalgia took over your entire being. That's hard to do when you feel so rotten—very hard. As the disease progresses, many people retract into some inner sanctuary that conserves strength only for essential activities that can't be shoved aside. Such a move is logical but ultimately counterproductive. Far better to streamline unavoidable chores by trimming wasted effort while still retaining everything that lends charm to life. Energy conservation is necessary, but only a modest beginning.

> I found that there were activities I had stopped doing long ago, such as playing the piano and sewing, that really make me feel good...If I am sad or stressed, perhaps experiencing early warning signs of an approaching flare, I make sure to spend some time involved in such an activity. It makes me feel better and my life feels enriched.
>
> —*Mary Ellen Copeland, coauthor,* Fibromyalgia and Chronic Myofascial Pain Syndrome[3]

Start by deciding what you really enjoy doing and what makes you feel good. You have to provide some time for your partner and children, but of similar importance, what do you particularly love to do? What makes you feel better? Is it just anticipating a particular activity? Possibly it's gardening, painting, reading, or solving crossword puzzles. Do you like strolling in the evening or just sitting quietly in the morning sun sipping a cup of coffee? Choose something so wonderful that it usually makes you lose track of time.

Make a list of all the things that were important to you when you still felt well enough to do them. If you love watching your son play soccer, jot it down. Logging on to a newsgroup that serves the needs of others may be to your liking; that's a major joy to include. Going to the library, art museums, concerts in the park...which of these pastimes do you miss? Many music schools and colleges provide plays and entertainment at reasonable prices in a less rigid setting. Maybe you haven't considered these lately.

Finish the list and get a calendar with unusually big spaces. For each day, make a simple entry. Write in what you plan to do for yourself. It might be working in the garden for whatever time you can safely expend, or going in the afternoon to watch your daughter practice softball. It could be a morning trip to a farmer's market or renting a movie you've been meaning to see. If it's an outdoor activity, you could run out of steam; have a standby book you've always wanted to read or download a favorite movie or television show that always makes you laugh.

It's true that life isn't just made up of fun time. So you'll have to add a chore or two to the daily schedule. At least they also give the satisfaction of a mandatory job completed. Pick a single item for each day from your list: changing bed sheets, cleaning out the car, or organizing the refrigerator. Marketing and errands could be necessities for another day. Con yourself into thinking that vacuuming is part of your exercise program.

Every day, try with all your might to satisfy your plan. If you can muster the discipline, you'll start getting in touch with the wonderful person you were and still are. Even if no one else praises your effort, pat yourself on the back for the strides you've made. Life will be enriched and more meaningful to you. You'll subdue some of your recent demons and gain respect for your steadfast resolve. You're now a doer, not just a viewer. Mounting confidence will smooth your interactions with friends, family, and even doctors. Your new focus is on the road ahead, and you're now unstoppable on your drive to health.

I had a couple days where I worked outside shoveling dirt, which to anyone else is no big deal, but for me, it's a miracle. We all experience it when it dawns on us we are doing something we never dreamed we would do again or are shocked when we push on and realize the next day we don't feel like a truck ran over us. For me it was like a dream—I asked myself several times, "Did I just do that?" I've noticed since starting the protocol I find myself doing pretty strenuous work. It will start that I need to do something like clean the bathtub and then I see something else that needs to be scrubbed and then move to something else gradually, and before I know it, I've been cleaning house for a couple hours. I still can't plan ahead but I am grateful for these hours.

—*Dana, Texas*

Conclusion

One Author's Last Word

R. Paul St. Amand, M.D.

IF YOU'VE READ this far, from beginning to end, despite your overstrained brain focus, fatigue, aches, and pains, I'm impressed. As Claudia and I were writing these pages, I wondered how to end this book—as I've said in our previous editions. This time I wonder how well you've grasped the significance of our recent, collaborative research. Indeed there now exists vindication for all that you've experienced these many years. That includes the times you were told to get a life or get to a psychiatrist. Those lucky enough to have been diagnosed have possibly accumulated a polypharmacy of symptom-suppression medications. Or worse, got hooked on one or more of the narcotics. Now you know it will be possible to get rid of them.

We're still serving the same formula we've offered in previous years: painful reversing cycles mixed with fatigue, cognitive intrusions, and reacquaintance with past symptoms. We've instructed you to give up all teas and some of your favorite cosmetics and hair products. If you're hypoglycemic or overweight, we've told you that you need to stop eating pasta, potatoes, and sugary desserts. And we need you to trust us.

Presented with a well-detailed medical history, many more physicians are suspecting fibromyalgia earlier and becoming adept at confirming the diagnosis. There is a significant surge in awareness since we first started writing about the illness. Yet too many people must still self-diagnose by gleaning data from the Internet or from convoluted TV advertisements.

It still takes diligence and persistence to find a well-versed physician who will strive sufficiently to make you better. Some of them remain unaware and uninformed, or they scoff at our protocol. That, too, is changing. More enlightened or curious doctors might willingly allow you to be their special guinea pig and wait for you to self-assess results. In this instance, you become the teacher, and by reporting your success, you may soften the destiny for other patients. Your doctor might even be sufficiently curious to seek out the multiple swollen places displayed in such predictable patterns. It's unlikely that you'll find a doctor who will accept the shortcut method we've described for diagnosing hypoglycemia. If the opportunity presents itself, remind the physician that you're suffering the same acute adrenaline symptoms diabetics get with insulin overdoses. The treatment is black and white so you can treat yourself. We've outlined what you can eat and drink and what you must assiduously avoid. It's all very straightforward and has continued to work for my patients over the past fifty years. Sure, total reversal requires perfect dietary discipline for about two months. Muster your willpower and allow yourself no excuses: Approach the diet with a positive attitude and remind yourself that there is no alternative method.

Another 30 percent of you are carbohydrate intolerant though not actually hypoglycemic. You'll have to recognize that fact on your own, curtail your cravings, and try either the liberal or the strict diet for a few weeks. You should feel a swell of energy within a few days and a slower decline in irritable bowel symptoms just by changing the way you eat. As you persevere, you won't need a professional to remind you that consuming excess carbohydrates doesn't serve you well.

A few of you are wondering: *How can I possibly do all of this?* Unfortunately, you're not alone. We've grown accustomed to hearing from those who can't accept the price paid for reversal. Hypoglycemics are usually successful because rewards are so swift in coming. Fighting fibromyalgia is tougher and benefits more slowly reaped. Yet the majority of you will adopt the protocol. We hope you can muster enough reserves to pay the highway toll for the road to your destination—health.

Very few professionals will give you the requisite warnings about salicylates; that's something you'll have to learn for yourself. Identifying and avoiding them will be your responsibility, so prepare to do some homework. That's the hardest part, but it must be done. The initial search demands time and patience. Once completed, even currently safe products may change and demand meticulous label reviews before buying replacements.

We're well aware of some who have failed on our protocol. Yet when we can get to them, we almost invariably find the reason is either blocking or insufficient dosage. One failure is far too many so please persevere to find the problem. Use the resources at www.fibromyalgiatreatment.com to check your products first. If you find nothing that could be blocking, then raise your dose.

The intensity of the reversal cycles will vary for each of you. When it seems most difficult, it may help to remember a few facts:

- You weren't well before you started, and were probably getting sicker.
- You'll likely feel worse initially, but since guaifenesin has no significant side effects, intense cycling pain means the drug is working.
- It took you time to develop full-blown fibromyalgia. It will take less to get rid of it, but it will surely take time.

- Your first good hours will tell you that your body is capable of recovery. Bunch a few good days together and you'll become a strong advocate for our protocol.
- We define happiness as freedom from pain—mental and physical. There are such days ahead for you.

Each of us who has conquered the disease owes something to those still sick. As wonderful as it is to get a person well, we remain saddened for those who will never learn about our protocol. As long as we receive e-mails and letters detailing lifelong struggles with pain, fatigue, and relationships, our victory is not complete and our job is not yet done. We hope this book will provide the initiating impetus for human chain letters. As you get well, you progressively incur a debt, and you should plan how to repay it. You can only do that by helping others who are still searching for the path you've already walked. Please, reach out and take someone by the hand.

> Those who say it is impossible should get out of the way of those who are doing it.
>
> —*Chinese proverb*

Technical Appendix

R. Paul St. Amand, M.D.

This technical supplement is intended primarily for medical personnel who are familiar with fibromyalgia. Herein we describe the disease, our theory as to the cause, and our treatment for its reversal. The following paragraphs are offered in support for our perceptions of the disturbed physiology and biochemistry that produce the illness.

The syndromes of fibromyalgia, chronic fatigue, myofascial pain, and chronic candidiasis are variants of a complex spectrum that should be merged under one name. Dominantly affected areas and differing pain thresholds greatly alter clinical presentations and lead to that disparate nomenclature. The name *fibromyalgia* infers pain in muscles and fibers. *Energopenia* (dearth of energy) would be a more unifying term to describe the underlying pathology.

When visiting physicians, patients usually focus on their currently worst and omit less-disturbing symptoms. The following is a compilation of potential presenting complaints: musculoskeletal pain (any muscle, tendon, ligament, joint, leg or foot cramps, restless legs, numb or tingling limbs-digits-face); brain (fatigue, irritability, depression, apathy, nervousness, anxiety, insomnia, suicidal ideation, impaired memory and concentration, heightened sensitivity to light, sounds, and odors sufficient to induce nausea or headaches); irritable bowel (nausea, gas, bloating, cramps, pain, constipation, diarrhea); genitourinary (dysuria, urgency, pungent urine, bacterial or interstitial cystitis, vulvodynia); dermatologic (rashes: hives, eczema, pruritic vesicles, acne, rosacea, seborrheic or neurodermatitis, red or clear maculopapules; brittle nails, dry hair with premature loss, paresthesias, allodynia, itching, purpura); head, eye, ear, nose, and throat (variably located headaches, dizziness or imbalance, vertigo, dry and irritated eyes, conjunctivitis, blepharitis, dark circles in the lower eyelids, crusty discharges and morning grit, blurred vision, nasal congestion and excess mucus, postnasal drip, abnormal tastes, painful tongue, scalded mouth, tinnitus or low-pitched sounds); and miscellaneous (weight gain, low-grade fever, water retention, and allergies, including late-onset hayfever or asthma).

Symptoms usually begin spontaneously; patients sometimes attribute onset to stress, infection, surgery, or trauma. Yet by taking a careful history, we can often jostle memories into recalling symptoms such as the misnomer of growing pains in childhood. Symptoms are initially cyclic and interspersed with good days. Progressively, serious incapacity prevails without significant respite. My fifty-year observations strongly suggest that unresolved fibromyalgia deteriorates into osteoarthritis. Older family members relate many past symptoms, but joint pains dominate. When examined, they display the same physical lesions as fibromyalgia.

We have long contended that fibromyalgia is a multigenetic disease, and we now offer supporting data. Errant genes have been identified on scattered chromosomes. Missense mutations are surfacing in up to 40 percent of our study patients. Feng recently reported our collaborative genetic findings.[1] Research is ongoing and another (the fifth) gene is the subject of another paper in preparation. We have diagnosed patients aged two and others with late onset in their seventies. Along with symptom variations, this reflects the interplay of dominant and recessive genes. There is equal frequency in prepubertal boys and girls, but a strong female preponderance (85 percent) in adulthood. Asymptomatic males still remain carriers so that either parent may transmit mutant genes.

- Fifty years ago we began treating fibromyalgia (then nameless) with uricosuric agents. Twenty years ago we found the potent, therapeutic value of the barely uricosuric guaifenesin[2] that we have now used for over ten thousand patients. Cyclic clearing reproduces prior symptoms reminiscent of purging gout. With medication, lesions reverse using various dosages determined by patient responsiveness. The cumulative dosages of longer-acting guaifenesin are as follows: 300 mg twice daily favorably affects 20 percent of patients; 600 mg twice daily, 80 percent; 1,800 mg daily, 90 percent. We add short-acting tablets (400 mg) in whatever increments are needed for the remaining 10 percent to bypass some of the cytochrome effects. Particularly destructive is CYP-450 3A4, which attacks long-acting medications owing to their long transit in the gut and delayed absorption. Over one hundred drugs and supplements may raise its level and thereby force dosage adjustments. Short-acting guaifenesin circumvents some of that assault owing to rapid absorption. By combining long- with short-acting drug, we bypass some cytochrome exposure and yet obtain protection for nearly twenty-four hours.

- Individual genetic responsiveness determines dosages and time needed for recovery. Even the slowest responders clear a minimum of one year of accumulated debris for every two months of treatment. Lower-dosage patients greatly accelerate the process. Improvement is initially expressed in hours, later in days, and eventually in weeks.

Like other uricosuric agents, renal effects of guaifenesin are totally blocked by salicylates. This compound is readily absorbed through the skin, oral or intestinal mucosa,[3,4] and a portion concentrates in the proximal renal tubules. All plants manufacture salicylates as a defense mechanism to heal their wounds, signal other plants, repel pests, or kill soil organisms.[5] Lotions containing botanicals such as aloe, castor oil, camphor, and mint family members found in muscle balms, mouthwashes, lozenges, or candies deliver salicylates systemically within seconds.[6] Conjugating liver capacity that renders food sources harmless is limited and is readily overwhelmed by plant concentrates.[7]

Our physical examination is more thorough than the limited search for eleven-out-of-eighteen tender points recommended by the American College of Rheumatology. We search for swollen tissues and sketch our findings on a body caricature. An image results that depicts the shapes, sizes, and locations of lesions. These so-called body maps are objective because we ignore subjective expressions of pain and so avoid the pitfall of variable pain thresholds. We remap patients on all subsequent visits and are thereby able to document sequential reversal of the illness. Certain tissues are preferentially affected: The earliest lesions appear near the elbows, followed by the sternomastoid and trapezial areas. Spastic muscle bundles of the left thigh (vastus lateralis and rectus femoris) are present in 100 percent of adults and reliably validate the diagnosis. Those same lesions dependably clear within one month in compliant patients on an adequate dosage of medication.

These steadily contracted muscles, tendons, and ligaments are working tissues. Only a fundamental biochemical aberration could force fibromyalgic cells into such unrelenting overdrive. Theories seeking to explain the illness should take into account both the plethora of symptoms arising from excitable and non-excitable tissues, and the ubiquitous, palpable abnormalities.

Since plasma uric acid levels were consistently normal, my success using uricosuric agents to treat this new entity forced me to implicate an anion other than urate. Cumulative data strongly point to a faulty metabolism of inorganic phosphate (P_i). Tissue excesses would evoke no inflammatory response, but could induce system-wide biochemical misadventures. Using probenecid or guaifenesin, our limited urinary studies showed a steep increase in twenty-four-hour excretion of phosphate. Uricosuric agents and guaifenesin equally promote lysis of dental calculus and cyclically normalize defective fingernails. Both structures are mineralized with calcium phosphate.

Studies other than our own support our theory. Exercise fatigue is attributed to lactic acid accumulation and consequent cellular acidification. However, muscles recycle lactate for energy production; lowering pH augments fiber sensitivity to calcium and promotes contraction. Both actions increase endurance. In a study of maximal wrist-flexion exercises, pH froze at 6.2 but exhaustion prevailed only after a ninefold increase in intracellular diprotonated phosphate (H_2PO_4)[8] Thus, two anions are required to buffer the H^+ assault on pH and to avoid myocyte apoptosis. The unrelenting sinew contractions of fibromyalgia are akin to a twenty-four-hour, continuous exercise yielding excess H^+ and the need for even more offsetting P_i intervention in mitochondria. Since ATP production is reduced by P_i accumulations, fatigue must follow as per the following formula:

$$\Delta G = \frac{ATP}{ADP + P_i} \ (\Delta G = energy\ change)\ (P_i = inorganic\ phosphate)$$

Many papers have addressed the energy deprivation of fibromyalgia; we refer to only a few. Bengtsson and Henriksson biopsied swollen and tender areas in trapezii and found a 20 percent reduction in ATP as well as the phosphocreatine reservoir for high-energy phosphates. The situation was actually worse because normal tissue was included and tested from the cored specimens.[9] Adjacent and unaffected muscle tissues were barely altered. This was confirmed by Lindman[10] and

Strobel,[11] who found increased P_i, decreased phosphocreatine, and low pH in contracted spinal erector muscles of fibromyalgics using 31P magnetic resonance spectroscopy.[11] Other studies support this, including one that tested patients at rest.[12] Low ATP in platelets and erythrocytes has also been reported by Bazzichi.[13] A similar state exists in neutrophils from chronic fatigue patients (to us, fibromyalgia) as determined by Myhill, who coined the term *ATP profile*.[14]

The P_i to PCr ratio is an accepted measure of fatigue and cellular energy availability. The depressed PCr cited above and high intracellular AMP and ADP reported in other studies testify to metabolic fatigue. Increases in plasma pyruvate, but low or normal lactate status, have been shown, reflecting intact anaerobic metabolism. High pyruvate suggests a fully operative glycolytic pathway that, for whatever reason, does not properly segue into the effective, aerobic sequences of the Krebs cycle.

Ingested P_i is 80–90 percent absorbed via dedicated receptors in the small intestine. The proximal renal tubules respond to bodily requirements either by reabsorbing it from glomerular filtrates or by measured excretion of surpluses. We postulate a basic tubular defect as well as other, chromosome-scattered, genetic aberrations that alter tissue rapport. The disharmony of fibromyalgia could certainly arise from pathologic retention of inorganic phosphate when it accumulates sufficiently to impose near-hibernation function on intracellular organelles. As described above, we implicate excess H_2PO_4 as prime suspect for the body-wide dearth of ATP and the exhaustion of fibromyalgia. Phosphate is heavily concentrated and energized in mitochondria by triple-bonding with adenosine to form ATP. Though phosphate successfully binds matrix hydrogen, it also leads to cellular fatigue by blocking egress of H^+ to the outer chamber and thus creates a proton deficit in that space. Such matrix trapping obstructs the mandatory to-and-fro H^+

migration through the inner membrane, the chemical cascade that is essential for ATP production. Accumulated matrix H^+ lowers pH, which attracts more phosphate and increases formation of diprotonated P_i.

ATP can be exported from muscles and platelets to sites that currently require higher energy expenditure. This support must falter in fibromyalgics since it barely meets energy demands and, too often, not at all. Tiny energy surpluses do occasionally arise and permit bursts of activity. Such free spending soon results in erratic deficits that account for rapidly shifting symptoms. Other high-energy phosphate suppliers (ITP,[3] GTP[3]) may likewise stumble when saddled with the accelerated metabolism of fibromyalgia. High energy demands from the stresses of healing infections, accidents, surgical damage, and emotional upsets can be final insults that initiate attacks.

The ultimate intracellular messenger, calcium, drives cells to perform their specialized functions. The intensity of cytosolic and organelle blushes or full flushes reflect the demand of incoming signals. Tiered impulses permit graded efforts as exemplified to the extreme by rigor mortis. Calcium enters cells to buffer the negatively charged P_i^2. ATP-driven pumps must then extrude calcium from cells or force storage into mitochondria and endoplasmic reticula to halt cellular activity. ATP-depleted fibromyalgics insufficiently man the pumps and fail to restore a mandatory calcium-free cytosol. Continuous goading by such residual calcium induces unrelenting tissue work and further exhausts an ever-dwindling energy supply. That is the only logical explanation for the unrelenting tissue spasm found on examination. *Sustained cytosol calcium levels permit neither complete brain-muscle-tendon-ligament relaxation* nor full rest for nonexcitable tissues. Since physiologic dilutions must be maintained, water is internalized through coentry of sodium and chloride. Palpable lesions are mainly due to intracellular water retention.

Swelling presses on nerves, causing malfunction expressed as a host of sensations such as pain, paresthesias, and allodynia.

As patients become progressively more sedentary, the body responds by destroying up to 80 percent of what it interprets as surplus mitochondria. Carbohydrate craving follows in a futile attempt to generate energy. Its metabolites have difficulty connecting into the fewer remaining, dysfunctional mitochondria. Residual glucose releases insulin, which abets its conversion to fat, subsequent storage, and weight gain. Insulin wreaks further havoc by stimulating renal reabsorption of phosphate. It is driven into myocytes and adipocytes along with water, and there combines with glucose, trapping it for local consumption.

Body-wide secretions try to eject the offending ions as phosphoric acid. Tears may burn and desiccate, leaving crystals, the morning sand. Salivary outflows produce a scalded oral mucosa, bad or metallic tastes, lingual irritation, and finally precipitate out as dental calculus. Amorphous urinary sediments are composed of calcium phosphate, oxalate, or carbonate. These precipitate in the bladder and, upon urination, abrade the trigone and urethral mucosa to cause dysuria. The denuded surfaces also facilitate bacterial invasion and repeated bladder infections. This added to frequency, urgency, bladder muscle spasms, and lower abdominal pain lead to the diagnosis of interstitial cystitis. The vaginal mucosa and muscles are likewise irritated as reflected by vulvitis, vestibulitis, bacterial or fungal infections, and dyspareunia.

Other mucosal surfaces in the eye, lids, or mouth may also suffer acidic burns. The integument is often affected, causing paresthesias, allodynia, defective nails (chipping or peeling), and poor hair texture and growth. Mast cells malfunction and add to systemic discomfort by releasing cytokines (eotaxin, MCP-1, TNF alpha, IL-6, etc.) into the epidermis, bronchial, intestinal, vaginal, and bladder mucosas.[15] Among those secretions are histamine, which induces itching and various rashes, and heparin, which accounts for the easy bruising seen in 80 percent of fibromyalgic women.

Though nondiagnostic and difficult to reproduce, other aberrations have been reported: *decreased* growth hormone, IGF-1, serotonin, free ionic Ca^{2+}, calcitonin, free urinary or salivary cortisol and a weak cortisol response to ACTH, certain amino acids, neuropeptide Y, defective T cell activation, poor TSH response to TRH; *increased* serum prolactin, mast cells that release their contents such as histamine, heparin, and multiple cytokines; elevated homocysteine and substance P in cerebrospinal fluid, and plasma angiotensin converting enzymes. A report by Zhang, others, and us recently revealed twenty-three elevated cytokines and chemokines. These seemingly neutralize each other and thereby avoid inflammation. Ten were reduced or normalized by guaifenesin.[16] Accumulating findings underscore the likelihood of a fundamental, metabolic error that is erratically and variably imposed upon selected tissues.

HYPOGLYCEMIA

Steady fuel consumption of overworked tissues demands energy replenishment frequently reflected as sugar craving. Carbohydrates generate very little, however, since ATP production is impaired downstream. Especially patients from families with diabetes mellitus or dysregulated beta-cell function evoke exaggerated insulin responses. They suffer episodes of hypoglycemia or *glucopenia,* the preferred term for tissue glucose deprivation especially in the brain. Genter and Ipp studied twenty young, healthy subjects during glucose tolerance testing. They sampled blood every ten minutes and measured counterregulatory hormone releases. Nine suffered acute epinephrine effects despite what seemed acceptably normal glucose levels.[17] Individual thresholds vary for instigating corrective neuroendocrine responses. Recurrent bouts alter set points and initiate countermeasures only at lower glucose levels.[18] Restriction of high-glycemic-index foods restores normal signaling within two weeks.[19]

The acute symptoms are flagrant: tremors; clamminess; pounding, fluttering, or rapid heart; headaches; weakness; irritability; anxiety; intense hunger; faintness; even panic attacks—all induced by counterregulatory surges of epinephrine. They last about twenty minutes and typically strike one to four hours postprandially or nocturnally. Were such complaints described by insulin-dependent diabetics, physicians would unhesitatingly diagnose hypoglycemia without challenging them to an unreliable glucose tolerance test. They are collectively diagnostic of glucopenia and should not be attributed to fibromyalgia. The chronic symptoms cannot be separated from fibromyalgia. They include: fatigue, irritability, nervousness, depression, insomnia, impaired memory and concentration, irritable bowel syndrome, water retention, and aching. All facets of hypoglycemia, acute or chronic, totally regress by close adherence to a low-carbohydrate diet.

Many fibromyalgics gain weight, some possibly owing to lassitude, but perhaps more from the loss of mitochondria as mentioned above. The body does not feed unused, expendable structures. Additionally, the surviving organelles are inefficient, and they struggle to produce basic survival requirements of ATP. The energy-starved brain and various hormones encourage carbohydrate consumption. That evokes insulin surges but also suppression of glucagon: a perfect milieu for weight gain. Malonyl CoA is enhanced to promote the conversion of glucose to fatty acids, and insulin triggers storage of triglyceride.

Aerobic exercises as simple as walking restore mitochondria in red muscle fibers (type I), those most affected in fibromyalgia. Such resurrected organelles increase energy production, burn calories, and facilitate weight reduction. Anaerobic workouts benefit primarily the less-affected white fibers (type II), which contain far fewer mitochondria.

TREATMENT SUMMARY

In summary, this paper is long in theory but it is based on many facts. Guaifenesin is highly successful for treating fibromyalgia, but is totally ineffective if salicylates gain entry from whatever portal. Even relatively tiny amounts found in cosmetics, toothpastes, and botanicals lodge in the proximal renal tubule and negate drug benefits. Genetic makeup determines dosage, susceptibility to blocking, and cytochrome recruitment. Hypoglycemia and carbohydrate intolerance cause confusion if not properly addressed and wrongly suggest inadequate control of fibromyalgia. During improvement, patients should begin aerobic exercising and thereby restore mitochondria. Adherence to our protocol must be meticulous, or there will be no reversal of the disease. Physicians who deviate from this design do disservice to their patients and condemn them to failure.

It is our mission to disseminate information gleaned by a single physician and a fifty-five-year experience. Our protocol uses a nontoxic, over-the-counter drug that works to mitigate an innate metabolic error. Most research focuses on obtunding symptoms and ignores the root cause of the illness. We offer the only currently successful protocol for reversing fibromyalgia. We hope to wean physicians and patients away from symptomatic "treatments," that promote polypharmacy with the use of habituating or addicting drugs.

REFERENCES

1. J. Feng, Z. Zhang, W. Li, R. P. St. Amand, et al., "Missense Mutations in the MEFV Gene Are Associated with

Fibromyalgia Syndrome and Correlate with Elevated IL-1 beta Plasma Levels," *PLoS One*, December 2009.

2. *Physicians' Desk Reference* (Montvale, NJ: Medical Economics, 1999). Entry for Humibid, p. 1698.

3. R. Winter, *A Consumer's Dictionary of Cosmetic Ingredients* (New York: Crown Trade Paperbacks, 1994).

4. J. R. Taylor and K. M. Halprin, "Percutaneous Absorption of Salicylic Acid," *Archives of Dermatology* III, no. 6 (June 1974): 740–43.

5. T. P. Delaney, et al., "A Central Role of Salicylic Acid in Plant Disease Resistance," *Science* 266, November 18, 1994.

6. J. R. Brubacher and R. S. Hoffman, "Salicylism from Topical Salicylates: Review of the Literature," *Journal of Toxicology* 34, no. 4 (1996): 431–36.

7. A. S. Yip, W. H. Chow, Y. T. Tai, and K. L. Cheung, "Adverse Effect of Topical Methylsalicylate Ointment on Warfarin Anticoagulation: An Unrecognized Potential Hazard," *Postgraduate Medical Journal* 66, no. 775 (May 1990): 367–79.

8. J. R. Wilson, K. K. McCully, D. M. Mancini, B. Boden, and B. Chance, "Relationship of Muscular Fatigue to pH and Diprotonated Pi in Humans: a 31P-NMR Study," *Journal of Applied Physiology* 64 (June 1988): 2333–39.

9. A. Bengtsson and K. G. Henriksson, "The Muscle in Fibromyalgia: A Review of Swedish Studies," *Journal of Rheumatology* 16, supplement 19 (November 1989): 144–49.

10. R. Lindman, M. Hagberg, K. A. Angqvist, K. Soderlund, E. Hultman, and L. E. Thornell, "Changes in Muscle Morphology in Chronic Trapezius Myalgia," *Scandinavian Journal of Work, Environment, & Health* 17 (1991): 347–55.

11. E. S. Strobel, M. Krapf, M. Suckfull, W. Bruckle, W. Fleckenstein, and W. Muller, "Tissue Oxygen Measurement and 31P Magnetic Resonance Spectroscopy in

Patients with Muscle Tension and Fibromyalgia, *Rheumatology International* 16 (1997): 175–80.

12. J. H. Park, P. Phothimat, C. T. Oates, M. Hernanz-Schulman, and N. J. Olsen, "Use of P-31 Magnetic Resonance Spectroscopy to Detect Metabolic Abnormalities in Muscles of Patients with Fibromyalgia," *Arthritis & Rheumatism* 41, no. 3 (March 1998): 406–13.

13. L. Bazzichi, G. Giannaccini, I. Betti, et al. "ATP, Calcium and Magnesium Levels in Platelets of Patients with Primary Fibromyalgia," *Clinical Biochemistry* 41, no. 13 (September 2008): 1084–90.

14. S. Myhill, N. Booth, and J. McLaren-Howard, "Chronic Fatigue Syndrome and Mitochondrial Dysfunction, *International Journal of Clinical and Experimental Medicine* 2 (2009): 1–16.

15. S. Enestrom, A. Bengtsson, and T. Frodin, "Dermal IgG Deposits and Increase of Mast Cells in Patients with Fibromyalgia," *Scandinavian Journal of Rheumatology* 26, no. 4 (1997): 308–13.

16. Z. Zhang, G. Cherryholmes, A. Mao, C. Marek, J. Longmate, M. Kalos, R. P. St. Amand, and J. E. Shively, "High Plasma Levels of MCP-1 and Eotaxin Provide Evidence for an Immunological Basis of Fibromyalgia," *Journal of Experimental Biology and Medicine*, June 2008.

17. P. Genter and E. Ipp, "Plasma Glucose Thresholds for Counterregulation After an Oral Glucose Load, *Metabolism* 43, no. 1 (January 1994): 98–103.

18. A. Hvidberg, et al., "Impact of Recent Antecedent Hypoglycemia on Hypoglycemic Cognitive Dysfunction in Nondiabetic Humans," *Diabetes* 45, no. 8 (1996).

19. J. Eisinger, A. Plantamura, and T. Ayavou, "Glycolysis Abnormalities in Fibromyalgia," *Journal of the American College of Nutrition* 13, no. 2 (1994): 144–48.

Notes

Chapter 1. An Invitation to Join Us and Find Your Way Back to Health

1. Frederick Wolfe, "The Fibromyalgia Problem," *Journal of Rheumatology* 24, no. 7 (1997): 1247–49.

2. W. R. Gowers, "A Lecture on Lumbago: Its Lessons and Analogues," *British Medical Journal* 1 (1904): 117–21.

3. Frederick Wolfe, "The Fibromyalgia Problem," *Journal of Rheumatology* 24, no. 7 (1997): 1247–49.

4. F. Wolfe, H. A. Smythe, and M. B. Yunus, "Criteria for the Classification of Fibromyalgia," *American College of Rheumatology* 33 (1990): 160–72.

5. The Copenhagen Declaration, "Consensus Document on Fibromyalgia," *Lancet* 240 (September 12, 1992). Incorporated into the ICD on January 1, 1993.

6. F. Wolfe, J. Anderson, and D. Harkness, "The Work and Disability Status of Persons with Fibromyalgia," *Journal of Rheumatology* 24 (1997): 1171–78.

Chapter 2. The Fibromyalgia Syndrome: An Overview of Symptoms and Causes

1. A. Bengtsson and K. G. Henriksson, "The Muscle in Fibromyalgia: A Review of Swedish Studies," *Journal of Rheumatology* 16, supplement 19 (November 1989): 144–49.

Chapter 3. Guaifenesin: How and Why It Works

1. *Physicians' Desk Reference* (Montvale, NJ: Medical Economics, 1999). Entry for Humibid, 1698.

2. C. M. Ramsdell, A. E. Postlewaite, and W. Kelley, "Uricosuric Effect of Glyceryl Guaiacolate," *Journal of Rheumatology* 1, no. 1 (1974): 114–16.

3. Julia Lawless, *The Encyclopedia of Essential Oils* (Lanham, MD: Barnes & Noble, 1992), 106.

4. *Physicians' Desk Reference for Herbal Medicines* (Montvale, NJ: Medical Economics, 1998).

5. *Physicians' Desk Reference* (Montvale, NJ: Medical Economics, 1999). Entry for Humibid, 1698.

Chapter 4. The Fly in the Ointment: Aspirin and Other Salicylates

1. P. Morra, W. R. Bartle, and S. E. Walker, "Serum Concentrations of Salicylic Acid Following Topically Applied Salicylate Derivatives," *Annals of Pharmacotherapy* 9 (September 1996): 935–40.

2. *Science Journal*, November 18, 1984.

3. A. R. Swain, S. P. Dutton, and A. S. Truswell, "Salicylates in Foods," *Journal of the American Dietetic Association* 85 (August 1998): 950–59.

Chapter 5. Patient Vindication

1. Z. Zhang, G. Cherryholmes, A. Mao, C. Marek, J. Longmate, M. Kalos, R. P. St. Amand, and J. E. Shively, "High Plasma Levels of MCP-1 and Eotaxin Provide Evidence for an Immunological Basis of Fibromyalgia," *Journal of Experimental Biology and Medicine* 233 (2008): 1171–80.

2. J. Feng, Z. Zhang, W. Li, X. Shen, W. Song, C. Yang, F. Chang, J. Longmate, C. Marek, R. P. St. Amand, T. G. Krontiris, J. E. Shively, and S. S. Sommer, "Missense Mutations in the MEFV Gene Are Associated with Fibromyalgia Syndrome and Correlate with Elevated IL-1 beta Plasma Levels," *PloS One* 4(12):e8480. doi:10.10.1371/journal.pone.0008480, December 30, 2009.

Chapter 6. Hypoglycemia, Fibroglycemia, and Carbohydrate Intolerance

1. P. Genter and E. Ipp, "Plasma Glucose Thresholds for Counterregulation After an Oral Glucose Load," *Metabolism* 43, no. 1 (January 1994): 98–103.

2. Janette Brand Miller, "International Tables of Glycemic Index," *American Journal of Clinical Nutrition* 62 (1995): 871–90.

3. Robert C. Atkins, *Dr. Atkins' New Diet Revolution* (New York: M. Evans and Co., Inc., 1992); Richard K. Bernstein, *Dr. Bernstein's Diabetes Solution* (New York: Little, Brown and Co., 1997).

Chapter 8. The Brain Symptoms: Chronic Fatigue and Fibrofog

1. Harvey Moldofsky, "Nonrestorative Sleep and Symptoms After a Febrile Illness in Patients with Fibrositis and Chronic Fatigue Syndromes," *Journal of Rheumatology* 16, supplement 19 (1989): 150–53.

Chapter 11. Genitourinary Syndromes

1. J. J. Yount and J. J. Willems, "New Direction in Medical Management of Vulvar Vestibulitis," *Vulvar Pain Newsletter* (Fall 1994): 5–7.

Chapter 12. Dermatologic Symptoms

1. S. Enestrom, A. Bengtsson, and T. Frodin, "Dermal IgG Deposits and Increase of Mast Cells in Patients with Fibromyalgia: Relevant Findings or Epiphenomena?" *Scandinavian Journal of Rheumatology* 26, no. 4 (1997): 308–13.

Chapter 14. Pediatric Fibromyalgia

1. Origin unknown. The guaiacum entry is from an old book sent to us from a patient in Washington State.

Chapter 15. Medical Band-Aids: Currently Promoted Treatments for Fibromyalgia—What You Don't Know Can Hurt You

1. Frederick Wolfe, "The Fibromyalgia Problem," *Journal of Rheumatology* 24, no. 7 (1997): 1247–49.

2. Robert Bennett, "Q & A with Robert Bennett, M.D.," *Fibromyalgia Network Newsletter* (October 1998): 13.

3. Don L. Goldenberg, "A Review of the Role of Tricyclic Medications in the Treatment of Fibromyalgia Syndrome," *Journal of Rheumatology* 16, supplement 19 (1989): 137–40.

4. Marcia Angell and Jerome P. Kassirer, "Alternative Medicine: The Risks of Untested and Unregulated Remedies," *New England Journal of Medicine* 339, no. 12 (September 17, 1998): 839–41.

5. Nortin M. Hadler, "Fibromyalgia: La Maladie Est Morte. Vive la Malade!" *Journal of Rheumatology* 24, no. 7 (1997): 1250–51.

6. Frederick Wolfe, "Disability and Distress in Fibromyalgia," *Journal of Musculoskeletal Pain* 1 (1993): 65–87.

Chapter 16. Coping with Fibromyalgia: What Will Help While Guaifenesin Helps Your Body Heal?

1. Devin J. Starlanyl, *The Fibromyalgia Advocate* (Oakland, CA: New Harbinger Publications, 1998), 227.

2. Ibid., 169.

3. Devin J. Starlanyl and Mary Ellen Copeland, *Fibromyalgia and Chronic Myofascial Pain Syndrome: A Survival Manual* (Oakland, CA: New Harbinger Publications, 1996), 161.

Resources

Part I. The Plan for Conquering Fibromyalgia

CHAPTER 1. AN INVITATION TO JOIN US AND FIND YOUR WAY BACK TO HEALTH

CHAPTER 2. THE FIBROMYALGIA SYNDROME: AN OVERVIEW OF SYMPTOMS AND CAUSES

Associations

The Arthritis Foundation: www.arthritis.org,
   (800) 283-7800.
The National Fibromyalgia and Chronic Pain Association:
   www.fmcpaware.org

Books

Marek, Claudia Craig, *The First Year: Fibromyalgia. An
   Essential Guide for the Newly Diagnosed* (New York: Da
   Capo Press, 2003).
Russell, I. Jon, *The Fibromyalgia Syndrome: A Clinical Case
   Definition for Practitioners* (Oakland, CA: New Harbinger
   Publications, 2004).
Starlanyl, Devin J., and Mary Ellen Copeland, *Fibromyalgia
   and Chronic Myofascial Pain Syndrome*, 2d edition
   (Oakland, CA: New Harbinger Publications, 2001).

Websites

Dr. St. Amand's website for the guaifenesin protocol: www
.fibromyalgiatreatment.com.

Devin Starlanyl's website: http://homepages.sover.net/
~devstar/.

The National Fibromyalgia Association's website: www
.fmcpaware.org. Many articles and features. (The NFCPA
accepts support from pharmaceutical companies.)

ProHealth: www.prohealth.com. This website has a newsletter
and an archive of articles about fibromyalgia.

Newsletter

The Fibromyalgia Treatment Forum: Claudia Marek,
Editor, P.O. Box 64339, Los Angeles, CA 90064; www
.fibromyalgiatreatment.com. Annual subscription $28.00.

CHAPTER 3. GUAIFENESIN: HOW AND WHY IT WORKS

Guaifenesin Sources

Marina del Rey Pharmacy: www.fibropharmacy.com, (800)
435-2330 or (310) 823-5311.

ProHealth: www.prohealth.com, (800) 366-6056.

CHAPTER 4. THE FLY IN THE OINTMENT: ASPIRIN
AND OTHER SALICYLATES

Salicylate-Free Products

Cleure Products: www.cleure.com, (888) 883-4276 (U.S. only)
or (805) 981-7600 (U.S. and international), customersupport@
cleure.com. Dental products, personal care products, and
makeup. All sales benefit The Fibromyalgia Treatment Center.
Everything is salicylate-free and gluten-free and made from
USA ingredients. No fragrances, gluten, or SLS.

Illuminaré Cosmetics: www.illuminarecosmetics.com, (866)
999-2033 or (916) 939-9888. High-quality mineral makeup
and lip products.

Easy Quick Check for Products

The ingredients listed below are what you cannot use. If you do not see one of these on the label, you can use the product.

No salicylate, salicylic acid

No oil, gel, or extract with the name of any plant (except corn, rice, oats, wheat, and soy, which you can use)

No chemicals with names that include the following syllables: SAL, CAMPH, MENTH

Sunscreens: No octisalate, homosalate, mexoryl, or meradimate

Vitamins: No bioflavonoids—quercetin, hesperiden, or rutin

Products with flavors (toothpaste, dental floss, hard candies, cough drops): No mint of any kind or menthol

No pycnogenol, bisabol, or balsam (barks)

Marina del Rey Pharmacy: www.fibropharmacy.com, (800) 435-2330 or (310) 823-5311. Dental products, personal care products, guaifenesin, and vitamins.

Tanner's Tasty Paste: www.tannerstastypaste.com, (866) 838-2789. Mint-free toothpastes for children with fluoride.

Tom's of Maine: www.Tomsofmaine.com, (800) 367-8667. Use mint-free flavors only.

To Check Products You Already Have

Drugstore products: Ingredients are listed at www.drugstore.com.

Higher-end products: Ingredients are listed at www.beauty.com or www.ulta.com.

Products normally sold by dermatologists: www.dermadoctor
.com or www.skinstore.com.

You can also contact individual manufacturers for a list of
ingredients in their products. For example: www.olay.com
or www.aveeno.com. You may have to use the "contact us"
button and request them.

CHAPTER 6. HYPOGLYCEMIA, FIBROGLYCEMIA, AND CARBOHYDRATE INTOLERANCE

The Hypoglycemia Support Foundation: www.hypoglycemia
.org.

Support Group for HG and the Guai Protocol: www
.fibromyalgiatreatment.com.

Books

St. Amand, R. Paul, and Claudia C. Marek, *What Your
Doctor May* Not *Tell You About Fibromyalgia Fatigue* (New
York: Warner Books, 2003), www.fibromyalgiatreatment
.com.

Taubes, Gary. *Good Calories, Bad Calories: Why We Get Fat*
(New York: Knopf, 2010), www.garytaubes.com.

Williamson, Miryam Erlich. *Blood Sugar Blues: Overcoming
the Hidden Dangers of Insulin Resistance* (New York: Walker
and Co., 2001).

All books by Robert Atkins, M.D., contain information about insulin, blood sugar, and carbohydrates. Recipes and resources are available online from www.atkins
.com. All recipes for the Induction Diet are suitable. For
the rest, check individual ingredients against Dr. St.
Amand's "Foods to Strictly Avoid" list. The Atkins information line is (800) 6-ATKINS.

Low-Carb Recipes

Most low-carb recipes are geared for weight loss. Therefore, it's important for hypoglycemics to make sure they contain none of the ingredients that will trigger low blood sugar. Use Dr. St. Amand's "Foods to Strictly Avoid" list to scan recipes to see if they are suitable.

Baker, Judy Barnes, *Carb Wars, Sugar Is the New Fat* (Snohomish, WA: Duck in a Boat, 2007), www.carbwarscookbook .com for her blog with recipes.

McCullough, Fran, *Living Low Carb* (New York: Little, Brown and Co., 2000).

———, *The Low Carb Cookbook* (New York: Hyperion, 1997).

Diabetes

Bernstein, Richard K., *Dr. Bernstein's Diabetes Solution* (New York: Little, Brown and Co., 1997), www.diabetes-book .com.

David Mendosa: www.mendosa.com. Many articles and a newsletter.

CHAPTER 7. THE PROTOCOL

Basic Treatment Information and Updates

Dr. St. Amand's website: www.fibromyalgiatreatment.com.

The Fibromyalgia Treatment Forum Newsletter: Claudia Marek, Editor, P.O. Box 64339, Los Angeles, CA 90064. $28/year

Guaifenesin

Mucinex (long-acting guaifenesin with a short-acting layer): 600 mg tablet. Available in all stores. Discount pharmacies or www.amazon.com have the best prices generally.

Marina del Rey Pharmacy: www.fibropharmacy.com, (800) 435-2330 or (310) 823-5311. Sells all types of guaifenesin, long and short acting, including compounded dye-free guaifenesin in 300 mg and 600 mg strengths. Ships worldwide.

ProHealth: www.prohealth.com, (800) 366-6056. Sells various types of guaifenesin. www.prohealth.com. Ships worldwide.

Support Group

Join our support group via Dr. St. Amand's website: www .fibromyalgiatreatment.com.

Book

Hoey-Sanders, Chantal, *I Have Fibromyalgia But It Doesn't Have Me* (Bloomington, IN: Balboa Press, 2011), www .chantalhoeysanders.com.

Part II. Distinguishing the Many Faces of Fibromyalgia

CHAPTER 8. THE BRAIN SYMPTOMS: CHRONIC FATIGUE AND FIBROFOG

CHAPTER 9. MUSCULOSKELETAL SYNDROME

The American Pain Society: www.painfoundation.org, (888) 615-7246.

National Headache Foundation: www.headaches.org, (888) 643-5552.

Migraine Headaches

The American Migraine Foundation: www .migrainefoundation.org, (856) 423-0043.

Restless Leg Syndrome

Restless Leg Foundation: www.rls.org, (507) 287-6465.

Book

Davis, Clair, *The Trigger Point Therapy Workbook,* 2d edition (Oakland, CA: New Harbinger Publications, 2004).

CHAPTER 10. THE IRRITABLE BOWEL SYNDROME: FIBROGUT

Information and Support
Irritable Bowel Self Help and Support Group: www.ibsgroup.org.
International Foundation for Functional Gastrointestinal
 Disorders: www.aboutibs.org, (888) 964-2001.

CHAPTER 11. GENITOURINARY SYNDROMES

Websites for Information, Products, and Support
The Interstitial Cystitis Association: www.ichelp.org,
 (800) 435-7422.
The Interstitial Cystitis Network: www.ic-network.com,
 (707) 538-9442.
The National Vulvodynia Association: www.nva.org,
 (301) 299-0775.
The Vulvar Pain Foundation: www.thevpfoundation.org,
 (336) 266-0704.

Products
Prelief: www.prelief.com.
Emu oil: Wild Rose Emu Ranch, Clover Quinn, www
 .wildroseemu.com, (406) 363-1710.
Glad Rags: www.gladrags.com, (800) 799-4523.

Low-Oxalate Diet Resources
The Vulvar Pain Foundation: www.thevpfoundation.com.

Treatment
John J. Willems, M.D.: (619) 554-8690.
Scripps Clinic and Research Foundation: 10666 N. Torrey
 Pines Road, La Jolla, CA 92037.

CHAPTER 12. DERMATOLOGIC SYMPTOMS

The American Academy of Dermatology: www.aad.org,
 (866) 503-7546.

CHAPTER 13. HEAD, EYE, EAR, NOSE, AND THROAT SYNDROME

TMJ: The TMJ Association, www.tmj.org, (414) 259-3223.

Dry eye syndrome: Maskin, Steven, M.D., *Reversing Dry Eye Syndrome* (New Haven: Yale University Press, 2007).

Dental problems, dry mouth: Stay, Flora, D.D.S., *The Fibromyalgia Dental Handbook* (New York: Da Capo Press, 2003). Her website also contains articles and resources: www.cleure.com.

Sensitivities: Heller, Sharon, *Too Loud, Too Bright, Too Fast, Too Tight: What to Do if You Are Sensory Defensive in an Overstimulating World* (New York: Perennial Currents, 2003).

CHAPTER 14. PEDIATRIC FIBROMYALGIA

Starlanyl, Devin J., and Mary Ellen Copeland, *Fibromyalgia and Chronic Myofascial Pain Syndrome*, 2d edition (Oakland, CA: New Harbinger Publications, 2001).

Williamson, Miryam Erlich, *Fibromyalgia: A Comprehensive Approach* (New York: Walker and Sons, 1998).

Some helpful information specific to children can be found at: www/fmscommunity.org/pediatric.

Part III. Strategies for the Road Back

CHAPTER 15. MEDICAL BAND-AIDS: CURRENTLY PROMOTED TREATMENTS FOR FIBROMYALGIA—WHAT YOU DON'T KNOW CAN HURT YOU

Books

Angell, Marcia, M.D., *The Truth About Drug Companies* (New York: Random House, 2004).

Jacobs, Greg, and Herbert Benson, *Say Good Night to Insomnia: The Six-Week, Drug-Free Program Developed at Harvard Medical School* (New York: Owl Books, 1999).

The National Sleep Foundation website: www
.sleepfoundation.org, (703) 243-1697.
Information about supplements (potency and purity): www
.consumerlab.com.

**CHAPTER 16. COPING WITH FIBROMYALGIA: WHAT WILL HELP
WHILE GUAIFENESIN HELPS YOUR BODY HEAL?**

Alexander Technique: www.alexandertechnique.com, (217)
367-6956.
American Academy of Physical Medication and
Rehabilitation: www.aapmr.org, (312) 464-9700.
American Massage Therapy Association: www.amtamassage
.org, (877) 905-0577.
American Physical Therapy Association: www.apta.org,
(800) 999-2782.
Curves International: www.curves.com, (800) 848-1096.
Feldenkrais Foundation: www.feldenkrais.com, (866)
333-6248.
Pilates: www.pilates.com, (800) 745-2837.
Men with Fibromyalgia: www.menwithfibro.com.

Index

adrenaline (epinephrine), 112, *113*, 114
alcohol, 123, 128, 215, 226, 250, 251, 303, 322
allergies, 66, 91, 92, 186, 206, 213–14, 244, 248, 262, 264, 374. *See also* hives
  percentage of FMS patients affected (table), 268
American College of Rheumatology, 9, 28–29, 376
Angell, Marcia, 311, 338
antianxiety drugs, 213, 248, 308, 319
antidepressants, 216, 227–28, 239, 294, 297, 305–8, 310, 319, 323, 354
antiseizure drugs, 308–9
anxiety, 45, 53, 62, 105, 111, *113*, 114, 118, 120, 121, 155, 182, 185, 186, 326, 347, 373, 382
  percentage of FMS patients affected (table), 180
Arthritis Foundation, 151–52, 356, 362
aspirin (and products containing), 9, 74–75, 76, 77, 79, 80, 81, 82, 286, 297, 299
asthma, 28, 50, 70, 245, 374
Atkins, Robert, 148
ATP (adenosine triphosphate), x–xi, 33–35, *36*, *37*, 38, 57, 59, 136, 377–79, 382
  musculoskeletal syndrome and, 193, 200

bad breath, 54, 264–65
Begoun, Paul, 92

Benadryl, 228, 238, 243, 247, 248, 285, 316, 324
Bernstein, Richard, 148
bladder infection, 10, 23, 27, 121, 153, 220–29, *223*, *237*, 380. *See also* interstitial cystitis
  antibiotics and, 224
  cystitis, 222, 224–25
  cystoscopy and, 224, 226
  honeymoon cystitis, 222, 224
  percentage of FMS patients affected (table), 221
bloating, 27, 105, 121, 155, 202, 204, 206, 208, 210, 215, 307, 373
bodywork and massage, 200, 362–64
  Alexander Technique and Bowen Therapy, 363
  Feldenkrais Method, 363
  Rolfing caution, 363
Butler, Robert, 328

caffeine, 123, 124, 157
calcium, 140
  dental tartar and, 42, 45
  guaifenesin and, 69
  musculoskeletal syndrome and, 198
  phosphates and, 35, *37*, 38, 41, 57, 59
  role in FMS, 38, 48–49, 69, 77, 193, 379
  supplements, 49, 227, 238, 240
  unloading of, 55
  in urine, 221